Otolaryngology: Head and Neck Surgery

Otolaryngology: Head and Neck Surgery

Edited by **Sam Hurd**

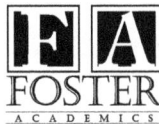

FA FOSTER
ACADEMICS

New Jersey

Published by Foster Academics,
61 Van Reypen Street,
Jersey City, NJ 07306, USA
www.fosteracademics.com

Otolaryngology: Head and Neck Surgery
Edited by Sam Hurd

International Standard Book Number: 978-1-63242-433-4 (Hardback)

Contents

Preface

Over the recent decade, advancements and applications have progressed exponentially. This has led to the increased interest in this field and projects are being conducted to enhance knowledge. The main objective of this book is to present some of the critical challenges and provide insights into possible solutions. This book will answer the varied questions that arise in the field and also provide an increased scope for furthering studies.

Otolaryngology is one of the oldest specialties of medical science that focuses on diseases related to ear, nose and throat. There is a long list of diseases that can be treated with the help of this discipline; some of the broader categories are head and neck oncologic surgery, facial plastic and reconstructive surgery, otology, neurotology, sleep medicine, pediatric otorhinolaryngology and voice disorders. This book includes some of the vital pieces of work being conducted across the world, on various topics related to this discipline. The various studies that are constantly contributing towards advancing technologies and evolution of this field are examined in detail. It is an essential guide for both academicians and those who wish to pursue this discipline further.

I hope that this book, with its visionary approach, will be a valuable addition and will promote interest among readers. Each of the authors has provided their extraordinary competence in their specific fields by providing different perspectives as they come from diverse nations and regions. I thank them for their contributions.

Editor

Our Experience with Embryonal Rhabdomyosarcoma Presenting as Aural Polyp

Anoop Attakkil, Vandana Thorawade, Mohan Jagade, Rajesh Kar, Dnyaneswar Rohe, Reshma Hanowate, Devkumar Rangaraja, Kartik Parelkar

Department of ENT, Grant Medical College & Sir J.J. Hospital, Mumbai, India
Email: fasttrack2317@gmail.com

Abstract

Aural polyps are a common clinical entity encountered by otorhinolaryngologist in daily practice. Polyps are frequently seen in paediatric patients, usually inflammatory in nature. In children rhabdomyosarcomas (RMS) can mimic all the cinical features of chronic suppurative otitis media which usually present as external auditory canal mass or polyp. Here we present a case where a male child presented with recurrence of polyp in left ear which was finally diagnosed as embryonal rhabdomyosarcoma which is a rare and invariably fatal disease in children. Through this article we intend to highlight the failures and delay committed in attaining diagnosis in this patient in spite of multispecialty evaluation involving repeated imaging and histopathological correlation. Our experience with embryonal rhabdomyosarcoma throws light on the high vigilance required in handling the aural polyps in pediatric population as early diagnosis and treatment are the key elements for successful outcomes.

Keywords

Embryonal Rhabdomyosarcoma, Aural Polyp, CSOM

1. Introduction

Aural polyps are well-circumscribed, soft, fleshy masses frequently found in the external auditory canal (EAC) of patients. They are usually inflammatory and suggest active middle ear disease presenting with ear discharge and hearing loss. Most commonly, polyps originate from middle ear mucosa and protrude into the external meatus through a tympanic membrane perforation [1]. The presence of a temporal bone malignancy must be considered, however, in any patient presenting with an aural polyp [1].

Rhabdomyosarcomas are highly aggressive locally destructive, malignant neoplasms of the soft tissue. The most common site involved by rhabdomyosarcoma is orbit followed by oral cavity and pharynx (29%), the face and neck region (24%) [2]; involvement of the ear and temporal bone with rhabdomyosarcoma is uncommon [3]. Rhabdomyosarcomas account for 5% to 15% or all childhood neoplasm and for 30% of temporal bone sarcomas. They are the most common malignant neoplasms of the temporal bone in childhood [4]. But the clinical presentation of this aggressive tumor mimics chronic suppurative otitis media which is a common clinical entity. The dilemma in diagnosis is often due to this close resemblance that results in the delay in diagnosis. Embryonal rhabdomyosarcoma of the middle ear is a rare and invariably fatal disease in children [5] distinct from other embryonal rhabdomyosarcomas of the head in its clinical presentation, prognosis and response to therapy. Early diagnosis and appropriate multimodality therapy holds key in the successful treatment of this rapidly growing tumor.

We present a case of embryonal rhabdomyosarcoma in a child which presented as polyp in the ear whose diagnosis was delayed in spite of the radiological and pathological evaluation. We intend to highlight the pitfalls in diagnosis that we are committed and hope that this case report may help the clinicians to attain an early and prompt diagnosis while dealing with these aggressive neoplasms. Our case report also reviews the histopathology, staging and treatment of embryonal rhabdomyosarcoma in brief.

2. Case Report

A 7 years old male child presented to a peripheral hospital with blood stained ear discharge and mass in the left ear which was accidentally noticed following a fall (**Figure 1**). He had no history of vertigo, decreased hearing or cranial nerve palsies at the time of presentation. Polypectomy was done and histopathological report showed granulation tissue consisting capillary sized vascular channels, mixed inflammatory infiltrate.

Following this the patient had recurrence of the polyp in the same ear with in twenty days. Computerised tomography (CT) scan of brain & temporal bone was done which showed extensive soft tissue collection in the left external auditory canal, middle ear with rarefaction of the left petrous temporal bone suggestive of infective aetiology with bilateral otomastoiditis. Patient presented to our department with the same complaints. On examination, reddish polypoidal mass was filling the left external auditory canal with no mastoid tenderness. Tympanomastoid exploration of the left ear showed polypoidal tissue filling the antrum and middle ear which was removed *in toto*. Histopathological examination of the specimen done at two different centres reported nonspecific pyogenic inflammatory lesion of the left mastoid antrum. Patient developed left lateral rectus palsy 10 days following the surgery and ear discharge. MRI brain with CT temporal bone was done that showed ill defined contrast enhancement in petrous temporal bone on Left side with extension into infratemporal fossa suggestive of inflammatory/infective changes which was also seen in left EAC and middle ear cavity. There was

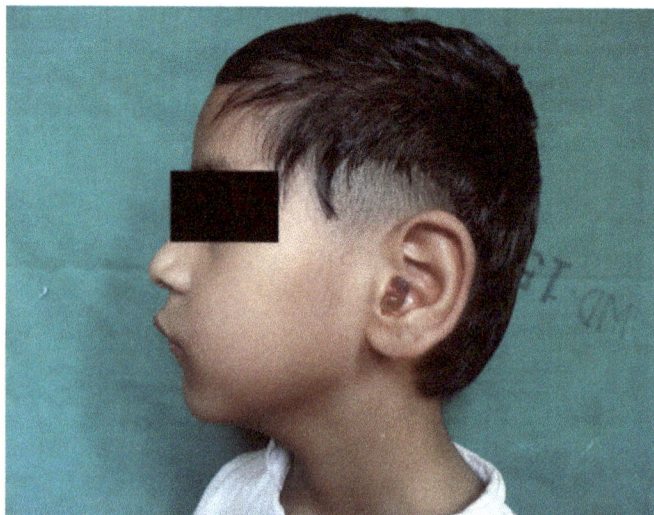

Figure 1. Showing the polypoidal mass protruding from the left EAC.

also osteomyelitis of petrous bone. Neurologist advice was sought for and given osteomyelitis of temporal bone as provisional diagnosis; patient was started on intravenous Meropenem for 2 weeks according to pus culture and sensitivity report of the ear discharge. But the patient failed to show any improvement. Since there was osteopenia noted on the petrous temporal bone suggestive of tuberculosis, patient was started on anti Koch's treatment as advised by the paediatrician.

Patient's neurological signs worsened. He developed loss of general sensation over left half of forehead with deviation of angle of mouth with in next ten days. Meanwhile the recurrence of polypoidal tissue from left EAC was noted. He then developed House Brackmann grade four left lower motor neuron facial nerve palsy and left abductor palsy (**Figure 2**). MRI brain (plain + contrast) was repeated that showed inflammatory soft tissue in the left petrous temporal bone with extension into the left carotid canal, left meckel's cave, along the left sixth nerve and clivus, left cavernous sinus (**Figure 3**).

The biopsy of the mass was repeated and the histopathological examination showed the presence of strap cells showing rhabdomyoblastic differentiation, loosely arranged but with condensation beneath the epithelium (cambium layer) suggestive of embryonal rhabdomyosarcoma confirmed by immunohistochemistry (**Figure 4**). There was no CSF spread or distant metastasis. Patient was given chemo radiotherapy according to IRS-IV (Intergroup rhabdomyosarcoma study) protocol, falling into intermediate risk group. Patient was given induction chemotherapy with Vincristine + Ifosfamide + Etoposide + Mesna (VIE regimen) followed by radiotherapy and maintenance chemotherapy with Vincristine + Dactinomycin + Cyclophosphamide (VAC regimen). Total duration of chemoradiotherapy was 36 weeks. Patient tolerated the treatment well and is on follow up for last one year.

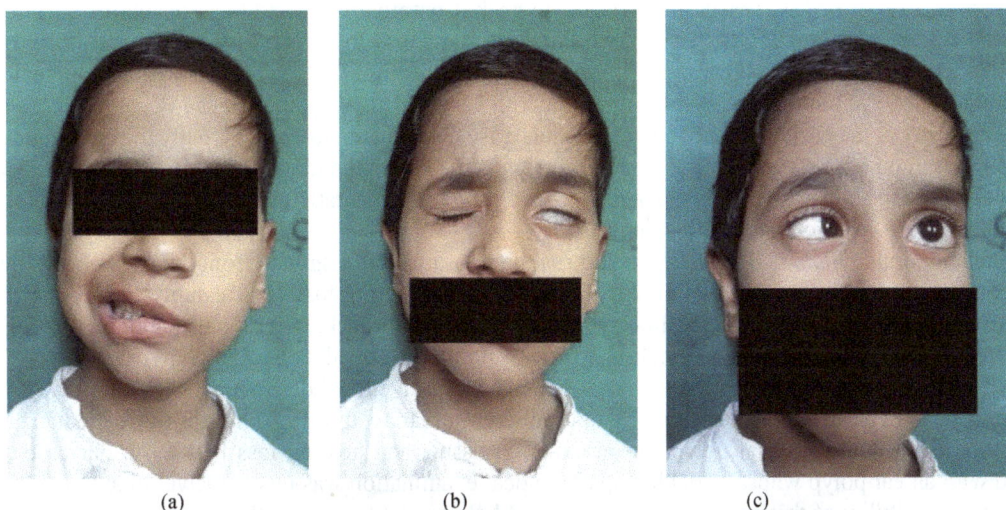

(a) (b) (c)

Figure 2. (a) (b) Showing left lower motor neuron facial palsy; (c) Showing left abductor palsy.

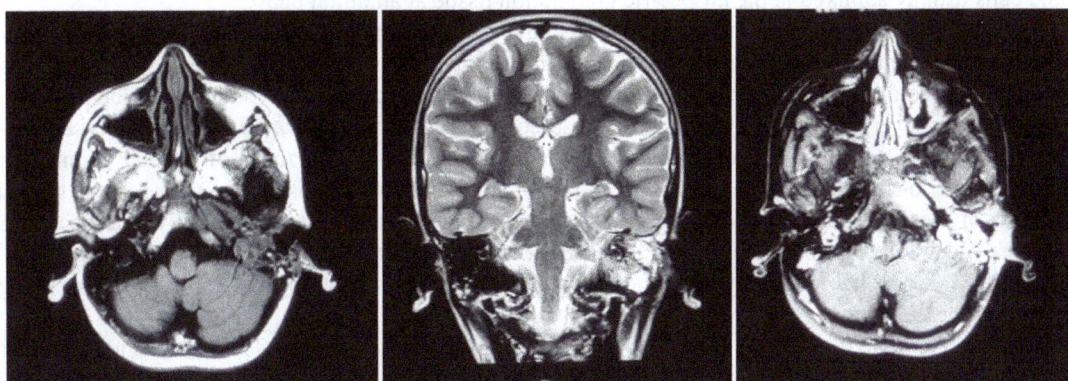

Figure 3. MRI Brain (plain + contrast) T1 & T2 weighted images showing enhancing soft tissue in the left petrous temporal bone with extensions.

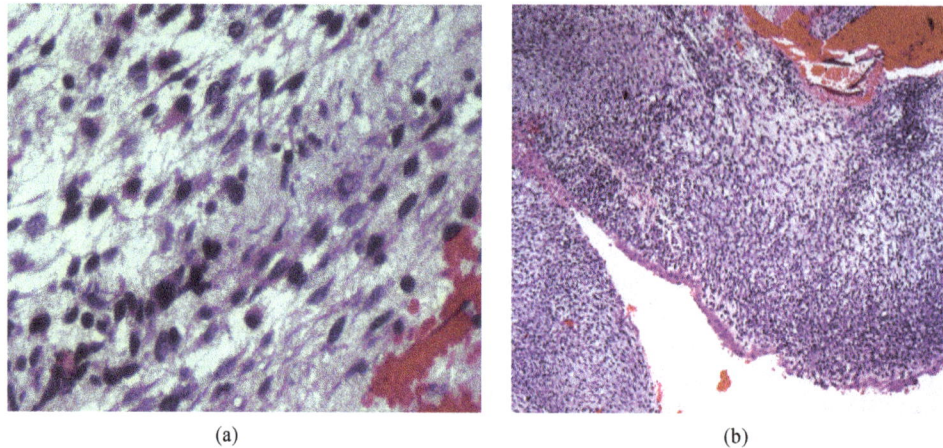

(a)   (b)

Figure 4. (a) Strap muscles showing rhabdomyoblastic differentiation; (b) Showing the arrangement of the cells beneath the cambium layer.

3. Discussion

Although comprising a large percentage of paediatric temporal bone tumours, temporal bone sarcomas are rare and represent less than 5% of all temporal bone malignancies with rhabdomyosarcoma the most common variety [1]. Forty percent of RMSs present in the head and neck. Commonly affected locations in the head and neck are the orbit, middle ear, oral cavity, nasopharynx and infratemporal fossa [4]. In the head and neck, rhabdomyosarcomas are divided into 3 categories: orbital (23%), parameningeal (56%) and nonparameningeal (21%). Parameningeal denotes tumors that develop near the skull base and adjacent meninges [4].

The majority of the auricular rhabdomyosarcomas arise from the middle ear [1]. Only the embryonal subtype of rhabdomyosarcoma is recognized as the one occurring at the external auditory canal [6]. The majority of tumours present before the child are 12 years old, and the average age at presentation is 4.4 years [1]. Rhabdomyosarcomas are slightly more common in boys than in girls [7].

In the temporal bone, it is hypothesized that rhabdomyosarcomas originate from the malignant transformation of myocytes residing in the stapedial or tensor tympani muscles. Four histological subtypes have been described: embryonal, alveolar, pleomorphic and botryoid. In the head and neck, embryonal rhabdomyosarcomas are the most frequently encountered histological subtype (85%) followed by alveolar rhabdomyosarcomas (15%) [4].

The natural history of RMS in the temporal bone is aggressive local destruction with a propensity for distant metastases [1]. The primary presenting symptoms are similar to those of chronic otitis media: purulent and bloody otorrhea, otalgia, canal polyp and granulation tissue, and hearing loss [1]. As in our case patient presented with an ear polyp whose initial histopathological examination was inconclusive. In a case of recurrent ear polyp, the possibility of this aggressive tumour should always be tumour as the early detection makes the prognosis better. Only a high index of suspicion and clinical correlation will help the pathologist to identify the round cells usually admixed in the unspecific granulation tissue at an initial phase.

The diagnosis of rhabdomyosarcoma and the subtype is confirmed by histopathological examination. The characteristics of this polypoid tumour are those of rhabdomyoblasts and primitive mesenchymal cells showing a variable degree of skeletal muscle differentiation loosely arranged but with condensation beneath the epithelium (cambium layer) [6]. Embryonal rhabdomyosarcomas are so-named because of their remarkable evocation of developing skeletal muscle. As such they are characterized by variable zones of condensation that produce alternating foci of hypocellularity and hypercellularity. Like embryonic muscle, the dense zones typically contain areas of more overt myogenesis, whereas loose areas more closely resemble primitive mesenchyme and lie in a loose gelatinous matrix [8]. The immunohistochemistry markers desmin and myogenin yields clue to subclassification embryonal rhabdomyosarcomas usually stain in a more heterogeneous fashion with myogenin as shown in our case (**Figure 5**).

The staging of RMS depends on the type of RMS (embryonal or alveolar), the TNM stage and the clinical group. According to these three variables, they can be classified as low risk, intermediate risk, high risk groups whose 5 year survival rates are respectively 90%, 60% - 80%, 20% - 40% [7]. Our patient was diagnosed as an intermediate risk group and was given chemo radiotherapy. The types of treatment that can be used for RMS include

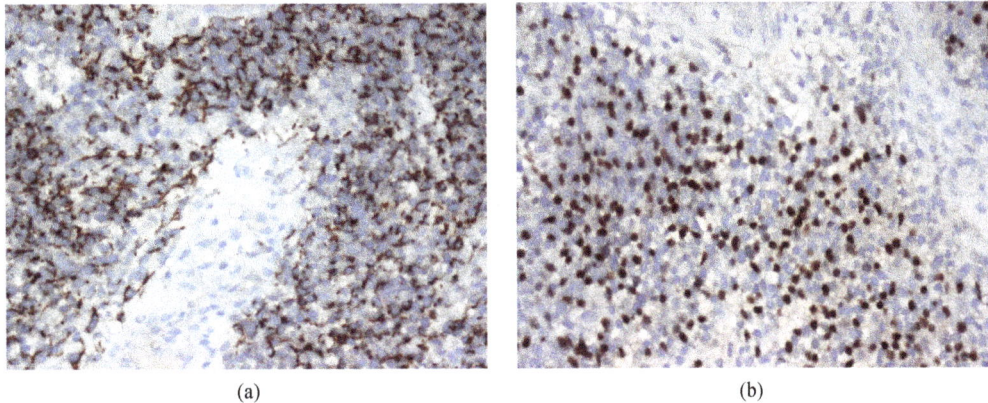

(a)   (b)

Figure 5. (a) The tumor cells showing immunoreactivity with desmin; (b) The tumor cells showing immunoreactivity with myogenin.

surgery, chemotherapy, radiation therapy or high-dose chemotherapy and stem cell transplant (very rarely). Chemotherapeutic regimen usually includes Vincristine + Ifosfamide + Etoposide + Mesna (VIE regimen) and Vincristine + Dactinomycin+ Cyclophosphamide (VAC regimen).

4. Conclusion

In this case report, we have described in detail the clinical course that patient went through and the delay in diagnosis that occurred in spite of the repeated radiological and histopathological evaluation. Though the temporal bone sarcomas are rare, only an approach with high clinical suspicion helps in diagnosing the disease at an early stage. We hope that this case report will guide the clinicians to approach the cases of recurrent ear polyp with high vigilance.

References

[1] Decker, B.C., Gulya, A.J. and Glasscock, M.E. (2003) Glasscock-Shambaugh Surgery of the Ear. Vol. 1, 5th Edition, PMPH, 353-755.

[2] Carol, J.M. and Richard, J.H. (2010) Pediatric Head and Neck Malignancies. In: Paul, W.F., Ed., *Cummings Otolarymgology Head & Neck Surgery*, Vol. 3, Mosby, Philadelphia, 2835-2849.

[3] Chao, C.K., Sheen, T.S., Shau, W.Y., Ting, L.L. and Hsu, M.M. (1999) Treatment, Outcomes, and Prognostic Factors of Ear Cancer. *Journal of the Formosan Medical Association*, **98**, 314-318.

[4] Bambakidis, N.C., Megerian, C.A. and Spetzler, R.F. (2009) Surgery of the Cerebellopontine Angle. PMPH USA Ltd., 261-262.

[5] Potter, G. (1966) Embryonal Rhabdomyosarcoma of the Middle Ear in Children. *Cancer*, **19**, 221-226. http://dx.doi.org/10.1002/1097-0142(196602)19:2<221::AID-CNCR2820190213>3.0.CO;2-G

[6] Barnes, L. (2005) Pathology and Genetics of Head and Neck Tumours IARC. WHO Classification of Tumours Series, Volume 9 of World Health Organization Classification of Tumours, IARC Press, 335.

[7] http://www.cancer.org/acs/groups/cid/documents/webcontent/003136-pdf.pdf

[8] Parham, D.M. and Ellison, D.A. (2006) Rhabdomyosarcomas in Adults and Children. An Update. *Archives of Pathology Laboratory Medicine*, **130**, 1454-1465

Hearing Disability in Colombia Self-Perception and Associated Factors 2002-2008

Augusto Peñaranda[1], Sandra Martínez[2], María Leonor Aparicio[3], Juan Manuel García[1], Clemencia Barón[3]

[1]Departamento de Cirugía, Grupo Implante Coclear, Fundación Santa Fe de Bogotá, Bogotá, Colombia
[2]Centro de Estudios e Investigación en Salud, CEIS, Fundación Santa Fe de Bogotá, Bogotá, Colombia
[3]Grupo Implante Coclear, Fundación Santa Fe de Bogotá, Bogotá, Colombia
Email: augpenar@gmail.com

Abstract

Introduction: Hearing disability is a condition that affects normal ear function, as much in adulthood as in the first years of life. According to the 2005 Census, 6.3% of the Colombian population has some type of disability, of which 17.4% have hearing limitations, including those with hearing devices. Elucidating the conditions of this population and identifying the factors related to hearing disability will permit the management of strategies from different sectors to mitigate the consequences associated with this limitation. Objective: To estimate the self-perception of hearing disability in Colombia and to determine the factors associated with this limitation. Materials and Methods: The present study is cross-sectional, based on the analysis of secondary information obtained from the Registry for Localization and Characterization of Persons with Disability (RLCPD) during the 2002-2008 period. Socio-demographic and healthcare variables were analyzed. Results: 13.6% (102,648/750,377) of the population reported hearing limitations even with the use of special hearing devices. 43.52% (44,041) of people over 3 years of age could neither read nor write. 29.39% (30,145) of people who reported this limitation are not affiliated to any sort of health insurance system. Factors found to be associated with hearing limitations were: socioeconomic stratus (OR: 1.33; CI 95% 1.25; 1.42), illiteracy (OR: 1.44; CI 95% 1.42; 1.46) and lack of affiliation to a health insurance system (OR: 1.03; CI 95% 1.01; 1.04). Conclusion: People registered with hearing disability live under vulnerable conditions; among them, most/the majority pertained to a segment of the population with low economic resources and had difficulty obtaining/accessing work, education and healthcare services.

Keywords

Disability, Hearing Loss, Perception, Health Services, Equity in Health

1. Introduction

Hearing disability, or profound neurosensory hypoacusia, or profound deafness, is a condition that affects inner ear function, as much in adulthood as in the first years of life. It can be acquired from, and the principal causes are, infections such as Rubella, Toxoplasmosis, or Meningitis (it can also present at birth due to genetic disorders); however, close to 30% of registered cases are from unknown causes [1].

Depending on the grade and type of hearing loss and the time in life in which it appears, the effects that it will have over language development and the wellbeing of the individual are different. It is estimated that one of every 1000 live births can present profound neurosensory deafness requiring auditory and language rehabilitation [2]. Each year approximately 5000 children in the United States are born with bilateral hearing loss; it is estimated that the prevalence is between 1 in 900 to 1 in 2500 [3]. When there are high risk factors, the incidence of hypoacusia grows between 20 to 40 in 1000 [4].

The frequency of deafness in Colombia has not been clearly established [5]; the World Health Organization (WHO) estimates that 1 in 1000 newborns suffer from profound deafness and that this rate may be as high as 5 in 1000 newborns if all degrees of hypoacusia are included [6]. According to the 2005 Census, 6.3% of the Colombian population has some degree of disability and of these, 17.4% present hearing limitations even with the use of special devices and 13.2% present speech limitations [7].

In any case, early identification of the hearing deficit, followed by an appropriate intervention, will reduce the impact of this disability in each age group, with respect to the ability to communicate and socialize.

The objective of our study is to estimate the self-perception of hearing disability in Colombia according to the information in the Register for the Localization and Characterization of Persons with Disability (RLCPD), and to identify the factors associated with this limitation, in order to highlight social, educational, and health services which could lead to the re-integration, control, and recovery of persons with auditory disability.

2. Materials and Methods

The present study is cross-sectional, based on analysis of secondary information from the RLCPD, carried out by the Administrative Department of National Statistics (DANE), which has been conducted since 2002 and includes information up to 2008. This information allows the identification of the population with disability in all age groups, with the purpose of establishing plans and strategies to improve their situation [8]. Local governors and mayors are in charge of leading the process of registration in their territory in such a way that after informative campaigns in their corresponding territories, persons that perceive themselves as disabled sign up to be registered, and those who are already included in the disability register are subsequently interviewed [8].

The register covers the entire country; since the basic sources of information are the municipalities, however, there exist differences in the degree of registration within the various territories as it is dependent on the participation and will of the local governors and mayors [8]. It should be noted that this register is included within the framework of the International Classification of Functionality, Incapacity, and Health (CIF) [8].

The total number registered for 2002-2008 was 750,277 persons with any degree of auditory disability, of which 102,648 report having permanent hearing limitations even with the use of special hearing devices. In the case of duplicate registrations, the oldest case was discarded. Information was analyzed according to question #30 in the registry: "In your daily activities, do you present permanent difficulties with hearing, even with the use of special hearing devices", since it allows identification of the population that perceives itself with some hearing disability which interferes with their daily activities, in spite of the use of devices to improve hearing.

A descriptive frequency analysis was carried out on the different variables analyzed in the questionnaire such as age, sex, family characteristics, home characteristics, education, work, origin of the disability, and health services, among others. Subsequently, a bivariate analysis was performed, and a statistical regression model was established where the dependent variable was self-perception of hearing disability and the independent variables were sex, age, ethnicity, family characteristics, health services, etc., and those variables which showed an association of p < 0.10 in the bivariate analysis, or which were considered important for analysis within the model. A p value of 0.05 was considered significant, with confidence intervals calculated at 95%. Statistical analysis was conducted with Stata 9.0.

3. Results

Self-perception of hearing disability: According to the RLCPD, 13.6% of the persons registered with hearing disability reported hearing limitations even with the use of special hearing devices (102,648/750,377).

3.1. Socio-Demographic Characteristics

A slight predominance was observed in women 50.35% (51,681) over men 49.65% (50,967). Of the 32 departments in the country, the majority of registrations were in Bogotá, with 20.96% (this city is considered a department in the registry), followed by Valle del Cauca 8.79%, Nariño 8.41%, Antioquia 7.52%, Tolima 6.21%, and Cundinamarca 5.74%, with all other departments constituting 42.18%.

Analysis by age showed the following distribution: 0 to 19 years, 17.58% (18,044); 20 to 49, 21.86% (22,432); and 50 and older 60.56% (62,149). The majority belonged to socioeconomic stratus 1, 2, 3 or without stratus (98.86%). By ethnic group, 93.0% (94,225) consider themselves "Mestizos", 3.71% (3755) of African descent, 2.96% (2995) as indigenous, 0.2% (202) "Raizals", 0.1% (104) "Palenqueros", and 0.03% (36) "Gypsies"/ "Roma". **Table 1** details the main sociodemographic characteristic of persons that consider themselves with

Table 1. Principal socio-demographic characteristics of persons who self-perceive with hearing limitations even with the use of special hearing limitations.

Category		n	%
Condition of the household	Their own home	52,065	53.06
	Another person's home, not paying	23,629	24.08
	Renting or subletting	20,839	21.24
	Other	1589	1.62
Principal activity in the last 6 months	Unable to work, without pension	32,957	35.15
	Housework	20,831	22.21
	Employed	11,997	12.79
	Other activity	8451	9.01
	Studying	6932	7.39
	Unable to work, with pension	3794	4.05
	Self-sustainment	3206	3.42
	Searching for employment	3244	3.46
	Pensioned	1592	1.70
	Receiving rent	769	0.82
Dependents	Yes	15,802	16.57
	No	79,542	83.43
Socioeconomic stratus	04/05/2006	1166	1.14
	1-2-3, no stratus	101,176	98.86
Healthcare affiliation	Yes	72,065	70.88
	No	29,604	29.11
Knows how to read and write (older than 3 years)	Yes	57,158	56.48
	No	44,041	43.52
Requires the permanent help of another person	Yes	42,179	58.9
	No	60,447	41.1

hearing limitations even with the use of special hearing devices.

7.46% of persons registered with this limitation live alone; this percentage increased following/after 60 years of age. 16.57% are dependent on another person upon analyzing this variable it was observed that within the last 6 months only 31.49% of these persons were employed 58.90% of those registered particularly in extreme age groups (younger than 10 and older than 60 years), indicated the need for permanent help from another person, this person being a member of the household in 88.98% of cases. Moreover, with respect to education, 43.52% of persons older than 3 years can neither read nor write, and the principal reason for which people of school age are not in school is because of disability (36.04%). Information about/ according to level of education and age can be found in **Table 2**.

3.2. Origin of the Disability

Of the total number of persons with a self-perceived hearing limitation 37.36% (37,309) do not know the origin of their limitation; of those that do 62.64% (65,263) attribute it to general illness 42.24% (27,565), followed by complications in childbirth or pregnancy 17.67% (11,532), genetic mutations 14.19% (9258) and accidents 13.44% (8769), as seen in **Table 3**.

Since the RLCPD examines in great depth the origins of work disability, accidents, and difficulties in obtain-

Table 2. Level of education and age of persons who self-perceive with hearing limitations even with the use of special hearing devices.

Maximum level of education	3 to 5		6 to 10		11 to 15		16 to 20		21 to 25		26 and older	
	n	%	n	%	n	%	n	%	n	%	n	%
None	1131	70.20	1694	33.54	1539	25.53	1514	31.87	1330	38.14	32,532	41.96
Preschool	477	29.61	989	19.58	355	5.89	151	3.18	98	2.81	1508	1.94
Primary	0	1.92	2346	46.45	3141	52.11	1549	32.61	986	28.28	34,889	45.00
Secondary	0	0.00	19	0.38	986	16.36	1457	30.67	914	26.21	7179	9.26
University	0	0.00	0	0.00	7	0.12	79	1.66	159	4.56	1429	1.84
Total	1611	100	5051	100	6028	100	4750	100	3487	100	77,537	100

Table 3. Origin of limited hearing in persons that self-perceive with hearing limitations even with the use of special hearing devices.

Their Disability is due to	Hearing limitations even with the use of special hearing devices	
	n	%
General illness	27,565	42.24
Complications during pregnancy or childbirth	11,532	17.67
Genetic disorder	9258	14.19
Accident	8769	13.44
Other	4356	6.67
Occupational disease	1591	2.44
Difficulty in providing health services	1155	1.77
Use of psychoactive drugs	401	0.61
Natural disaster	155	0.24
Self-inflicted injury	481	0.74
Total	65,263	100

ing of healthcare services, it is notable that those that attribute their hearing disability to workplace illness, 61.47% (943) indicated that this was due to physical conditions and workplace safety. Of the 8769 persons who attributed the origin of their disability to accidents, 58.47% (5118) attribute it to traffic accidents, and of the 1155 people that attribute the origin of their disability to slow or deficient medical attention, 59.66% attribute it to slow or deficient medical attention.

3.3. Healthcare

29.11% (29,604) of persons who reported hearing limitations are not affiliated with any type of health insurance system; the majority of those with affiliation to a health insurance service belong to the subsidized group 52.18% and fewer to the contributory group 17.18%. 58.27% of registered persons have not received guidance in how to manage their disability; however, 64.61% have been prescribed special aides, prosthetics, or permanent medications, although only 51.92% actually use them. It is necessary to note that 83.54% of the population believes they still need special help.

82.99% of persons indicate that they are not recovering from their disability, but those that have recovered attribute it principally to health services 39.11%, the help of God 26.98%, and the support of their family 20.63%.

Only 25.80% of persons who perceive themselves with hearing limitations have been subject to speech therapy and 10.40% to occupational therapy. Persons that currently do not receive rehabilitation services (60.14%), 62.98% indicated that this was due to lack of funds.

3.4. Factors Associated with Limited Hearing

The bivariate analysis shows that people that perceive themselves with hearing limitation are more likely to belong to a low socioeconomic stratus (OR: 1.51; CI 95% 1.33 - 1.59), not be affiliated to a health insurance system (OR: 1.05; CI 95% 1.03 - 1.07), live alone (OR: 1.32; CI 95% 1.28 - 1.35), can neither read nor write (OR: 1.45; CI 95% 1.43 - 1.47), require the permanent help of another person (OR: 1.20; CI 95% 1.19 - 1.22), do not know the origin of their disability (OR: 1.11; CI 95% 1.11 - 1.13), or have not worked in the last 6 months (OR: 1.28; CI 95% 1.26 - 1.31), as shown in **Table 4**. In so far as the origin of the/their disability, it was observed that

Table 4. Associated factors in person who self-perceive with hearing limitations even with the use of special hearing devices.

Variable	Bivariate			Multivariate	
	Reference	OR	CI 95%	OR	CI 95%
Socioeconomic stratus	1, 2, 3 or no stratus	1.41	1.33 - 1.50	1.33*	1.25 - 1.42
Sex	Female	0.9	0.88 - 0.91	-	-
Healthcare affiliation	No	1.05	1.03 - 1.07	1.03*	1.01 - 1.04
Knows how to read and write	No	1.45	1.43 - 1.47	1.44*	1.42 - 1.46
Requires the permanent help of another person	Yes	1.2	1.19 - 1.22	-	-
Currently lives alone	Yes	1.32	1.28 - 1.35		
Currently attends an educational institution	No	1.28	1.25 - 1.3	-	-
Knows the origin of their disability	No	1.11	1.1 - 1.13	-	-
By occupational disease	Physical conditions or workplace safety	1.59	1.42 - 1.77	-	-
By accident	Travel or work	1.06	1.02 - 1.11	-	-
Is recovering from their disability	No	1.49	1.47 - 1.52	-	-
Currently uses special help	No	1.36	1.34 - 1.38	-	-
Has receive guidance in the management of their disability	No	1.3	1.28 - 1.32	-	-
Currently uses a rehabilitation center	No	1.2	1.18 - 1.22	-	-
Has received health care in the last year	No	1.18	1.16 - 1.20	-	-
Has worked in the last 6 months	No	1.28	1.26 - 1.31	-	-

workplace illness (OR: 1.59; CI 95% 1.42 - 1.77) and accidents (OR: 1.06; CI 95% 1.02 - 1.11) were associated with limited hearing.

In the multivariate analysis, socioeconomic stratus (OR: 1.33; CI 95% 1.25 - 1.42), illiteracy (OR: 1.44; CI 95% 1.42 - 1.46), and not being affiliated with the healthcare system (OR: 1.03; CI 95% 1.01 - 1.04) continued to be factors associated with limited hearing.

4. Discussion

Because communication permits socialization and autonomy of individuals, hearing deficiency impacts society in an important way from economic and psychosocial perspectives [9]. The present study shows that the group of persons registered who perceive themselves with hearing limitations, including those with the use of special hearing devices, belong to the poorest segment of the population and is composed principally of those above 60 years of age, although there exists an important group between 10 and 19 years (11.26%). The rates of illiteracy, affiliation with a health insurance system, and deficient working conditions show inequality in each of these sectors, affecting the physical, mental, and social well-being of this population and their families.

This limitation has greater impact on young people due to it affecting the education process and the capability of entering the workforce. Given the demographic conditions of the country, a large percentage of people with limited hearing are expected, especially in older adults (It is anticipated, given the demographic conditions of the country, that there will be a large percentage of people with limited hearing, especially in older adults) [10]. Hearing limitation causes communication difficulties in both sexes, which can lead to stigmatization and isolation [11].

Self-perception of limited hearing found within the registry was 13.6%; however it should be noted that according to the 2005 census it was 17.4%, and that in countries such as Brazil and Cuba values from 4.4% to 4.6%, respectively, have been reported [12] [13]. This information should be analyzed with caution, since the register is specialized to measure only the population that self-perceives with hearing disability. The principal limitation of this study is that since it uses secondary information whose procurement depends on the assistance of local governors and mayors [8], there exists a selection bias in certain municipalities or departments where there is greater interest in characterizing the population as disabled and thus does not necessarily reflect all of the disabled population. In addition to using an instrument that identifies self-perception of disability (in this case hearing disability), it is recommended that future investigations estimate hearing disability with the use of audiometric tests.

Several factors are of note with respect to health services: 1) the small percentage of persons who have recovered due to "other help" different from the social healthcare security system, demonstrate failures in the care of this population, and 2) the small percentage of persons who received occupational therapy and speech therapy services highlight the same drawback. It is possible that this situation is related to the low rate of affiliation in the population to a health insurance system, as well as the low availability of these services in isolated and difficult to reach areas. Additionally, it is possible that the doctor-patient relationship is impeded due to difficulties in communication [14] [15].

In so far as the causes of limited hearing, the following are known: hereditary or congenital disease, infections during pregnancy, other infections, complications in the perinatal period, otitis media, noise, trauma, cerebrovascular disease, and old age, among others [16] [17]. The present study shows that general illness, complications related to pregnancy and childbirth, as well as genetic disorders and accidents were the most frequent. The available information did not permit a deeper analysis of said causes, but important information was obtained regarding occupational disease, consumption of psychoactive drugs, accidents, and difficulties in accessing health services, due to the instrument giving said information. In so far as hearing disability by occupational disease, 2.44% of those that knew the origin of their disability attributed it to this cause. In Colombia, neurosensory deafness placed third in occupational disease between 2001 and 2003 and fell to fourth in 2004. Only since 2006 has the country had the "Guide for the Care of Hypoacusia Induced by Noise in the Workplace", which presents recommendations to workers exposed to noise [18], as well as the legal framework for hypoacusia, specifically Resolution 8321 of 1983 of the Ministry of Health, where the norms for protection and conservation of healthcare are dictated [19]. This is in contrast to some countries where hypoacusia by workplace illness is considered a serious problem, possibly due to legislation specific to the production of noise [20].

In so far as the factors associated with self-perception of hearing limitation, even with the use of special hearing devices, our study found correlations with low socioeconomic stratus, illiteracy, and the lack of affiliation to a healthcare system, showing the inequity of these persons; several studies have shown that inequalities exist in the socioeconomic level and the use of health insurance services among persons with hearing disability [21] [22]. However, taking into account that the RLCPD does not provide homogenous coverage of the departments of the country, it does not necessarily reflect the factors associated with this limitation in the Colombian population. With respect to the consumption of psychoactive drugs, different studies have shown weak correlations between the use of tobacco and sudden deafness in those that consume more than 20 cigarettes daily (OR: 1.28; CI 0.77 - 2.13). Moreover, the risk grows in those that consume more than 2 servings of alcohol per day (OR: 1.92; CI 1.12 - 3.29) [23]. According to the RLCPD less than 1% of persons who knew the origin of their disability attributed it to use of psychoactive drugs, and of these 74.5% use socially accepted psychoactive drugs (tobacco, alcohol).

The vascular origin hypothesis is plausible because the cochlea is highly vascularized such that it has similar risk factors to other vascular diseases such as coronary disease and infarction [23] [24]. This shows the risk of suffering from this limitation in a society that permits the use of licit drugs such as alcohol and tobacco.

We wish to highlight that although the country has passed the Law 982 of 2005 [25], which expresses the right to identification and early intervention in hearing loss, as well as the right for the hearing disabled to access education and employment, the law has not yet been instated, despite the efforts of different sectors [26]. The law also requires important modifications such as the implementation of auditory screening with the latest technology in those younger than 1 year, and early intervention programs to mitigate the risk of the social, educational, health, and psychological consequences that go along with hearing loss.

5. Conclusion

The present study reveals the inequality, injustice, and social imbalance in the group of people that self-perceive with hearing limitations even with the use of special hearing devices, showing that sustainable and political interventions are required, especially in health, education and employment, which will eliminate barriers so that these people have the same opportunities as other Colombians. The state must invest greater effort so that these people can access health, rehabilitation, and education services to facilitate their integration and to not perpetuate these conditions.

Acknowledgements

We thank the Administrative Department of National Statistics (DANE) for providing the information from the Register for the Localization and Characterization of Persons with Disability.

Declaration of Conflict of Interest

The authors declare that they present no conflict of interest.

Financing

The present study was financed by the Unidad Médico-quirúrgica de Otorrinolaringologia S.A.

General Considerations

The present study was not submitted to the Ethical Committee, due to it being a study based on the use of secondary sources, that did not have access to the identity of the subjects, and that did not present a risk to the integrity of those persons.

References

[1]   García, J.M., Penaranda, A., Barón, C. and Campos, S. (2004) The Fundacion Santafe de Bogota-Colombia Cochlear Implant Program: A Five year Experience. In: Cohen, N. and Waltzman, S., Eds., *Cochlear Implants*, Thieme Medical Pub., New York, 337-339.

[2]   Peñaranda, A. and Megaglia, A. (2007) Predisposing Factors in the Perception of Speech. In: Peñaranda, A., García, J., Pinzón, M., Eds., *Manual de otorrinolaringología*, AMOLCA, Bogotá, 212-223.

[3]   Thompson, D., McPhillips, H., Davis, R., Lieu, T., Homer, C. and Helfand, M. (2001) Universal Newborn Hearing Screening: Summary of Evidence. *JAMA*, **286**, 2000-2010. http://dx.doi.org/10.1001/jama.286.16.2000

[4]   Stein, K. (1999) Factors Influencing the Efficacy of Universal Newborn Screaning. *Pediatric Clinics of North America*, **46**, 95-105. http://dx.doi.org/10.1016/S0031-3955(05)70084-5

[5]   Comisión de regulación en salud. CRES. (2011) http://www.cres.gov.co/Portals/0/ConsultaCiudadana/IMPLANTE%20COCLEAR.pdf

[6]   Perez, R., Arriagada, M., Aviles, M., Palma, J. and Valenzuela, M. (2006) Maternal and Perinatal Factors Associated with Hearing Loss. *Rev Colomb Obstet Ginecol.* [Online], **57**, 201-206.

[7]   Carrasquilla, G., Martínez, S., Latorre, M., García, S., González, C., Rincón, C., *et al.* (2009) Disability in the Context of the General System of Social Security in Colombia: Guidelines, Epidemiology and Economic Impact. Bogotá.

[8]   Departamento Administrativo Nacional de Estadística (2006) Preliminary Results of the Implementation of the Data for Localization and Characterization of People with Disabilities. National Consolidated to July 2006. Departamento Administrativo Nacional de Estadística, Ministerio de Educación Nacional, Bogotá.

[9]   Bittencourt, Z. and Hoehne, E. (2009) Quality of Life of Deaf People's Relatives Assisted in a Rehabilitation Center. *Ciência Saúde Coletiva*, **14**, 1235-1239.

[10] Gething, L. (2000) Ageing with Long-Standing Hearing Impairment and Deafness. *International Journal of Rehabilitation Research*, **23**, 209-215. http://dx.doi.org/10.1097/00004356-200023030-00011

[11] Mackenzie, I. and Smith, A. (2009) Deafness the Neglected and Hidden Disability. *Annals of Tropical Medicine & Parasitology*, **103**, 565-571. http://dx.doi.org/10.1179/000349809X12459740922372

[12] de Castro, S., Galvão, C., Carandina, L., Azevedo, M., Goi, M. and Goldbaum, M. (2008) Visual, Hearing, and Physical Disability: Prevalence and Associated Factors in a Population-Based Study. *Cadernos de Saúde Pública*, **24**, 1773-1782.

[13] Cobas, M., Zacca, E., Morales, F., Icart, E., Jordán, A. and Valdéz, M. (2010) Epidemiological Characterization of People with Disabilities in Cuba. *Revista Cubana de Salud Pública*, **36**, 306-310.

[14] Scheier, D. (2009) Barriers to Health Care for People with Hearing Loss: A Review of the Literature. *Journal of the New York State Nurses' Association*, **40**, 4-10.

[15] Steinberg, A., Barnett, S., Meador, H. and Wiggins, E. (2006) Health Care System Accessibility Experiences and Perceptions of Deaf People. *Journal of General Internal Medicine*, **21**, 260-266. http://dx.doi.org/10.1111/j.1525-1497.2006.00340.x

[16] Isaacson, B. (2010) Hearing Loss. *Medical Clinics of North America*, **94**, 973-988. http://dx.doi.org/10.1016/j.mcna.2010.05.003

[17] García, F., Peñaloza, Y. and Poblano, A. (2003) Hearing Disorders as a Problem of Public Health in Mexico. *Anales de otorrinolaringología Mexicana*, **48**, 20-29.

[18] Ministerio de Protección Social (2006) Guía de Atención Integral Basada en la Evidencia para Hipoacusia Neurosensorial Inducida por Ruido en el Lugar de Trabajo (GATI-HNIR). http://www.epssura.com/guias/guia_ved.pdf.

[19] Ministerio de Salud (1983) Resolution 8321/1983 by Which Dictate the Rules on Protection and Conservation of the Hearing of Health and Well-Being of People, Cause of the Production and Emission of Noise. Ministerio de Salud, Bogotá.

[20] Fuente, A. and Hickson, L. (2011) Noise-Induced Hearing Loss in Asia. *International Journal of Audiology*, **50**, 3-10.

[21] Boss, E., Niparko, J., Gaskin, D. and Levinson, K. (2011) Socioeconomic Disparities for Hearing-Impaired Children in the United States. *The Laryngoscope*, **121**, 860-866. http://dx.doi.org/10.1002/lary.21460

[22] Kubba, H., MacAndie, C., Ritchie, K. and MacFarlane, M. (2004) Is Deafness a Disease of Poverty? The Association between Socio-Economic Deprivation and Congenital Impairment. *International Journal Audiology*, **43**, 123-125. http://dx.doi.org/10.1080/14992020400050017

[23] Mieko, N., Nobuo, A., Tsutomu, N., Tomoyuki, H., *et al.* (2001) Smoking, Alcohol, Sleep and Risk of Idiopathic Sudden Deafness: A Case-Control Study Using Pooled Controls. *Journal of Epidemiology*, **11**, 81-86. http://dx.doi.org/10.2188/jea.11.81

[24] Zuñiga, J., Espinoza, C. and Martínez, C. (2008) Sudden Hearing Loss. One Year Experience. *Revista de otorrinolaringología y cirugía de cabeza y cuello*, **68**, 255-262.

[25] Congreso de la República de Colombia (2005) 982 Law of 2005 Which Lays down Rules Aimed at Equal Opportunities for Deaf and Deafblind and Enacting Other Provisions. Congreso de la República de Colombia, Bogotá.

[26] INSOR (2008) Clínica Rivas, Universidad Nacional de Colombia, Fundación Santa Fe de Bogotá. Working Paper on Chapter IX of the 982 Law 2005, Bogotá. (Unpublished)

3

Cochlear Implantation in Patients with Eosinophilic Otitis Media

Masahiro Takahashi[1*], Yasuhiro Arai[1], Naoko Sakuma[1], Daisuke Sano[1],
Goshi Nishimura[1], Takahide Taguchi[1], Nobuhiko Oridate[1], Satoshi Iwasaki[2],
Shin-Ichi Usami[3]

[1]Department of Otorhinolaryngology Head and Neck Surgery, Yokohama City University School of Medicine, Yokohama, Japan
[2]Department of Otorhinolaryngology, International University of Health and Welfare, Mita Hospital, Tokyo, Japan
[3]Department of Otorhinolaryngology, Shinshu University School of Medicine, Nagano, Japan
Email: [*]masa12_1@yokohama-cu.ac.jp

Abstract

It is known that cochlear implantation for deaf patients with eosinophilic otitis media (EOM) is safe and can provide good speech perception. However, the best timing of implant surgery in patients with EOM is not yet known. The aim of this case report is to suggest the appropriate timing of the surgery in EOM patients with deaf. Cochlear implantation was indicated in two patients with EOM. One underwent cochlear implantation in the absence of any ear discharge. In the other case, implant surgery was delayed for three years due to persistent ear discharge. No complications related to implant device or skin flap were observed in either case. The speech recognition score after implantation was good in the first case and poor in the second case. Perioperative complications were manageable even in the patient with persistent ear discharge. However, the delay in implant surgery due to the persistent ear discharge resulted in a poor speech recognition score. Early implantation should be considered even in EOM patients with ear discharge, although the presence of active middle ear inflammation is regarded as one of the contraindications for implantation according to the current Japanese guidelines.

Keywords

Eosinophilic Otitis Media, Cochlear Implantation, Speech Recognition

---

[*]Corresponding author.

1. Introduction

Eosinophilic otitis media (EOM) is an intractable middle ear disease with eosinophil-enriched middle ear effusion [1] [2]. The most common characteristic of EOM is the presence of highly viscous mucoid middle ear effusion enriched with eosinophils, although the mechanism of eosinophil accumulation in the middle ear has not yet been determined. The deterioration of bone conductive hearing level (BCHL) is more frequently observed in patients with EOM than that in those with chronic otitis media (COM) [3], with 47% of EOM patients showing deterioration in BCHL and 6% developing profound hearing loss [4]. It has been reported that cochlear implantation is safe and provides good speech recognition for EOM patient with deafness [5].

We experienced two cases of EOM in which the patients required cochlear implant. The patients showed different speech recognition scores after implantation, and we herein discuss the reason for this difference.

2. Case

Case 1. A 53-year-old female was referred to our hospital for the investigation on progressive bilateral sensorineural hearing loss. Thirty years previously, she had been diagnosed with bilateral chronic otitis media (COM). She was also diagnosed with chronic sinusitis without nasal polyposis, and she had been treated with steroid inhalation therapy for bronchial asthma. At the age of 49, bilateral profound sensorineural hearing loss was detected. On pathological examination, the middle ear mucosa contained numerous eosinophils and she was diagnosed with EOM according to the 2011 diagnostic criteria [6]. Pure tone audiometry showed bilateral profound hearing loss (**Figure 1**). Her speech recognition score was 10% (Japanese monosyllable list) in both ears. Temporal bone computed tomography (CT) and magnetic resonance imaging (MRI) showed no low density tissue in mastoid or tympanic cavities (**Figure 2(a)**). No ossification of the cochlea was evident (**Figure 2(b)**). As she did not present with any ear discharge, we recommend cochlear implantation. After systemic administration of a corticosteroid (dexamethazon 2 mg/day × 7 days), we performed cochlear implantation through the round window approach with miryngoplasty in her left ear. As no ossification of the cochlea was observed, flex electrode arrays (Med-EL Flex[28]) were used and inserted completely. No complications in relation to the implant device or skin flap were observed during a three-year follow-up. In spite of postoperative oral steroid administration, the tympanic membrane was re-perforated and ear discharge recurred at six months post-surgery (**Figure 3**). Even

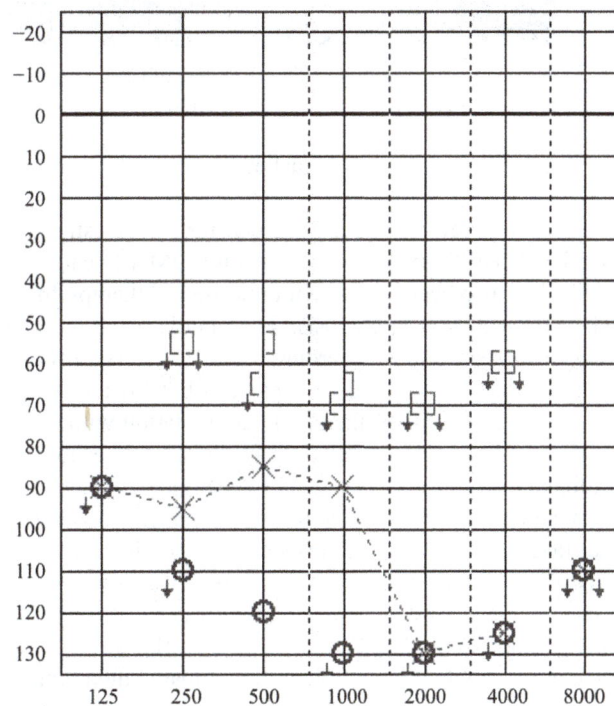

Figure 1. Preoperative pure tone audiometry of Case 1.

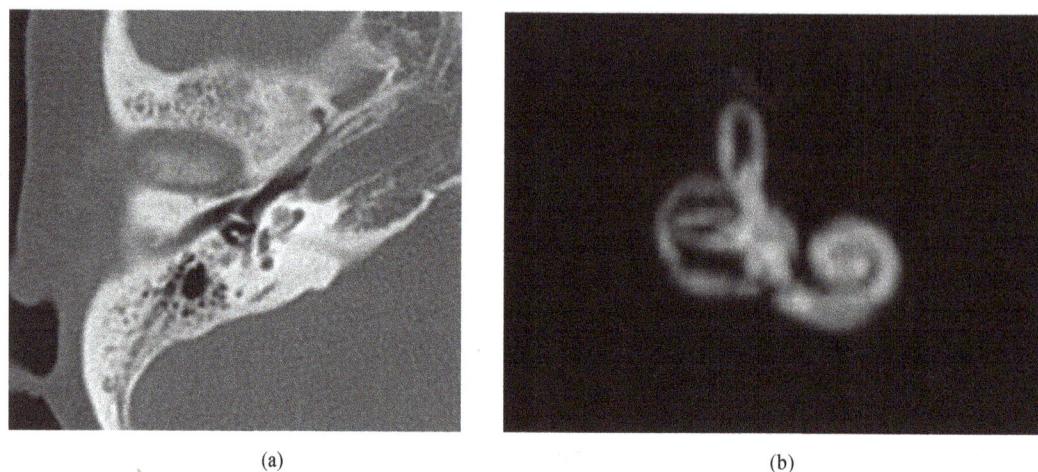

(a)   (b)

Figure 2. (a) Preoperative CT of Case 1. No low density tissue in mastoid and tympanic cavity; (b) Preoperative 3D MRI of Case 1. Ossified cochlea was not evident.

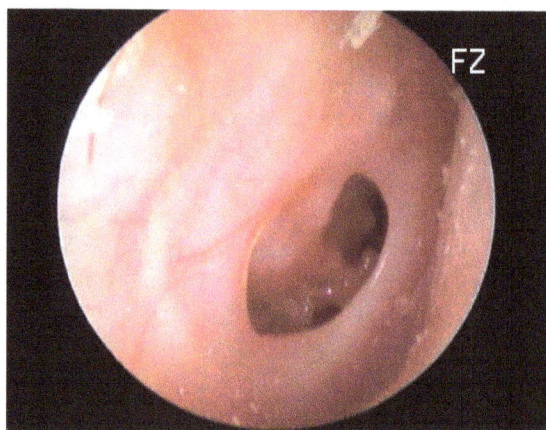

Figure 3. The right tympanic membrane of Case 1 was reperforated and ear discharge was recurred.

under such conditions, her speech recognition score reached 92 % (Japanese monosyllable list) at three years after surgery.

Case 2. A 65-year-old female was referred to our hospital for the investigation on progressive bilateral sensorineural hearing loss. She had been diagnosed with bilateral COM 12 years previously and she had been suffering from ear discharge. She had also been treated with oral steroid therapy for bronchial asthma. She was also diagnosed with chronic sinusitis with nasal polyposis. The middle ear viscous discharge contained numerous eosinophils and she was diagnosed with EOM according to the 2011 diagnostic criteria [6]. Temporal bone CT showed low density areas in the mastoid and tympanic cavities but MRI showed no ossification of the cochlea (**Figure 4(a)**, **Figure 4(b)**). In spite of anti-IgE therapy in combination with oral steroids, an anti-histaminergic agent and leukotriene receptor antagonist administration, her hearing threshold was gradually deteriorated, and she developed bilateral profound hearing loss at the age of 70 (**Figure 5**). Her speech recognition score was 20% (Japanese monosyllable list) in both ears. As the middle ear discharge was persistent, we decided not to perform the cochlear implant at that time. 3 years later, she insisted on receiving a cochlear implant since she could not hear at all with hearing aids. The electrode array (Med-EL Flex[28]) was inserted into the scala vestibule in her left ear as ossification of the scala tympani was found during the surgery. Myringoplasty was also performed in her left ear. No complications in relation to the implant device or skin flap were observed during a two-year follow-up. In spite of postoperative oral steroid administration, the tympanic membrane was re-perforated and ear discharge recurred three months post-surgery (**Figure 6**). Her speech recognition score was 20% (Japanese monosyllable list).

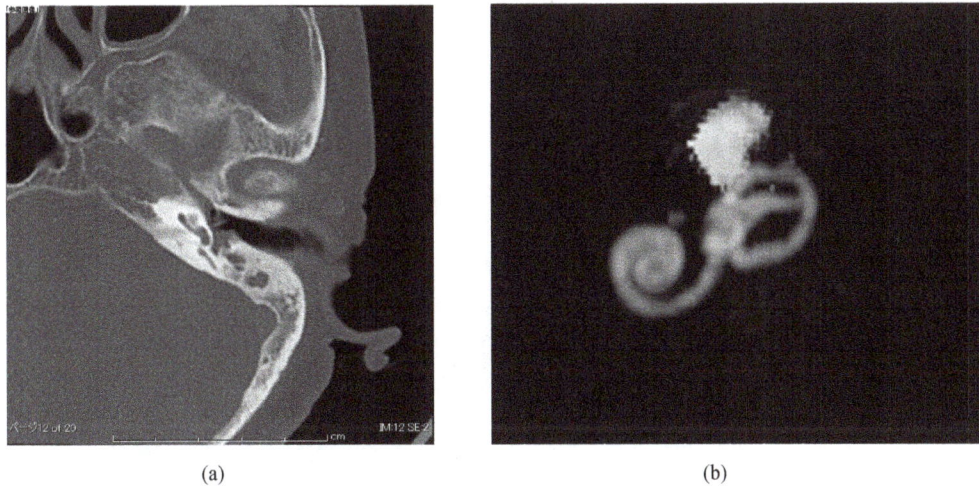

(a)   (b)

Figure 4. (a) Preoperative CT of Case 2. Low density area in mastoid and tympanic cavity; (b) Preoperative 3D MRI of Case 2. Ossified cochlea was not evident.

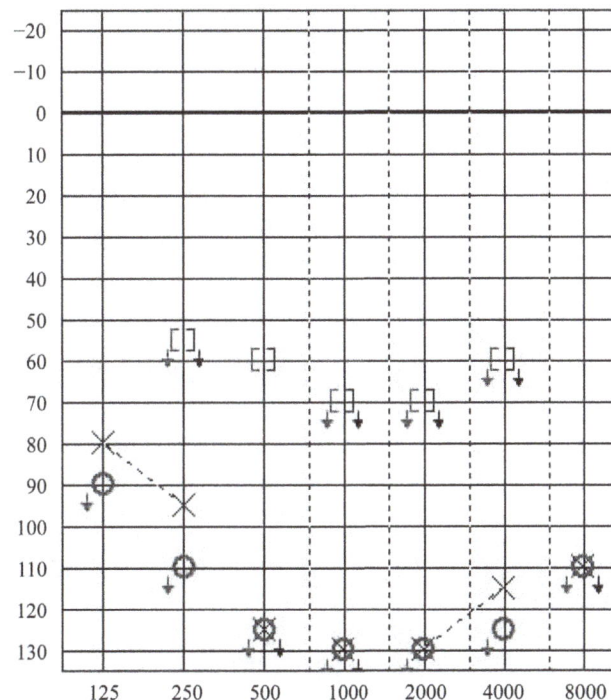

Figure 5. Preoperative pure tone audiometry of Case 2.

3. Discussion

EOM causes marked damage to sensorineural hearing, with the rate of BCHL loss being about ten times greater than that for chronic suppurative otitis media [3]. High-tone hearing loss, in particular, is more frequent and more severe in EOM patients than in COM patients [7], with 47% of EOM patients showing deterioration in BCHL, and 6% developing bilateral profound hearing loss according to the clinical survey of EOM in Japan [4]. The cause of deterioration in BCHL in cases of EOM remains unclear, but significantly higher concentrations of eosinophil cationic protein (ECP) and IgE have been detected in the middle ear effusion of EOM patients than in that of control patients [8]. Further, numerous eosinophil infiltrations were in the scala tympani, as well as severe morphological damage to the cochlea, the organ of Corti and the stria vascularis was observed in the prolonged topical stimulation animal model and is thought to be the cause of the deterioration in BCHL [9].

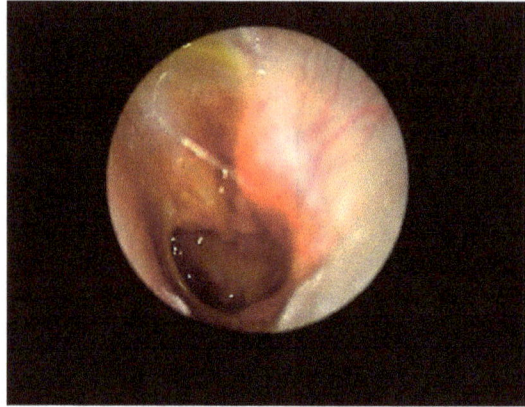

Figure 6. The left tympanic membrane of Case 2 was re-perforated and ear discharge was recurred.

Patients with EOM and profound sensorineural hearing loss are considered to be good candidates for cochlear implantation, and the results of speech recognition testing after implantation have shown marked improvements [5].

However, the speech recognition scores after implantation were quite different between the two cases we experienced. We selected a single-staged cochlear implant in these cases, because a planned-staged (such as mastoidectomy and tympanoplasty) cochlear implant can lead to cochlear ossification [10] and subsequently, to poor results in terms of speech perception after implantation. For cochlear implantation in patients with COM, obliteration and isolation of the middle ear cavity by closure of the external ear canal is required to control the ear discharge [11]. The characteristic of ear discharge of EOM is completely different from that of COM. Appropriate management of EOM for cochlear implant surgery is not yet determined, but the most important event in the perioperative period is thought to be the management of ear discharge.

As we believe that it is difficult to manage the clinical condition of EOM itself, one of options involving closure of the tympanic membrane and external auditory canal at the time of implant surgery was not adopted. Instead, by adding myringoplasty to cochlear implantation, we managed to control short-term postoperative ear discharge. However, in both patients, the tympanic membrane was eventually re-perforated and ear discharge recurred despite postoperative oral steroid administration.

On the other hand, the speech recognition score after implantation differed markedly between the two cases, suggesting that postoperative ear discharge may not necessarily be associated with poor functional outcomes. In such circumstances, and in the light of the fact that no complications were observed during the perioperative period, early implantation could be taken into consideration in cases of deaf patients with EOM showing persistent ear discharge. Further accumulation of cases, however, is still needed to confirm the best timing and method of cochlear implantation in EOM patients with ear discharge.

The long-term results of cochlear implantation in EOM patients were another important issue, especially in patients with persistent ear discharge. It is difficult to manage the clinical condition of EOM, and long-term inflammation within the cochlea affects the cochlear structures, with organs including the organ of Corti, stria vascularis, and spiral ganglion showing signs of degeneration [12]. Although it has been reported that good speech recognition scores after implantation for patients with EOM were maintained for eight years [5], long-term observation is definitely needed to verify the benefits of cochlear implantation in EOM patients.

4. Conclusion

In conclusion, in cases where cochlear implantation is indicated for EOM patients, early implantation should be considered, even in patients with persistent ear discharge, as the perioperative complications are manageable and a delayed in cochlear implantation surgery due to the ear discharge may result in cochlear ossification and subsequent poor speech recognition scores.

Conflict of Interest

The authors declare that there is no conflict of interest.

References

[1] Tomioka, S., Kobayashi, T. and Takasaka, T. (1997) Intractable Otitis Media in Patients with Bronchial Asthma (Eosinophilic Ottis Media). In: Sanna, M., Ed., *Cholesteatoma and Mastoid Surgery*, CICI Edizioni International, Rome, 851-853.

[2] Nagamine, H., Iino, Y., Kojima, C., Miyazawa, T. and Iida, T. (2002) Clinical Characteristics of So-Called Eosinophilic Otitis Media. *Auris Nasus Larynx*, **29**, 19-28. http://dx.doi.org/10.1016/S0385-8146(01)00124-9

[3] Nakagawa, T., Matubara, A., Shiratsuchi, H., Kakazu, Y., Nakashima, T., Koike, K., Umezaki, T. and Komune, S. (2006) Intractable Otitis Media with Eosinophils: Importance of Diagnosis and Validity of Treatment for Hearing Preservation. *ORL*, **68**, 118-122. http://dx.doi.org/10.1159/000091215

[4] Suzuki, H., Matsutani, S. and Kawase, T. (2004) Epidemiologic Surveillance of "Eosinophilic Otitis Media" in Japan. *Otology Japan*, **14**, 112-117. (In Japanese)

[5] Iwasaki, S., Nagura, M. and Mizuta, K. (2006) Cochlear Implantation in a Patient with Eosinophilic Otitis Media. *European Archives of Oto-Rhino-Laryngology*, **263**, 365-369. http://dx.doi.org/10.1007/s00405-005-1006-2

[6] Iino, Y., Matsutani, S., Matsubara, A., Nakagawa, T. and Nonaka, M. (2011) Diagnostic Criteria of Eosinophilic Otitis Media, a Newly Recognized Middle Ear Disease. *Auris Nasus Larynx*, **38**, 456-461. http://dx.doi.org/10.1016/j.anl.2010.11.016

[7] Iino, Y., Usubuchi, H., Kodama, K., Takizawa, K., Kanazawa, T. and Ohta, Y. (2008) Bone Conduction Hearing Level in Patients with Eosinophilic Otitis Media Associated with Bronchial Asthma. *Otology Neurotology*, **29**, 949-952. http://dx.doi.org/10.1097/MAO.0b013e318185fb0d

[8] Iino, Y., Usubuchi, H., Kodama, K., Kanazawa, H., Takizawa, K., Kanazawa, T. and Ohta, Y. (2010) Eoshinophilic Inflammation in the Middle Ear Induces Deterioration of Bone—Conduction Hearing Level in Patients with Eosinophilic Otitis Media. *Otology Neurotology*, **31**, 100-104. http://dx.doi.org/10.1097/MAO.0b013e3181bc3781

[9] Matubara, A., Nishizawa, H., Kurose, A., Nakagawa, T., Takahata, J. and Sasaki, A. (2014) An Experimental Study of Inner Ear Injury in an Animal Model of Eosinophilic Otitis Media. *Acta Oto-Laryngologica*, **134**, 227-32. http://dx.doi.org/10.3109/00016489.2013.859395

[10] Himi, T., Harabuchi, Y., Shintani, T., Yamaguchi, T., Yoshida, I. and Kataura, A. (1997) Surgical Strategy of Cochlear Implantation in Patients with Chronic Middle Ear Disease. *Audiology and Neurotology*, **2**, 410-417. http://dx.doi.org/10.1159/000259266

[11] Kojima, H., Sakurai, Y., Rikitake, M., Tanaka, Y., Kawano, A. and Moriyama, H. (2010) Cochlear Implantation in Patients with Chronic Otitis Media. *Auris Nasus Larynx*, **37**, 415-421. http://dx.doi.org/10.1016/j.anl.2010.01.009

[12] Keithley, E. and Haris, J. (1996) Late Sequelae of Cochlear Infection. *Laryngoscope*, **106**, 341-345. http://dx.doi.org/10.1097/00005537-199603000-00019

4

Prolonged Middle Ear Ventilation by Cartilage-Grommet Tympanoplasty

Kartik Parelkar, Smita Nagle, Mohan Jagade, Vandana Thorawade, Poonam Khairnar, Anoop Attakil, Madhavi Pandare, Rajanala Nataraj, Reshma Hanwate, Rajesh Kar

Department of ENT, Grant Government Medical College & Sir J J Group of Hospitals, Mumbai, India
Email: kartikparelkar@ymail.com

Abstract

In 1994, the American Otological Society reported favourable experience with composite cartilage shield tympanoplasty. The tragal cartilage with a grommet inserted in it was used for tympanoplasty in our patient with unilateral CSOM, supposedly because of severe chronic eustachian tube dysfunction. The marriage of cartilage tympanoplasty with grommet insertion was aimed to add the advantages and abolish the disadvantages of both the procedures. In 1990 Lary Hall first introduced the "long term ventilation of the middle ear" with a T-tube placed in the tragal cartilage perichondrium composite island graft. T-tube insertion in the cartilage has been described. But insertion of the Indian Sheperds grommet (ventilation tube) in the cartilage graft as described in this case and its technique are possibly the first of its kinds in literature. The report is aimed to ignite innovation of newer and better techniques of cartilage tympanoplasty.

Keywords

Tragal Cartilage, Grommet, Tympanoplasty

1. Introduction

The aim of tympanoplasty is to reconstruct the tympanic membrane and the sound conducting mechanism.

In 1990 Lary Hall first introduced the technique of cartilage T-tube tympanoplasty, the goal of placement of the permanent tube is to prevent repeated insertions of ventilating tubes, especially in children with severe and chronic secretory otitis media.

Chronic severe eustachian tube dysfunction is the main indication of cartilage shield T-tube tympanoplasty; such a situation most often is present in craniofacial abnormalities, downs syndrome, nasopharyngeal adenoid cystic carcinoma, previous head neck cancers involving the nasopharynx.

Also this technique can be used in cases with recurrences of chronic otitis media and history of multiple surgeries with chronic eustachian tube dysfunction as the possible eitiolgy. Recurrent long term middle ear effusion and atelectasis also can be managed by this method.

Prolonged middle ear ventilation is possible when a ventilation tube is inserted in the cartilage graft.

The possibility of grommet migration and displacement due to proliferation of the epithelial layer of tympanic membrane are reduced in this technique.

We would thus like to report our experience of cartilage-grommet tympanoplasty in this case.

2. Case Report

A 17-year-old male (**Figure 1**) with right ear discharge since 7 years presented to our out-patient department. The discharge was mucopurulent, non-foul smelling, intermittent and non-blood tinged. Patient had no active mucopurulent ear discharge since last 6 months.

On otoscopy right tympanic membrane showed large central perforation with a small tympanosclerotic patch in the anterosuperior quadrant while the left tympanic membrane was intact showing grade 4 retraction.

Patient had valsalva test and methylene blue dye test negative on both sides.

On tuning fork tests, Webers was lateralized to the right ear. Rinnes test was negative for the right ear.

Pure tone audiogram showed right ear mild to moderate conductive hearing loss.

Patient had right sided 2×2 cm sized lymph node over the right mastoid tip, no scalp infection.

FNAC (fine needle aspiration cytology) of which was suggestive of inflammatory cells.

Patient was taken up for right ear cartilage-grommet tympanoplasty after meticulous routine pre-anaesthetic investigations.

Tragal cartilage graft was harvested (**Figure 2**) with perichondrium on both sides. The margins of the perforation were freshened and tympanosclerotic patch was removed. Appropriate size and shape of the graft was fashioned. The antero-inferior quadrant of the graft was noted and marking for the site of grommet insertion made with methylene blue dye on a needle.

The perichondrium from over the lateral surface of the graft was raised all along its margins and a part of it over the grommet insertion site excised.

A small hole was made at the marked site with a cutting burr matching the approximate diameter of the grommet through which the grommet (0.75 mm internal diameter made of teflon) was inserted (**Figure 3**).

There was evidence of glue like secretion in the hypotympanum and retrotympanum which was suctioned out.

Post auricular Wildes incision was made, the lymphnode was dissected out and sent for HPR (s/o inflammatory cells, no evidence of tuberculous pathology).

Tympanomeatal flap was elevated and the cartilage-grommet graft placed in an underlay fashion (**Figure 4**), while the perichondrium over the lateral aspect was spread in an overlay manner except in the region of the grommet.

Gelfoam was kept in the EAC and the postauricular wound closed in layers. Post operative period was uneventful.

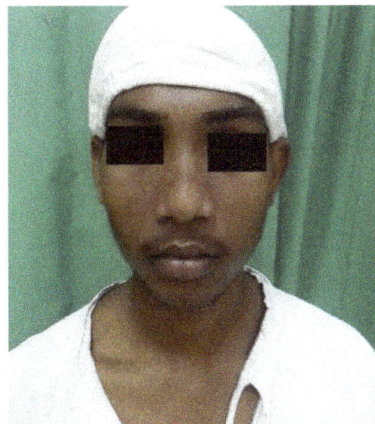

Figure 1. Case of right CSOM.

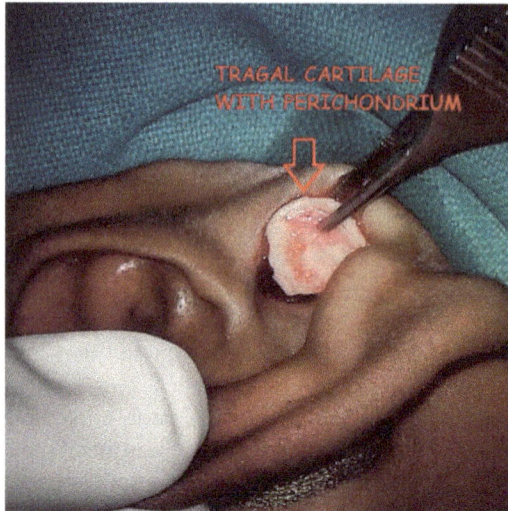

Figure 2. Tragal cartilage being harvested.

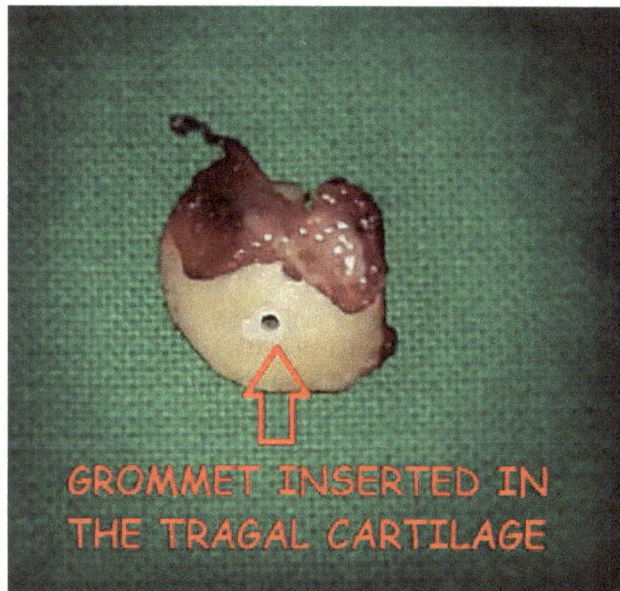

Figure 3. Composite tragal cartilage graft with inserted grommet.

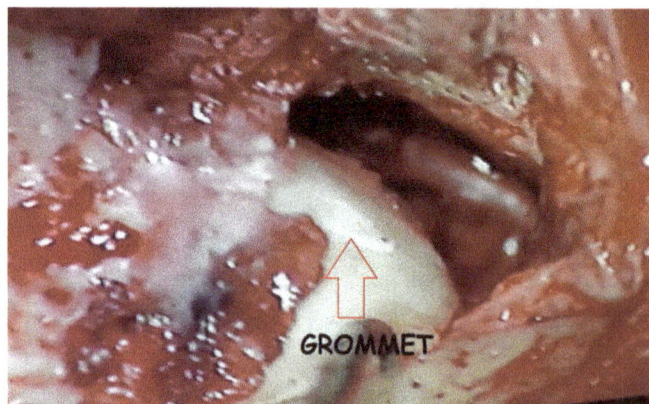

Figure 4. Cartilage-grommet graft being placed in underlay fashion.

3. Discussion

Since the introduction of tympanoplasty, in the fifties, by Zoellner [1] and Wullstein [2], numerous graft materials have been used for the closure of the defective membrane: skin, *fascia lata*, *temporalis fascia*, vein, perichondrium, *dura mater* [3]-[5].

Even today, *temporalis fascia* remains the most commonly used material for tympanic membrane reconstruction with a success rate of 93% - 97% in primary tympanoplasties [6].

In certain situations, such as recurrent perforation following myringoplasty, severe attical or posterior uncontrolled retraction pockets with cholesteatomatous formation, atelectasis of the tympanic membrane, fascia and perichondrium may undergo atrophy and subsequent failure, irrespective of the placement technique used [7].

In these patients, cartilage can be used as a grafting material on account of its increased stability and resistance to negative middle ear pressure, even in cases with chronic eustachian tube dysfunction [8].

It has been proved, both in experimental and clinical studies, that cartilage is well tolerated by the middle ear and shows long term survival [9] [10].

However, acceptance of routine reconstruction of the tympanic membrane with cartilage has been hampered by its reputation of sacrificing maximum hearing improvement, although various studies have shown that the hearing results are good, regardless of the thickness of the grafts [11]-[14].

Though in our case postauricular approach was used with a view to remove the lymph node over the mastoid tip, transcanal technique to harvest and place the composite tragal cartilage graft can be done. The transcanal technique is minimally invasive and sutureless one, with reduced hospital stay and better patient compliance.

Duckert, Muller, Malkielshi and Helms (1995) from university of Washington and university of Wirzburg have developed an interesting cartilage T-tube device to ventilate the tympanic cavity for prolonged period of time.

There are different methods of cartilage T-tube tympanoplasty *i.e.* Hall cartilage shield T-tube graft, Duckert cartilage graft, Dornhoffer graft and Elsheikh U-shaped cartilage perichondriun T-tube graft [15] [16].

In our technique a graft similar to the Duckert cartilage shield with a V-shaped notch to accommodate the handle of malleus was made.

Inserting the grommet in the cartilage graft is technically difficult, a pick can be used to gradually dilate a small hole made in the cartilage but in our experience an appropriate ossiculoplasty cutting burr is a better option to make the required hole for grommet insertion.

The cartilage shield T-tube tympanoplasty can effectively reverse atelectasis and provide prolonged middle-ear ventilation. The technique can be used safely and minimizes the risk of tympanic membrane perforation and other complications associated with prolonged middle ear intubation [16]. Patients undergoing tympanoplasty with this technique require long term follow-up though Dukert *et al*. (2003) have not found any extrusion of the tubes among 40 patients of their latest series.

The safety and efficacy of tympanoplasty in conjunction with anteriorly placed subannular T-tubes was examined by Elluru *et al*. [17].

Elsheikh et al compared the results for cartilage tympanoplasty with and without T-tube placement in those patients with atelectactic tympanic membrane though safe they found no particular advantage in primary insertion of ventilation tube in their study [18].

Reinsertion of the T-tube in case of extrusion can be done through the same hole in the cartilage and is relatively easy as risk of medializing the graft is reduced due to the increased rigidity of the graft.

However in our case as the grommet doesn't have flanges which can open up like the T-tube, hence resinsertion would be very difficult.

Closure of the ventilating tube by overlying cerumen can be managed by regular follow-up for cleaning and suctioning with a fine suction cannula.

There maybe chances of granulation tissue formation near the grommet site which can be managed by instillation of steroid containing drops.

Granulation tissue forms in 10% - 20% of cases (Danner and Dornhoffer, 2001), but it responds well to steroid containing drops and has never prompted tube removal.

Also coloured grommet would be a better option to use as it would be easier to visualize the grommet inserted in the cartilage both during the procedure and postoperatively.

Though only valsalva and methylene blue dye test along with the clinical and intra-operative findings (glue in middle ear) were used to suggest eustachian tube dysfunction as the possible eitiological factor for the chronic suppurative otitis media, it would be advisable to measure tubal patency and function by series of other tests as well.

Tympanometery and measurement of tubal function with deflation test and aspiration test should be done.

Our patient is on regular follow-up since 1 month postoperatively with no evidence of displacement of the grommet.

Pure tone audiogram will be repeated after 6 months and follow-up will be continued.

4. Conclusions

Tragal cartilage-grommet tympanoplasty requires specifications for patient selection. A defined set of tests pointing at eustachian tube dysfunction as a causative factor of the chronic suppurative otitis media are also required.

Through an attractive technique long term follow-up of patient and randomised control trials for this technique will help to establish its efficiency in cases requiring prolonged middle ear ventilation.

References

[1]   Zoellner, F. (1955) The Principles of Plastic Surgery of the Sound-Conducting Apparatus. *The Journal of Laryngology Otology*, **69**, 567-569.

[2]   Wullstein, H.L. (1952) Functional Operations in the Middle Ear with Split-Thickness Skin Graft. *Arch Otorhinolaryngol*, **161**, 422-435. http://dx.doi.org/10.1007/BF02129204

[3]   Heermann, H. (1960) Tympanic Membrane Plastic with Temporal Fascia. *Archiv für Ohren-, Nasen- und Kehlkopfheilkunde*, **9**, 136-139.

[4]   Shea, J.J. (1960) Vein Graft Closure of Eardrum Perforations. *The Journal of Laryngology Otology*, **74**, 358-362. http://dx.doi.org/10.1017/S002221510005670X

[5]   Preobrazhenski, T.B. and Rugov, A.A. (1965) The Employment of Preserved Dura Mater Graft in Tympanoplasty. *Vestnik Otorinolaringologii*, **5**, 38-42.

[6]   Sheehy, J.L. and Anderson, R.G. (1980) Myringoplasty. A Review of 472 Cases. *Annals of Otology, Rhinology Laryngology*, **89**, 331-334. http://dx.doi.org/10.1177/000348948008900407

[7]   Buckingham, R.A. (1992) Fascia and Perichondrium Atrophy in Tympanoplasty and Recurrent Middle Ear Atelectasis. *Annals of Otology, Rhinology Laryngology*, **101**, 755-758. http://dx.doi.org/10.1177/000348949210100907

[8]   Duckert, L.G., Muller, J., Makielski, K.H. and Helms, J. (1995) Composite Autograft "Shield" Reconstruction of Remnant Tympanic Membranes. *American Journal of Otolaryngology*, **16**, 21-26.

[9]   Yamamoto, E., Iwanaga, M. and Fukumoto, M. (1988) Histologic Study of Homograft Cartilage Implanted in the Middle Ear. *Otolaryngology—Head and Neck Surgery*, **98**, 546-551.

[10]   Hamed, M., Samir, M. and El Bigermy, M. (1999) Fate of Cartilage Material Used in Middle Ear Surgery Light and Electron Microscopy Study. *Auris Nasus Larynx*, **26**, 257-262. http://dx.doi.org/10.1016/S0385-8146(99)00012-7

[11]   Amedee, R.G., Mann, W.J. and Riechelmann, H. (1989) Cartilage Palisade Tympanoplasty. *American Journal of Otology*, **10**, 447-450.

[12]   Dornhoffer, J.L. (1997) Hearing Results with Cartilage Tympanoplasty. *The Laryngoscope*, **107**, 1094-1099. http://dx.doi.org/10.1097/00005537-199708000-00016

[13]   Gerber, M.J., Mason, J.C. and Lambert, P.R. (2000) Hearing Results after Primary Cartilage Tympanoplasty. *The Laryngoscope*, **110**, 1994-1999. http://dx.doi.org/10.1097/00005537-200012000-00002

[14]   Heermann, J. (1992) Autograft Tragal and Conchal Palisade Cartilage and Perichondrium in Tympanomastoid Reconstruction. *Ear, Nose & Throat Journal*, **71**, 344-349.

[15]   Hall, L.J. (1990) T-Tube with Tragus Cartilage Flange in Long Term Middle Ear Ventilation. *American Journal of Otology*, **11**, 454-457.

[16]   Duckert, L.G., Makielski, K.H. and Helms, J. (2003) Prolonged Middle Ear Ventilation with the Cartilage Shield T-Tube Tympanoplasty. *Otology & Neurotology*, **24**, 153-157. http://dx.doi.org/10.1097/00129492-200303000-00006

[17]   Elluru, R.G., Dhanda, R., Neely, J.G. and Goebel, J.A. (2001) Anterior Subannular T-Tube for Prolonged Middle Ear Ventilation during Tympanoplasty: Evaluation of Efficacy and Complications. *Otology & Neurotology*, **22**, 761-765. http://dx.doi.org/10.1097/00129492-200111000-00008

[18]   Elsheikh, M.N., Elsherief, H.S. and Elsherief, S.G. (2006) Cartilage Tympanoplasty for Management of Tympanic Membrane Atelectasis: Is Ventilatory Tube Necessary? *Otology & Neurotology*, **27**, 859-864. http://dx.doi.org/10.1097/01.mao.0000226288.96423.ed

5

Atrial Septal Defect and Left Recurrent Laryngeal Nerve Paralysis: A Case of Ortner's Syndrome and Literature Review

Andrew M. Vahabzadeh-Hagh[1], Catherine Yim[2], Jayson Fitter[1], Dinesh K. Chhetri[1]

[1]Department of Head and Neck Surgery, UCLA David Geffen School of Medicine, Los Angeles, USA
[2]Radiological Sciences, UCLA David Geffen School of Medicine, Los Angeles, USA
Email: AvahabzadehHagh@mednet.ucla.edu

Abstract

Introduction: Cardiovocal syndrome, or hoarseness resulting from vocal fold paralysis secondary to cardiovascular pathology, is commonly referred to as Ortner's syndrome. We present a brief overview of vocal fold paralysis, present an illustrative case of Ortner's syndrome, and provide a review of the pertinent literature. Here we aim to broaden one's differential for vocal fold paralysis, discuss its importance as pertains to cardiovascular pathology and outcomes, and highlight the difficulties in therapeutic planning for these unique patients. Methods: A case report and literature review. Results: A 26-year-old female with an atrial septal defect and pulmonary hypertension presented with 5 months of hoarseness. Laryngoscopy revealed left vocal fold paralysis. Imaging from the skull base to chest showed an enlarged pulmonary artery (PA) in the absence of other abnormalities. Literature review suggests that this left laryngeal nerve paralysis results from nerve compression within the aortopulmonary window, a triangle defined by the aortic arch, PA, and ligamentumarteriosum. Imaging in our patient over 8 months demonstrated an increase in PA size from 3.9 to 4.2 cm correlating with the onset of hoarseness. Conclusions: Importantly, hoarseness second ary to laryngeal nerve compression in cardiovascular disease may correlate with a poorer prognosis, *i.e.*, in thoracic aortic aneurysms and mitral valvestenosis. Awareness of vocal changes in the setting of cardiovascular disease improves diagnostic acumen in vocal foldparalysis.

Keywords

Ortner's, Cardiovocal, Vocalfoldparalysis

1. Introduction

Unilateral vocal fold paralysis (UVFP) primarily impacts a patient's voice, but may result in dysphagia as well as dyspnea. The etiologies for UVFP have evolved over time but continue to include the following leading causes: 1) iatrogenic/postsurgical, commonly with procedures involving the anterior cervical spine, carotid artery, and thyroid; 2) neoplastic, commonly with thyroid and lung neoplasms; 3) others including trauma, systemic disease (e.g. infectious, inflammatory, neurologic, cardiovascular, medication related); and 4) idiopathic, which is a small but persistent group of cases [1]. An uncommon cause of unilateral vocal fold paralysis may result from a cardiovascular disease, Ortner's syndrome, also known as cardiovocal syndrome. Originally described in 1897, Ortner's syndrome detailed a left VFP resulting from recurrent laryngeal nerve compression within the aortopulmonary window, a triangle defined by the aortic arch, pulmonary artery, and ligamentumarteriosum [2] [3]. This phenomenon was originally described in the setting of mitral stenosis, but has since been correlated with a broader list of cardiovascular pathology (**Table 1**). Here we present an illustrative case of a 26-year-old female with an atrial septal defect and hoarseness.

2. Case Report

A 26-year-old Hispanic female was referred to otolaryngology for 5 months of hoarseness. Nearly one-year prior she was in her usual state of health training for Navy boot camp when she developed a progressive productive cough. She was found to have pneumonia, but among her work-up an EKG demonstrated right ventricular hypertrophy prompting referral to a cardiologist. A transthoracic echo was performed which demonstrated pulmonary hypertension with a dilated right atrium and ventricle. Weeks later she developed significant and sudden dyspnea on exertion and her exercise tolerance drastically diminished. Ultimately she required hospital admission, during which extensive cardiovascular workup revealed pulmonary hypertension and a secundum type atrial septal defect. Approximately 4 months after her discharge she began to develop hoarseness. She was then seen and evaluated in the head and neck surgery clinic 5 months later.

In clinic, her voice was hoarse. She had a persistent non-productive cough but denied any respiratory difficulties above her baseline dyspnea secondary to her cardiac disease. She denied any dysphagia. Notably she had no other prior medical or surgical history and denied any tobacco or alcohol use. On exam her neck was flat and without lymphadenopathy. Flexible laryngoscopy demonstrated a paralyzed left vocal fold in the paramedian position. Imaging from the skull base to aortic arch showed an enlarged pulmonary artery (PA) in the absence of other abnormalities consistent with Ortner's syndrome (**Figure 1** [4], **Figure 2**). A retrospective look at her prior imaging demonstrated an increase in PA size from 3.9 to 4.2 cm over an approximate 8-month period correlating with the onset of hoarseness and the progression of her cardiovascular disease.

Table 1. Cardiovascular pathologies that may result in vocal fold paralysis.

Cardiovascular pathology	Ref.
Left ventricular failure secondary to HTN	[3]
Atrial septal defect (ASD)	
Eisenmenger's syndrome	
Patent ductusarteriosus (PDA)	
Primary pulmonary HTN (PPH)	
Pulmonary embolism (PE)	
Aortic arch pseudoaneurysm	[10]
Mitral stenosis (MS)	
Mitral regurgitation (MR)	
Atrial myxoma	
Left ventricle aneurysm	
Corpulmonale	
Rheumatic heart disease	[11]

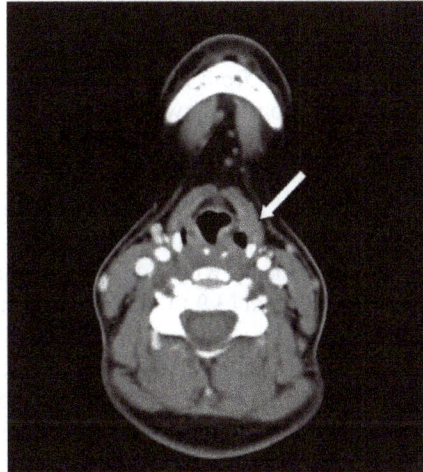

Figure 1. Axial CT with contrast at the level of the hypopharynx/supraglottis. Note the expansion of the left piriform sinus with air and medialization of the left aryepiglottic fold/false vocal fold (white arrow). CT evidence of VFP must not be confused with cervical neoplasms, arytenoid cartilage subluxation or fracture, or oblique imaging findings, all of which can mimic VFP.

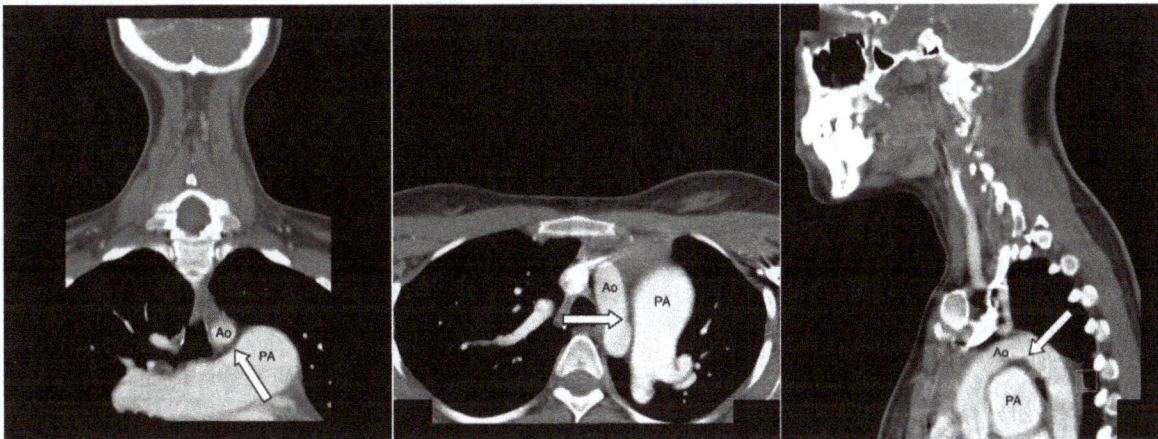

Figure 2. Cross sectional imaging of aortopulmonary window. White arrow denotes aortopulmonary window, the borders of which are defined by the aortic arch (Ao), pulmonary artery (PA), and ligamentumarteriosum, shown in coronal (left), axial (middle), and sagittal (right) sections.

The patient was deemed a high operative risk from a cardiovascular standpoint. Operative intervention including medializationthyroplasty and/or arytenoid adduction would likely have improved her dysphonia. In addition, we discussed the temporary benefits she could obtain from an injection laryngoplasty but she elected against this option. Given her mild symptoms, the possibility of recovering nerve function by addressing her cardiovascular disease, and her high operative risk, the risks of proceeding with a more definitive laryngeal intervention on aggregate outweighed the benefits. As such we elected to awaither cardiovascular treatment and recovery.

3. Discussion

Evaluation of dysphonia from UVFP begins with an auditory-perceptual evaluation, in which one may appreciate a hoarse or breathy voice. Laryngoscopy then provides direct visualization to confirm vocal fold paralysis or paresis. Imaging provides a means of determining the possible etiology. Imaging often begins with a chest X-ray but may include a CT or MRI typically from the skull base to aortic arch if the chest X-ray is unrevealing. High-resolution imaging allows for the assessment of any potential pathology along the course of the recurrent laryngeal nerve [1].

In this report we provide an example of a unique cardiovascular explanation for UVFP. Cardiovocal or Ortner's syndrome has been described in a wide array of cardiovascular pathologies that all result in encroachment upon the aortopulmonary window; **Table 1**. A report from Japan described two cases of pulmonary hypertension, one resultant from a longstanding PDA similar to our case, with new onset hoarseness. Here, cross sectional CT imaging was shown to be an easy and noninvasive method for confirming the cause of hoarseness [3]. In Ortner's syndrome secondary to pulmonary hypertension, CT imaging demonstrates an enlarged pulmonary truncus that exhibits cephalad displacement to be adjacent to the lower border of the aortic arch; namely, lying within the same tomographic plane. Autopsy studies by Fetterrolf and Norris showed that the distance between the aorta and the pulmonary artery within the aortopulmonary window is only 4 mm [5]. Hence, hoarseness in our patient corresponding to the dilation of her PA by 3 mm (3.9 to 4.2 cm) is a very reasonable and perhaps expected finding.

The presence of VFP in the setting of cardiovascular disease (e.g. aortic aneurysms, mitral stenosis) is regarded as a poor prognostic indicator. In the setting of VFP secondary to thoracic aortic aneurysms, some have used the development of VFP to influence the need for surgical intervention [6] [7]. Some have even suggested that all patients with select forms of cardiovascular disease be referred for laryngoscopy as part of their overall clinical evaluation [3] [8]. Cardiovocal syndrome provides the head and neck surgeon with a unique dilemma. Namely, these patients are high-risk surgical candidates with potentially reversible disease through correction of their underlying cardiovascular pathology. 2 of 4 patients with thoracic aortic aneurysms and 3 of 8 patients with distal aortic arch aneurysms had improvement or complete recovery in vocal fold mobility following cardiovascular treatment [6] [9]. Our patient was still undergoing cardiovascular evaluation in the setting of her progressive disease and undoubtedly was a high-risk surgical candidate currently compensating and functioning quite well despite her VFP. As such, we collectively decided to await possible cardiovascular intervention and recovery while clinically following her VFP.

4. Conclusion

Overall, it is important for the clinician to be aware that hoarseness in the setting of cardiovascular disease may be due to cardiovocal syndrome. CT imaging provides an efficient means for diagnosis and the therapeutic course must be well thought out in a multidisciplinary setting.

References

[1] Misono, S. and Merati, A.L. (2012) Evidence-Based Practice: Evaluation and Management of Unilateral Vocal Fold Paralysis. *Otolaryngologic Clinics of North America*, **45**, 1083-1108. http://dx.doi.org/10.1016/j.otc.2012.06.011

[2] Ortner, N. (1897) Recurrent Nerve Palsy in Patient with Mitral Stenosis (German). *Wiener Klinische Wochenschrift*, **10**, 753-755.

[3] Nakao, M., Sawayama, T., Samukawa, M., *et al.* (1985) Left Recurrent Laryngeal Nerve Palsy Associated with Primary Pulmonary Hypertension and Patent Ductus Arteriosus. *Journal of the American College of Cardiology*, **5**, 788-792. http://dx.doi.org/10.1016/S0735-1097(85)80413-7

[4] Paquette, C.M., Manos, D.C. and Psooy, B.J. (2012) Unilateral Vocal Cord Paralysis: A Review of CT Findings, Mediastinal Causes, and the Course of the Recurrent Laryngeal Nerves. *Radiographics*, **32**, 721-740. http://dx.doi.org/10.1148/rg.323115129

[5] Mulpuru, S.K., Vasavada, B.C., Punukollu, G.K. and Patel, A.G. (2008) Cardiovocal Syndrome: A Systematic Review. *Heart, Lung and Circulation*, **17**, 1-4. http://dx.doi.org/10.1016/j.hlc.2007.04.007

[6] Ishii, K., Adachi, H., Tsubaki, K., Ohta, Y., Yamamoto, M. and Ino, T. (2004) Evaluation of Recurrent Nerve Paralysis Due to Thoracic Aortic Aneurysm and Aneurysm Repair. *Laryngoscope*, **114**, 2176-2181. http://dx.doi.org/10.1097/01.mlg.0000149453.91005.ab

[7] Plastiras, S.C., Pamboucas, C., Zafiriou, T., Lazaris, N. and Toumanidis, S. (2010) Ortner's Syndrome: A Multifactorial Cardiovocal Syndrome. *Clinical Cardiology*, **33**, E99-E100. http://dx.doi.org/10.1002/clc.20646

[8] Subramaniam, V., Herle, A., Mohammed, N. and Thahir, M. (2011) Ortner's Syndrome: Case Series and Literature Review. *Brazilian Journal of Otorhinolaryngology*, **77**, 559-562. http://dx.doi.org/10.1590/S1808-86942011000500004

[9] Morales, J.P., Chan, Y.C., Bell, R.E., Reidy, J.F. and Taylor, P.R. (2008) Endoluminal Repair of Distal Aortic Arch Aneurysms Causing Aorto-Vocal Syndrome. *International Journal of Clinical Practice*, **62**, 1511-1514. http://dx.doi.org/10.1111/j.1742-1241.2006.01282.x

[10] Fennessy, B.G., Sheahan, P. and McShane, D. (2008) Cardiovascular Hoarseness: An Unusual Presentation to Otola-ryngologists. *Journal of Laryngology and Otology*, **122**, 327-328. http://dx.doi.org/10.1017/S0022215107008110

[11] Dolowitz, D.A. and Lewis, C.S. (1948) Left Vocal Cord Paralysis Associated with Cardiac Disease. *American Journal of Medicine*, **4**, 856-862. http://dx.doi.org/10.1016/0002-9343(48)90482-3

6

CSF Rhinorrhoea with Encephalocele through Sternberg's Canal: Our Experience

Reshma Hanwate, Vandana Thorawade, Mohan Jagade, Anoop Attakil, Kartik Parelkar, Madhavi Pandare, R. V. Natraj, Rajesh Kar

Department of ENT, Grant Government Medical College & Sir J J Hospital, Mumbai, India
Email: drreshma06@gmail.com

Abstract

Spontaneous cerebrospinal fluid rhinorrhoea with encephalocele restricted to the sphenoid sinus is rare clinical finding. As of today, only 17 cases encephalocele protruding through the Sternberg's canal and extending into the lateral recess of sphenoid sinus, have been described in literature. Patients presenting with this special clinical entity usually do not have any history of trauma, tumour or iatrogenic injury. Thus the lesions are considered to originate from a congenital bony defect in the lateral wall of the sphenoid sinus, first described by Sternberg in 1888 as the lateral craniopharyngeal canal (Sternberg's canal). In our experience each patient of spontaneous CSF rhinorrhea should have suspicion of intrasphenoid encephalocele though cribriform plate is a common site. Endoscopic transasnasal approach is one of the best modalities for such cases.

Keywords

CSF Rhinorrhoea, Sternberg's Canal, Encephalocele

1. Introduction

Spontaneous cerebrospinal fluid leaks with encephaloceles restricted to the sphenoid sinus are rare. As of today, only 17 cases protruding through the Sternberg's canal and extending into the laterals recess of sphenoid sinus, have been described in literature [1]-[3]. Associations among persisting Sternberg's canal, extensively pneumatised sphenoid sinuses, elevated intracranial pressure and obesity are discussed as possible reason for spontaneous CSF rhinorrhoea and encephaloceles in this region. Spontaneous sphenoidal encephaloceles are uncommon entities and the presence of lateral sphenoidal encephalocele is a rare congenital anomaly [4]. Cranial encephaloceles, herniation of intracranial meninges and brain tissue through a defect in the cranium or skull base, are rare conditions with an incidence of approximately 1 in 35,000 people, and are more common in the anterior cranial fossa than those in the middle one [3]-[7]. Basal encephaloceles represent up to 10% of them [7]. Intrasphenoidal encephaloceles are extremely rare findings. Temporal lobe herniation through a middle fossa defect into the lateral recess of the SS is even rarer than the medial localization, and it is probably the least common type of basal encephaloceles [6] [8]-[10].

2. Case Report

A 39-year-old, multiparous, obese female presented to our out patient departement with complain of spontaneous watery nasal discharge through nose associated with refractory headache since 9 months. $\beta2$ transferrin test was found to be positive. HRCT PNS (high resolution computed tomography of paranasal sinuses) (**Figure 1**) revealed the bony defect in the lateral wall of sphenoid sinus with soft tissue protruding through it, MRI (magnetic resonanace imaging) (**Figure 2**) showed herniation of brain tissue through the same with empty sella.

Following pre-aneasthetic fitness endoscopic examination of nasal cavity was done. Patient was posted for the repair of the defect by an endoscopic transnasal approach. Herniated brain tissue (**Figure 3**) was cauterised with angled bipolar cautery and removed. The defect was closed in TRIPLE LAYER fashion which consisted of fat tissue, tensor fascia lata and biological glue. The first layer *i.e.* fat tissue was by kept by Wormold bath plug technique. The triple layer technique offers the advantage of reconstituting the layers of the skull base and thus may reduce the long-term failure rates. The post operative period was uneventful. No recurrence was found after 6 months of interval.

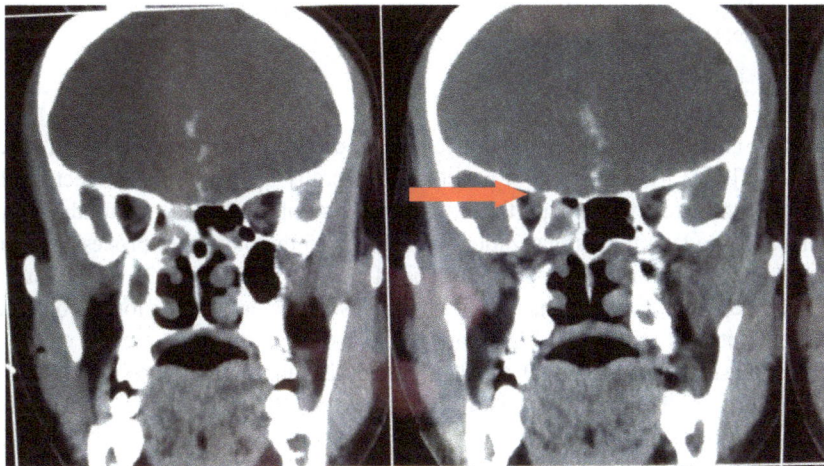

Figure 1. CT showing site of leak in sphenoid sinus.

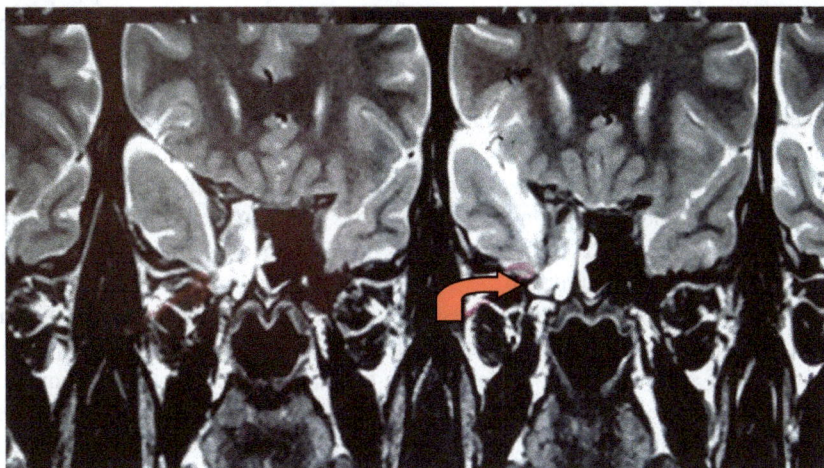

Figure 2. Encephalocele through defect.

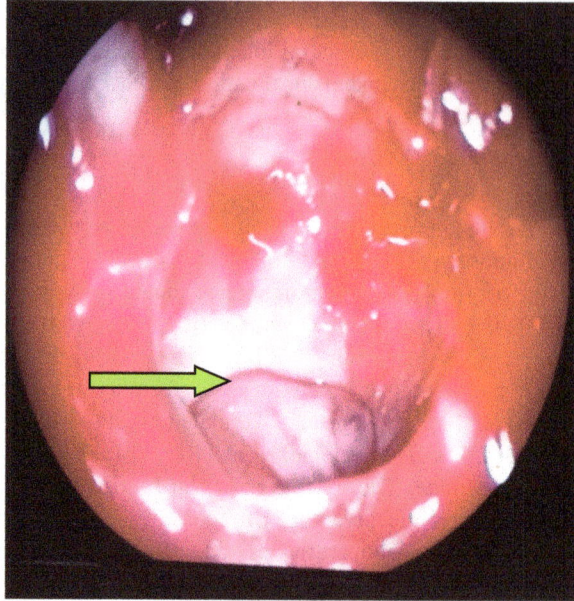

Figure 3. Endoscopic view of herniated brain tissue through defect.

3. Discussion

The sphenoid sinus (SS) is widely variable in its anatomy and degree of pneumatization. It reaches its full size during adolescence [7] [8] [11]. Anatomically it is extended laterally upto the line connecting the medial edges of the anterior opening of the vidian canal and the extracranial end of the foramen rotundum [7]. The lateral recess of the SS is an extensive lateral pneumatization of the SS into the pterygoid process, the great wing of the sphenoid bone or both, and it is also known as lateral type of sinus [7] [8] [11]-[13]. Rarely, it may extend up to the foramen ovale [14]. Lewin *et al.* found that 41 of 72 patients had lateral recess formation on at least one side and Barañano *et al.* found it in 35.3% of 1000 CT scans [8].

The sphenoid bone has several independent cartilaginous ossifiction centres, presphenoid and postsphenoid/ basisphenoid centers (body of the sphenoid bone), orbitosphenoids (lesser wings), and alisphenoids (greater wings). Union of these ossified components results in formation of the sphenoid bone [15] [16]. If the posterior portion of the bony fusion of the greater wings with the bone's body is incomplete, it creates a lateral cranio-pharyngeal canal, which was described by Sternberg in 1888. In the presence of a lateral recess of the SS, the Sternberg's canal can communicate with the SS after its pneumatization, acting as a possible site of origin of congenital encephaloceles. As the resistance to pneumatization at fusion plane is more, so sphenoidal defects at these planes are more likely to be congenital than acquired [10] [16]-[19]. Sternberg's canal has been reported in up to 4% of adults, but Barañano *et al.* found only one case in 1000 CT scan. Obesity may be the cause of CSF leak, increased weight increases intraabdominal and intrathoracic pressure which could lead to the development of benign intracranial hypertension [13] [17]. CSF rhinorrhea is the most common clinical manifestation of temporal encephaloceles through Sternberg's canal and other previously occult malformations of the skull base. The CSF drainage is generally intermittent and not voluminous and may be ignored by the patient for a long time until complicated by meningitis. Recurrent meningitis may also occur. Others signs and symptoms of this entity are chronic headache, seizures and vertigo.

Patients with encephaloceles within the lateral recess of the SS classically present with CSF rhinorrhea during adulthood, enhancing the importance of pneumatization of the SS in the pathogenesis [19]. Regarding neuroradiological investigations, CT scan is a noninvasive imaging technique which gives good bone detail and identifies the site of the skull base defect. CT cisternography consists of injecting intrathecal water-soluble contrast medium before the CT scan and then visualizing it at the level of the dural and skull base defect. Intermittent or inactive CSF leaks are usually associated with a high incidence of false-negative results and MR imaging may be a better choice in those patients [1] [10] [14] [19]. MR images are more informative for soft tissues like the encephalocele itself [2]. If radiological images may also show partial or complete opacity of the SS [3]. Then, the site of leak is confirmed at the time of surgery [9].

Persistent CSF leak is potentially lethal because it may lead to meningitis or brain abscess. Thus, repair of intrasphenoidal encephaloceles has two main objectives: prevention of CSF leak and to avoid central nervous system infection [2] [6] [13] [18].

Surgical treatment should be tailored to each patient. Endoscopic transnasal approaches are less invasive and do not require a large external incision and temporal lobe retraction, minimizing brain manipulation [2] [5] [9] [13] [17]-[20].

4. Conclusions

A persisting Sternberg's canal should be considered the source of spontaneous CSF leak with or without encephalocele in sphenoid sinuse with extensive lateral pneumatisation. Endoscopic repair of such leaks is very technically challenging. Nevertheless, endoscopic transnasal surgery is safe as no intraoperative complications occur in our patient. It is less traumatic than transcranial approaches providing a good access and view of the surgical field.

Endoscopic management of CSF leaks represents an early but elegant example of the evolution and effectiveness of transnasal endoscopic techniques in managing various sinonasal and skull base pathology.

References

[1]   Buchfelder, M., Fahlbusch, I., Huk, W.J. and Thierauf, P. (1987) Intrasphenoidal Encephalocele—A Clinical Entity. *Acta Neurochirurgica*, **89**, 10-15. http://dx.doi.org/10.1007/BF01406661

[2]   Blaivie, C., Lequeux, T., Kampouridis, S., Louryan, S. and Saussez, S. (2006) Congenital Transsphenoidal Meningocele: Case Report and Review of the Literature. *American Journal of Otolaryngology*, **27**, 422-444. http://dx.doi.org/10.1016/j.amjoto.2006.01.011

[3]   Schick, B., Brors, D. and Prescher, A. (2000) Sternberg's Canal—Cause of Congenital Sphenoidal Meningocele. *European Archives of Oto-Rhino-Laryngology*, **257**, 430-432. http://dx.doi.org/10.1007/s004050000235

[4]   Buchfelder, M., Fahlbusch, R., Huk, W.J. and Thierauf, P. (1987) Intrasphenoidal Encephaloceles—A Clinical Entity. *Acta Neurochirurgica*, **89**, 10-15. http://dx.doi.org/10.1007/BF01406661

[5]   Kwon, J.E. and Kim, E. (2010) Middle Fossa Approach to a Temporosphenoidal Encephalocele. Technical Note. *Neurologia Medico-Chirurgica*, **50**, 434-438. http://dx.doi.org/10.2176/nmc.50.434

[6]   Lopatin, A.S., Kapitanov, D.N. and Potapov, A.A. (2003) Endonasal Endoscopic Repair of Spontaneous Cerebrospinal Fluid Leaks. *Archives of Otolaryngology—Head and Neck Surgery*, **129**, 859-863. http://dx.doi.org/10.1001/archotol.129.8.859

[7]   Wang, J., Bidari, S., Inoue, K., Yang, H. and Rhoton Jr., A. (2010) Extensions of the Sphenoid Sinus: A New Classification. *Neurosurgery*, **66**, 797-816. http://dx.doi.org/10.1227/01.NEU.0000367619.24800.B1

[8]   Lewin, J.S., Curtin, H.D., Eelkema, E. and Obuchowski, N. (1999) Benign Expansile Lesions of the Sphenoid Sinus: Differentiation from Normal Asymmetry of the Lateral Recesses. *American Journal of Neuroradiology*, **20**, 461-466.

[9]   Tabaee, A., Anand, V.K., Cappabianca, P., Stamm, A., Esposito, F. and Schwartz, T.H. (2010) Endoscopic Management of Spontaneous Meningoencephalocele of the Lateral Sphenoid Sinus. *Journal of Neurosurgery*, **112**, 1070-1077. http://dx.doi.org/10.3171/2009.7.JNS0842

[10]   Schlosser, R.J. and Bolger, W.E. (2003) Significance of Empty Sella in Cerebrospinal Fluid Leaks. *Otolaryngology—Head and Neck Surgery*, **128**, 32-38. http://dx.doi.org/10.1067/mhn.2003.43

[11]   Rhoton Jr., A.L. (2002) The Sellar Region. *Neurosurgery*, **51**, S335-S374. http://dx.doi.org/10.1097/00006123-200210001-00009

[12]   Ciobanu, I.C., Motoc, A., Jianu, A.M., Cergan, R., Banu, M.A. and Rusu, M.C. (2009) The Maxillary Recess of the Sphenoid Sinus. *Romanian Journal of Morphology and Embryology*, **50**, 487-489.

[13]   Lai, S.Y., Kennedy, D.W. and Bolger, W.E. (2002) Sphenoid Encephaloceles: Disease Management and Identification of Lesions within the Lateral Recess of the Sphenoid Sinus. *The Laryngoscope*, **112**, 1800-1805. http://dx.doi.org/10.1097/00005537-200210000-00018

[14]   Devi, B.I., Panigrahi, M.K., Shenoy, S., Vajramani, G., Das, B.S. and Jayakumar, P.N. (1999) CSF Rhinorrhoea from Unusual Site: Report of Two Cases. *Neurology India*, **47**, 152-154.

[15]   Nemzek, W.R., Brodie, H.A., Hecht, S.T., Chong, B.W., Babcook, C.J. and Seibert, J.A. (2000) MR, CT, and Plain

Film Imaging of the Developing Skull Base in Fetal Specimens. *AJNR American Journal of Neuroradiology*, **21**, 1699-1706.

[16] Schick, B., Brors, D. and Prescher, A. (2000) Sternberg's Canal—Cause of Congenital Sphenoidal Meningocele. *European Archives of Oto-Rhino-Laryngology*, **257**, 430-432. http://dx.doi.org/10.1007/s004050000235

[17] Castelnuovo, P., Dallan, I., Pistochini, A., Battaglia, P., Locatelli, D. and Bignami, M. (2007) Endonasal Endoscopic Repair of Sternberg's Canal Cerebrospinal Fluid Leaks. *Laryngoscope*, **117**, 345-349. http://dx.doi.org/10.1097/01.mlg.0000251452.90657.3a

[18] Arai, A., Mizukawa, K., Nishihara, M., Fujita, A., Hosoda, K. and Kohmura, E. (2010) Spontaneous Cerebrospinal Fluid Rhinorrhea Associated with a Far Lateral Temporal Encephalocele—Case Report. *Neurologia Medico-Chirurgica*, **50**, 243-245.

[19] Wind, J.J., Caputy, A.J. and Roberti, F. (2008) Spontaneous Encephaloceles of the Temporal Lobe. *Neurosurgical Focus*, **25**, E11. http://dx.doi.org/10.3171/FOC.2008.25.12.E11

[20] Ohkawa, T., Nakao, N., Uematsu, Y. and Itakura, T. (2010) Temporal Lobe Encephalocele in the Lateral Recess of the Sphenoid Sinus Presenting with Intraventricular Tension Pneumocephalus. *Skull Base*, **20**, 481-486. http://dx.doi.org/10.1055/s-0030-1261261

7

Antibiotic Treatment for Chronic Rhinosinusitis after Endoscopic Surgery: How Long Should Macrolide Antibiotics Be Given?*

Motohiro Sawatsubashi#, Daisuke Murakami, Shizuo Komune

Department of Otolaryngology—Head and Neck Surgery, Graduate School of Medical Sciences, Kyushu University, Fukuoka, Japan
Email: #motohiro@gent.med.kyushu-u.ac.jp

Abstract

Background: The purpose of this study was to determine an appropriate period for macrolide antibiotic therapy, and to investigate whether this period could be shorter, for patients with chronicrhino sinusitis (CRS) after functional endoscopic sinus surgery (FESS). Methods: A retrospective analysis of 41 patients undergoing FESS for CRS was performed. All patients underwent pre-operative computed tomography (CT). Patients with fungal sinusitis, allergic fungal sinusitis, and eosinophilic sinusitis were excluded. After FESS, normalized sinus mucosa was confirmed by CT and endoscopy in all patients. Postoperative antibiotic therapy consisted of first-line and second-line regimens. Garenoxacin (GRNX), or clarithromycin (CAM, 400 mg/day) was used as the first-line regimens and low-dose macrolide therapy (CAM, 200 mg/day) was used as the second-line regimen and was prescribed at outpatient visits based on our clinical criteria. Results: Second-line antibiotic therapy (low-dose CAM) was not necessary in 12 of 41 (29%) patients, while it was prescribed in 29 of 41 (71%). The mean duration of low-dose CAM therapy after FESS was 36 days (range 7 to 122 days; median, 25 days). Patients who received second-line therapy (n = 29) were divided into two groups based on the choice of first-line therapy, a GRNX group (n = 13) and a non-GRNX group (n = 16). Those in the non-GRNX had longer periods of postoperative CAM therapy than those in the GRNX group. Conclusion: GRNX was associated with a shorter duration of low-dose macrolide therapy after FESS, and 29% of patients did not need any low-dose macrolide therapy postoperatively. Therefore, macrolide antibiotics should not be routinely prescribed after FESS.

---

*This study was partially presented at the 115th Annual Meeting of the ORL Society of Japan, Fukuoka, Japan, 17 May 2014.
#Corresponding author.

Keywords

Chronic Rhinosinusitis, Functional Endoscopic Sinus Surgery, Macrolide Therapy, Garenoxacin, Postoperative Antibiotic Therapy

1. Introduction

Antibiotics are routinely used by otolaryngologists to reduce the risk of postoperative infection in patients undergoing functional endoscopic sinus surgery (FESS). Antibiotic containing nasal packing can reduce postoperative infections [1]. The efficacy of postoperatively administered antibiotics, including macrolides, for patients with chronic rhinosinusitis (CRS) has been documented [2]. Previous studies have concluded that the sufficient period for low-dose macrolide treatment in CRS patients undergoing FESS should be long-term, *i.e.*, 3 to 6 months [3] [4]. However, consensus on how long patients should be given antibiotics after FESS is not established. In our experience, long-term macrolide administration is not necessary for all patients undergoing FESS for CRS. Furthermore, as antibiotic resistance is now a serious problem; some action is required [5] [6].

The purpose of this study is to examine the state of postoperative antibiotic treatment, especially low-dose macrolide therapy, and to determine the appropriate period of macrolide therapy after FESS for CRS.

2. Patients and Methods

The retrospective analysis included 41 patients (28 men, and 13 women) who underwent FESS for CRS at Kyushu University Hospital from April 2009 to October 2013. The mean age at the time of FESS was 59 years, with a range of 14 to 84 years. The diagnosis of CRS was based on a history of rhinosinusitis and the findings of endoscopy and computed tomography (CT) examinations. The patients were screened for allergy and cases with allergy were excluded. There were 20 patients who had sinusitis with polyp and 21 who had sinusitis without polyp. Cases of fungal sinusitis, allergic fungal sinusitis, eosinophil-related fungal rhinosinusitis including allergic fungal rhinosinusitis (AFRS) and eosinophilic sinusitis were not included in this study. All patients included in the study had responded poorly to medical treatments for more than 6 months. Preoperative CT was performed in all cases. The CT findings were summarized according to the Lund-Mackay score [7], which ranges from 0 to 24 (complete opacity of all sinuses), and the severity of sinus mucosal inflammation or fluid accumulation was scored as 0 (complete lucency), 1 (partial lucency), or 2 (completeopacity). The surgeries were performed under general or local anesthesia. All patients underwent FESS without extra-nasal approaches (Caldwell-Luc' procedure or canine fossa approach). The surgical interventions of the procedure were designed to remove the osteomeatal blockage and restore normal sinus ventilation and mucociliary function. The nasal cavity was decongested using gauze with lidocaine and epinephrine; subsequently 0.5 or 1 percent lidocaine with 1:100,000 epinephrine was injected at the level of the middle turbinate root and uncinate process. The uncinated process was removed in cases of middle meatal antrostomy. After widening of the antrostomy for the maxillary sinus, ethmoid cells, frontal sinus, and sphenoid sinus were opened if necessary based on the previous report [8].

Nasal and sinus saline irrigation was performed at the end of the surgery. If patients required nasal packing, the nasal cavity was minimally packed with chitin-coated gauze (Beschitin® F, Unitika Co., Ltd., Kyoto, Japan), that was to be removed within 1 to 2 days after surgery. Septoplasty prior to FESS was performed in 8 patients with severe nasal septal deviation. Nasal and sinus saline irrigation using a bulb syringe was recommended after discharge. Antibiotic prophylaxis (piperacillin 2 g IV or cefazolin 2 g IV) was given during surgery to all patients. Postoperative antibiotic therapy consisted of a first-line regimen and a second-line regimen. Garenoxacin (GRNX, 400 mg/day), or clarithromycin (CAM, 400 mg/day) was used as the first-line regimen during hospitalization, and low-dose CAM (200 mg/day) therapy was used as the second-line regimen during the outpatient period. The surgeon decided whether or not to perform the second-line regimen (low-dose CAM therapy) based on the following conditions;

1) Long-term sinusitis (more than one year);
2) Sinusitis with granulomatous inflammation;
3) Sinusitis with bleeding disorders;

4) Patients on antiplatelet or anticoagulant treatment;

5) Excessive bleeding during or after FESS;

6) Postoperative nasal packing in place for more than four days;

7) Patients with diabetes mellitus;

8) Patients on steroid treatment for chronic disease.

All patients underwent postoperative CT examination at three or four months after the FESS. Normalized mucosa in sinuses was postoperatively confirmed by CT and endoscopy in all patients. Patients were followed for 3 to 12 months postoperatively; the follow-up period ranged from 4 to 24 months (average, 12 months).

Statistical analysis was performed using the Mann-Whitney U test or Fisher's exact test for the duration of low-dose CAM. CT scores were compared using Cochran-Cox, Welch t, and Kruskal-Wallis H test. A P-value of <0.05 was considered statistically significant.

This research received no specific grant from any funding agency, commercial, or not-for-profit entity. The authors assert that all procedures contributing to this work comply with the ethical standards of the relevant national and institutional guidelines on human experimentation and with the Helsinki Declaration of 1975, as revised in 2008.

3. Results

The study of the patients was summarized in **Table 1**. The mean age at the time of FESS was 59 years, with a range of 14 to 84 years. Most cases of bacterial culture were *S. pneumonia*, *H. influenza*, and *S. aureus*, including PISP (penicillin G insensitive *Streptococcus pneumonia*), PRSP (penicillin-resistant *Streptococcus pneumonia*), and BLNAR (beta-lactamase-negative ampicillin-resistant). But the results of this study were not associated with the bacterial culture. Postoperative low-dose CAM therapy was given to 29 of 41 (71%) patients. The mean duration of low-dose CAM therapy after FESS was 36 days (range, 7 to 122 days; median, 25 days). CAM (400 mg/day) followed by low-dose CAM (200 mg/day) was used in 13 patients, and GRNX followed by low-dose CAM was used in 16 patients (**Table 2**, **Table 3**). Five patients received GRNX and no low-dose CAM (**Table 2**, **Table 3**), and 7 patients did not receive any postoperative antibiotics (control group, **Table 1**, **Table 2**). The duration of GRNX therapy varied from 2 to 7 days. There were no differences in CT scores among these groups (Cochran-Cox, Welch t, and Kruskal-Wallis H test, **Table 2**).

Table 1. Summary of the patients.

Post-Ope therapy		Gender		Polyp		Total
First-line	Second-line	Man	Women	With	Without	No. of case
CAM (200 mg/day)	CAM (100 mg/day)	8	5	3	10	13
GRNX	CAM (100 mg/day)	10	6	8	8	16
GRNX	None	4	1	4	1	5
None	None	6	1	5	2	7
Total		28	13	20	21	41

Abbreviations: CAM, clarithromycin; GRNX, garenoxacin.

Table 2. Postoperative therapy and CT score.

Post-Ope therapy		No. of case	CT Score					
First-line	Second-line		Min	Max	Median	Mean	SD	SE
CAM (200 mg/day)	CAM (100 mg/day)	13	2	15	6	7	4.5	1.2
GRNX	CAM (100 mg/day)	16	4	15	6	6.8	3.1	0.8
GRNX	None	5	2	11	6	6.2	3.5	1.6
None	None	7	3	10	6	6.1	2.4	0,9
Total		41	2	15	6	6.1	3.1	0.4

P > 0.05. Abbreviations: CAM, clarithromycin; GRNX, garenoxacin; CT, computed tomography (CT scores are by the Lund-Mackay System); SD, standard deviation; SE, standard error.

Table 3. Postoperative therapy and low-CAM period.

Post-Ope therapy		No. of case	Low-CAM period (days)					
First-line	Second-line		Min	Max	Median	Mean	SD	SE
CAM (200 mg/day)	CAM (100 mg/day)	13	7	122	21	46	46.9	13
GRNX	CAM (100 mg/day)	16	14	60	28	28	12	3
GRNX	None	5	0	0	0	0	0	0
None	None	7	0	0	0	0	0	0
Total		41						

Abbreviations: CAM, clarithromycin; GRNX, garenoxacin; SD, standard deviation; SE, standard error.

Postoperative low-dose CAM therapy was not necessary in 12 of 41 (29%) patients, all of whom exhibited normalized sinuses mucosa within 3 months.

The second-line, low-dose CAM therapy patients (n = 29) were divided into two groups based on the first-line antibiotic choice, a GRNX group (n = 16) and a non-GRNX group (n = 13).

The duration of low-dose CAM therapy ranged from 14 to 60 days (mean, 28 days) in the GRNX group and from 7 to 122 days (mean 46 days) in the non-GRNX group (**Table 3** and **Figure 1**). The duration of low-dose CAM therapy was longer in the non-GRNX group than in the GRNX group, but the difference was not statistically significant (Mann-Whitney U test, $P > 0.05$, **Figure 1**). All cases of the postoperative CT scores were finally 0 (zero).

4. Discussion

It has been found that prophylactic administration of antibiotics for patients undergoing FESS can decrease postoperative morbidity and reduce the risk of infection [9].

In the early 1990s in Japan, long-term low-dose erythromycin treatment was used primarily. Since then, the anti-inflammatory effect of macrolides in vitro has been well-documented [2] [3], and macrolide therapy is now the standard treatment for CRS after FESS in Japan. Although Japanese guidelines for CRS have recommended postoperative macrolide therapy in order to obtain a favorable outcome in sinus surgery, the appropriate duration of therapy is not obvious [10]. In 1995, the recommended duration for an effective long-term low-dose erythromycin treatment after FESS, varied from 3 to 6 months [3]. More recently (2013), it has been recommended that CRS patients with rhinorrhea or postnasal drip should be treated with low-dose CAM for 6 months after FESS [4]. However, some authors have reported shorter durations, such as 2 to 3 weeks, of postoperative antibiotic treatments [11]-[13]. In accordance with these reports, and based on our own experience, there have been patients showing favorable outcomes after surgery for CRS with no postoperative antibiotic treatment. Furthermore, in terms of increasing antibiotic resistance, patients undergoing FESS for CRS have usually undergone, repeated courses of antibiotic therapy before surgery, and a previous report has shown that up to 90% of CRS patients, undergoing FESS harbor penicillin-resistant bacteria, and 65% harbor cephalosporin-resistant species [5]. Therefore, concerns of an increasing incidence of macrolide-resistant bacterial strains should be taken seriously, and we believe that these concerns, should prompt reduced antibiotic utilization in patients with CRS after FESS.

In this retrospective study, first-line (CAM or GRNX) and second-line (low-dose CAM) postoperative antibiotic treatment regimens were established. Low-dose CAM therapy was prescribed as the second-line treatment at outpatient visits after FESS in patients for whom, the first-line may not work adequately, and it was not necessary in 29% of patients. The sinus mucosa was normalized within 3 months in all of those patients. This result indicates that patients should not routinely be given a prescription for CAM after FESS. Although previous reports have recommended a duration of 3 to 6 months for low-dose macrolide therapy [3] [4], in the present study the mean duration of low-dose macrolide therapy was about one month (36 days).

Garenoxacin (GRNX), a synthetic des-F (6)-quinolone, has been available since 2007 in Japan [14]. GRNX is reported to have anti-inflammatory activity along with strong antibacterial activity against both gram-positive and gram-negative bacteria. In one only study, the in vitro activity of GRNX against *Streptococcus pneumonia* was 32× that of levofloxacin and ciprofloxacin [15]. In the present study, patients who received GRNX as first-

Periods (days)   Periods (days)

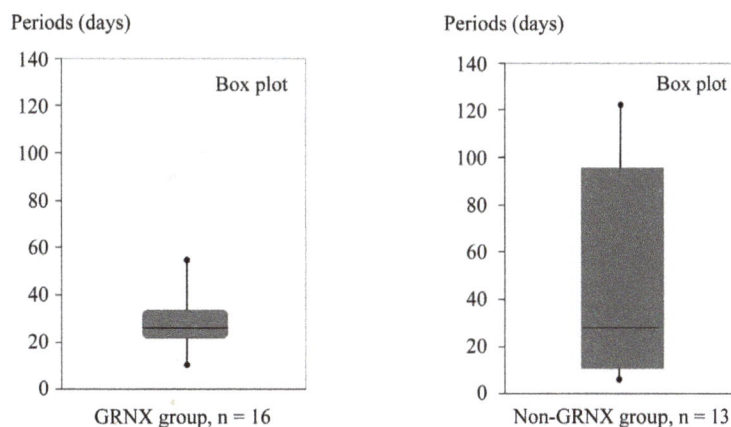

GRNX group, n = 16   Non-GRNX group, n = 13

Figure 1. Duration of low-dose clarithromycin (CAM) therapy after functional endoscopic sinus surgery (FESS) in garenoxacin (GRNX) and non-GRNX groups (box-plot). The duration of therapy was longer in the non-GRNX group, but the difference was not significant (P > 0.05).

line therapy after FESS had shorter periods of low-dose CAM therapy as outpatients, and 5 of 21 (24%) patients who received GRNX therapy received no low-dose CAM therapy. There were no patients in the GRNX group who received low-dose CAM therapy for more than 60 days. These results suggest that GRNX could be useful for permitting shorter durations of low-dose CAM therapy postoperatively in CRS patients undergoing FESS.

4. Conclusion

Because of a small number of patients and the retrospective study, this report was a preliminary result, but it showed that 29% of patients did not need low-dose CAM therapy after FESS. Therefore, CAM antibiotics should not be prescribed routinely after FESS. GRNX was associated with shorter durations of low-dose CAM therapy postoperatively. The duration of CAM therapy after GRNX ranged from 14 to 60 (mean, 28) days.

References

[1]   Bandhauer, F., Buhl, D. and Grossenbacher, R. (2002) Antibiotic Prophylaxis in Rhinosurgery. *American Journal of Rhinology*, **16**, 135-139.

[2]   Cervin, A. and Wallwork, B. (2007) Macrolide Therapy of Chronic Rhinosinusitis. *Rhinology*, **45**, 259-267.

[3]   Moriyama, H., Yanagi, K., Ohtori, N. and Fukami, M. (1995) Evaluation of Endoscopic Sinus Surgery for Chronic Sinusitis: Post-Operative Erythromycin Therapy. *Rhinology*, **33**, 166-170.

[4]   Nakamura, Y., Suzuki, M., Yokota, M., Ozaki, S., Ohno, N., *et al.* (2013) Optimal Duration of Macrolide Treatment for Chronic Sinusitis after Endoscopic Sinus Surgery. *ANS*, **40**, 366-372.

[5]   Shikani, A.H. (1996) Use of Antibiotics for Expansion of the Merocel Parking Following Endoscopic Sinus Surgery. *Ear, Nose Throat Journal*, **75**, 524-526.

[6]   Bhattacharyya, N. and Kepnes, L.J. (2008) Assessment of Trends in Antimicrobial Resistance in Chronic Rhinosinusitis. *Annals of Otology, Rhinology Laryngology*, **117**, 448-452. http://dx.doi.org/10.1177/000348940811700608

[7]   Lund, V.J. and Mackay, I.S. (1993) Staging in Rhinosinusitis. *Rhinology*, **107**, 183-184.

[8]   Kennedy, D.W., Zinreich, S.J., Shaalan, H., Kuhn, F., Naclerio, R., Loch, E.L. (1987) Endoscopic Middle Meatal Antrostomy: Theory, Technique, and Patency. *Laryngoscope*, **97**, 1-9. http://dx.doi.org/10.1288/00005537-198708002-00001

[9]   Bandhauer, F., Buhl, D. and Grossenbacher, R. (2002) Antibiotic Prophylaxis in Rhinosurgery. *American Journal of Rhinology*, **16**, 135-139.

[10]   Japan Rhinologic Society (2013) Japanese Guideline for Chronic Sinusitis. Vol. 4, Kanehara, Tokyo, 50-60.

[11]   Albu, S. and Lucaciu, R. (2010) Prophylactic Antibiotics in Endoscopic Sinus Surgery: A Short Follow-Up Study. *American Journal of Rhinology Allergy*, **24**, 306-309. http://dx.doi.org/10.2500/ajra.2010.24.3475

[12]   Jiang, R.S., Liang, K.L., Yang, K.Y., Shiao, J.Y., Su, M.C., *et al.* (2008) Postoperative Antibiotic Care after Functional

Endoscopic Sinus Surgery. *American Journal of Rhinology*, **22**, 608-612. http://dx.doi.org/10.2500/ajr.2008.22.3241

[13] Bhandarkar, N.D., Mace, J.C. and Smith, T.L. (2011) Endoscopic Sinus Surgery Reduces Antibiotic Utilization in Rhinosinusitis. *International Forum of Allergy Rhinology*, **1**, 18-22.

[14] Takahata, M., Shimakura, M., Hori, R., Kizawa, K., Todo, Y., *et al.* (2001) *In Vitro* and *in Vivo* Antimicrobial Activities of T-3811ME (BMS-284756) against Mycoplasma Pneumonia. *Antimicrobial Agents and Chemotherapy*, **45**, 312-315. http://dx.doi.org/10.1128/AAC.45.1.312-315.2001

[15] Ito, M., Maruyama, Y., Murono, S., Wakisaka, N., Kondo, S., *et al.* (2012) Efficacy and Safety of Garenoxacin in the Treatment of Upper Respiratory Tract Infections. *ANL*, **39**, 512-518.

8

An Unusual Maxillary Sinus Foreign Body and Its Endoscopic Assisted Removal

R. V. Nataraj, Mohan Jagade, Reshma Chavan, Rajesh Kar, Madhavi Pandare, Kartik Parelkar, Arpita Singhal, Kiran Kulsange

Department of Ear, Nose & Throat and Head & Neck Surgery, Grant Government Medical College, Mumbai, India
Email: nataraj.rv@gmail.com

Abstract

Foreign bodies in maxillary sinuses are uncommon. But the incidence is on a rise. Herewith we present a case of foreign bodies (glass pieces) in left maxillary sinus and bilateral nasolacrimal ducts, which is managed endoscopically.

Keywords

Maxillary Sinus, Foreign Body, Endoscopic Approach

1. Introduction

Foreign bodies are very frequently encountered entities in routine ENT practice, which warrant immediate removal. Most common types, which are brought to the surgeon's notice, involve the ear, nose and pharynx. The procedures for removal of most of such foreign bodies are fair and can be performed in the OPD, with help of local anesthesia.

Foreign bodies in paranasal sinuses are still an uncommon clinical condition and the procedures for removal are far more challenging. The most common causes of paranasal foreign bodies are iatrogenic (60%) or accidental (25%) [1] [2]. The iatrogenic causes include various dental, ophthalmic and otorhinolaryngologic procedures [1] [2]. History regarding any of the above mentioned procedures should raise the suspicion of a paranasal foreign body.

The maxillary sinus is most frequently involved (75%), followed by the frontal sinus (18%) [1] [2]. There have been cases of foreign body which have been introduced willingly into the maxillary sinus [3]. The foreign bodies can be of varying natures such as dental fillings, broken fragments of tooth and bones, pieces of glass, stones, gunshot pellets etc.

Removal of paranasal foreign body is always a challenge. But with advent of advanced diagnostic procedures and endoscopic assisted surgeries, such surgeries can be performed safely with relative ease.

Hereby we report a case of foreign bodies (glass particles) lodged in both nasolacrimal ducts and left maxillary sinus following an accident, with a barely visible scar over the nose.

2. Case Report

A healthy 25 years old male presented to ophthalmology OPD with complaints of watering of left eye. A CT DCG was advised and bilateral nasolacrimal ducts were found to be blocked with impacted foreign bodies, most probably pieces of glass. Past history revealed that, 3 months ago, the patient was involved in a road traffic accident in which his vehicle hit a tree. As a result of which, patient's face came in contact with the vehicle's windshield. This resulted in multiple abrasions and lacerations over his face. Though most wounds were superficial, a few lacerations, over left side of the nose and the ones just below the eyes were deep enough to warrant primary closure. The routine investigations including, non contrast CT scan brain, were found to be normal. The wounds were sutured and the patient was discharged.

As the patient also complained of recurrent headache, left nasal discharge and post nasal drip, the patient was referred to our OPD for evaluation and further management. Upon anterior rhinoscopic examination revealed mild septal deviation to right, hypertrophied inferior turbinates on both sides and purulent and foul-smelling discharge from left nostril but no foreign body or any other nasal pathology could be visualized. Left maxillary sinus tenderness could, also, be elicited. Oral cavity was examined for evidence of oroantral fistula but none could be found. A barely visible scar was seen over the face just below the left eye (**Figure 1** and **Figure 2**).

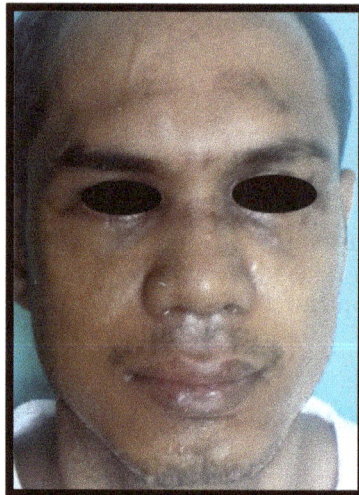

Figure 1. Patient with barely visible scar over his face.

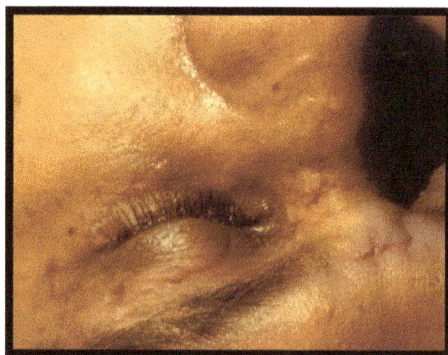

Figure 2. Close up of the scar.

Syringing test revealed immediate and watery regurgitation from left eye. CT PNS (plain and contrast) revealed mucosal thickening of left maxillary sinus and multiple irregular foreign bodies, most probably glass particles, in left maxillary sinus, blocking the left ostium. There was no evidence of any fistula or sinuses (**Figure 3** and **Figure 4**).

The patient was admitted and thoroughly investigated. Functional endoscopic sinus surgery and endoscopic dacrocystorhinostomy, in a single sitting, under general anesthesia were planned for the removal of the foreign bodies. Intra-operative findings revealed mucosa thickening in left maxillary sinus. Numerous small pieces of glass and three large irregular pieces of glass were found in the left maxillary sinus and ostia and one large piece of glass in each of the nasolacrimal duct (**Figure 5** and **Figure 6**).

Bilateral nasal packing was done and patient was given antibiotic coverage for 48 hours post-operatively. and CT scan of paranasal sinuses showed no remnant foreign bodies. Patient was re-evaluated after 1 month and he

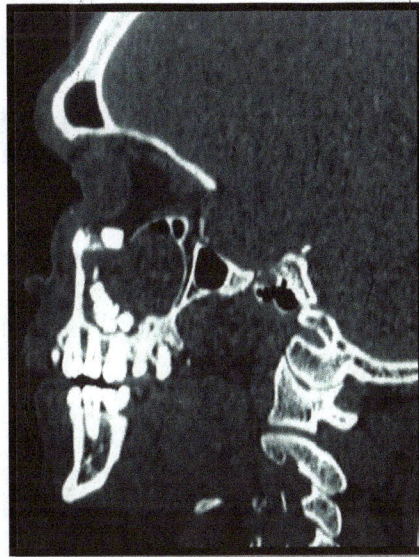

Figure 3. CT scan showing FB in left maxillary sinus and left NLD.

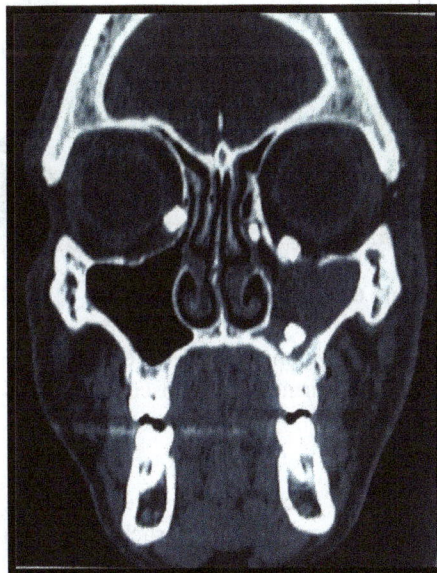

Figure 4. CT scan showing FB in bilateral NLD.

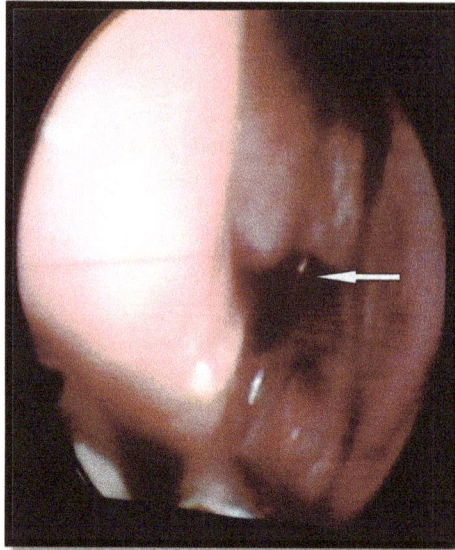

Figure 5. Endoscopic view of the FB.

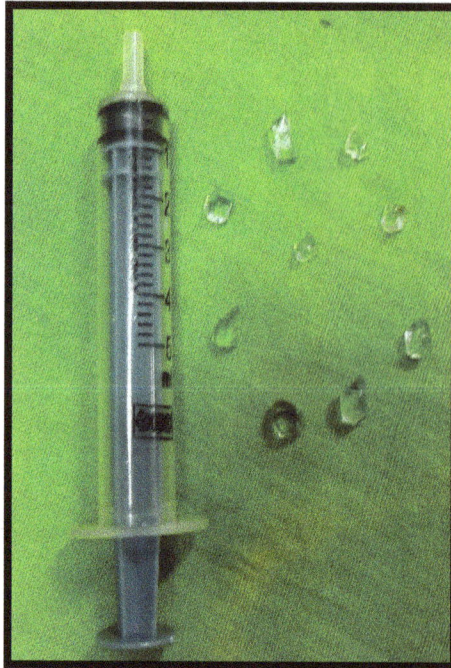

Figure 6. Glass pieces extracted.

underwent a diagnostic nasal endoscopy, which showed no evidence of residual foreign bodies. CT scan of paranasal sinuses was performed, which confirmed the endoscopic findings (**Figure 7**).

3. Discussion

Regardless of their origin, foreign bodies in maxillary sinus are a rare entity, especially in cases of unilateral sinusitis that is resistant to medical line of management. In such cases detailed history regarding long forgotten dental procedures and accidents needs to be elicited. Careful examination of the oral cavity is helpful to diagnose oroantral fistula. But absence of any fistula doesn't necessarily rules out foreign bodies as, more often than not, fistula heals leaving no evidence behind. The exact mechanism of how foreign body causes sinusitis is not

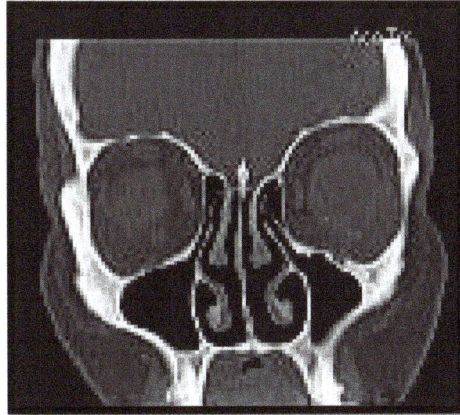

Figure 7. Post-operative CT scan.

known. However it has been postulated that foreign body causes chronic physical irritation of the mucosa leading to impaired cilliary movements and secondary infections. Foreign bodies can also obstruct the ostium leading to improper drainage. So removal of all the foreign bodies is necessary, even if they do not cause any symptoms [4].

Pre-operative CT scan is necessary for numerous reasons, chief amongst them being diagnostic. It not only shows the exact site, size and number of the foreign bodies but also detects the presence of any fistula. Site and size of the foreign bodies helps us in deciding between endoscopic approach and Caldwell-Luc procedure or combination of both. The most common procedure used is the endoscopic approach with a wide endonasal meatotomy. The advantages of functional endoscopic sinus surgery noted in literature include its less invasiveness, ability to fully visualize the antrum, a short recovery time and little or no risk of injury to the infraorbital nerve [5]-[8]. The potential problem of altered facial growth in children associated with the Caldwell-Luc operation is absent with this technique [9]. But in cases where the foreign body is too large or endoscopic approach fails, the surgery should be converted to an external approach using Caldwell-Luc procedure as it allows a much better visualization of the antrum. In recent literature a combination of Caldwell-Luc and endoscopic approach has been described as the gold standard procedure for treating various diseases of the maxillary sinus, including foreign body removal [5].

This case is unique and interesting for two reasons; first of all coexisting of both maxillary and nasolacrimal duct foreign bodies giving rise to symptoms of both chronic dacrocystitis and chronic sinusitis. Secondarily the route of entry of the foreign bodies is due to an accident, which left behind only a barely visible scar as evidence.

4. Conclusion

In cases of unilateral sinusitis and/or sinusitis not responding to any drug regime, possibility of a foreign body in maxillary sinus should be kept in mind. In literature, the most common cause of maxillary sinus foreign body is oroantral fistula. Detailed history focused upon any previous dental procedure or accident should be elicited. And pre-operative CT scan should be ordered. Even though endoscopic approach with wide meatotomy is the most preferred procedure, the surgeon should also be prepared for Caldwell-Luc approach and the need should rise. And efforts should be made to remove all the foreign bodies from the maxillary sinus, irrespective of the impact on the symptom profile of the patient.

References

[1] Krause, H.R., Rustemeyer, J. and Grunert, R.R. (2002) Foreign Body in Paranasal Sinuses. *Mund-, Kiefer- und Gesichtschirurgie*, **6**, 40-44. http://dx.doi.org/10.1007/s10006-001-0344-5

[2] Liston, P.N. and Walters, R.F. (2002) Foreign Bodies in the Maxillary Antrum: A Case Report. *Australian Dental Journal*, **47**, 344-346. http://dx.doi.org/10.1111/j.1834-7819.2002.tb00549.x

[3] Lima, M.M., Moreira, C.A., da Silva, V.C. and de Freitas, M.R. (2008) 34 Self-Inflicted Foreign Bodies in the Maxil-

lary Sinus. *Revista Brasileira de Otorrinolaringologia*, **74**, 948.

[4]   Mehra, P. and Murad, H. (2004) Maxillary Sinus Disease of Odontogenic Origin. *Otolaryngologic Clinics of North America*, **37**, 347-364. http://dx.doi.org/10.1016/S0030-6665(03)00171-3

[5]   Friedlich, J. and Rittenberg, B.N. (2005) Endoscopically Assisted Caldwell-Luc Procedure for Removal of a Foreign Body from the Maxillary Sinus. *Journal of the Canadian Dental Association*, **71**, 200-201.

[6]   Costa, F., Robiony, M., Toro, C., Sembronio, S. and Politi, M. (2006) Endoscopically Assisted Procedure for Removal of a Foreign Body from the Maxillary Sinus and Contemporary Endodontic Surgical Treatment of the Tooth. *Head Face Medicine*, **2**, 37. http://dx.doi.org/10.1186/1746-160X-2-37

[7]   Chandrasema, F., Singh, A. and Visavadia, B.G. (2010) Removal of a Root from the Maxillary Sinus Using Functional Endoscopic Sinus Surgery. *British Journal of Oral and Maxillofacial Surgery*, **48**, 558-589. http://dx.doi.org/10.1016/j.bjoms.2009.09.007

[8]   Hasbini, A.S., Hadi, U. and Ghafari, J. (2001) Endoscopic Removal of an Ectopic Third Molar Obstructing the Osteomeatal Complex. *Ear, Nose Throat Journal*, **80**, 667-670.

[9]   Wolf, G., Anderhuber, W. and Kuhn, F. (1993) Development of the Paranasal Sinus in Children. Implications of Paranasal Sinus Surgery. *Annals of Otology, Rhinology Laryngology*, **102**, 705-711. http://dx.doi.org/10.1177/000348949310200911

Role of Cartilage as a Graft Material for Tympanic Membrane and in Middle Ear Reconstruction

Anant Chouhan*, Bhuvnesh Kumar Singh, Praveen Chandra Verma

Department of ENT, JLN Medical College, Ajmer, India
Email: *dr.apschouhan@gmail.com

Abstract

Objective: The work was planned to evaluate the results of cartilage graft in the surgical treatment of chronic suppurative otitis media. Study Design: A prospective study. Materials and Methods: The present study was a prospective study of tympanoplasties and tympanomastoid surgeries performed on 100 patients. The main outcome measures were both anatomical and functional in form of graft incorporation and postoperative hearing function. Results: Cartilage was used as tympanic membrane and/or ossicle graft in the cases. There were no immediate postoperative or long term complications of surgery except for 10 cases in which there was a failure of graft uptake. There was a 7.6-decibel (dB) improvement in mean air conduction threshold post-operatively. A mean closure of average air bone gap of 8.4 decibels (dB) was noted which was statistically significant. Conclusion: The cartilage graft is a very effective option for the repair of the conducting mechanism of the ear with good take-up rates, less chances of rejection or extrusion and very few significant complications. The thickness of cartilage creates stiffness that is more resistant than the fascia to the anatomic deformities caused by negative middle ear pressure thus improving the long term integrity of the graft.

Keywords

Cartilage Graft, Pure Tone Audiometry, Air Bone Gap

1. Introduction

A dry and intact hearing apparatus is an essential prerequisite for normal hearing. In our clinical practice, we

---

*Corresponding author.

encounter a great deal of patients suffering from chronic suppurative otitis media (CSOM) leading to tympanic membrane perforations, retractions, atelectasis and cholesteatoma. Each of these conditions has a deleterious effect on some part of the sound conducting mechanism.

Cartilage is a reliable graft for tympanic membrane reconstruction [1]. Most frequently used grafting material is temporal fascia graft due to the ease of its accessibility at the surgical site. However, in situations such as advanced middle ear pathology, large perforations, atelectatic ears or retraction pockets, temporalis fascia may cause higher failure rates regardless of the surgical technique used [2] [3].

The earliest reconstructive surgeries of the hearing apparatus were tried in the 16th century. "Tympanoplasty" has been defined by the American Academy of Ophthalmology and Otolaryngology Subcommittee on Conservation of Hearing [4] as "A procedure to eradicate disease in the middle ear and to reconstruct the hearing mechanism, with or without tympanic membrane grafting."

The long term aim of middle ear reconstruction is to reconstruct the tympanic membrane and the sound conducting mechanism and to keep the ear dry. Since the introduction of tympanoplasty, in the fifties, by Zollner [5] and Wullstein [6] various graft materials and perforation closure techniques have been described since then such as temporal fascia [7], perichondrium [8], periosteum [9], vein [10], duramater [11] and cartilage [12] [13]. Cartilage is preferred because of its increased stability and resistance to middle ear pressure even in cases with chronic eustachian tube dysfunction. Utech, in 1959, first introduced cartilage in middle ear surgery [14]. The technique was then promoted by Prof. Heermann J. from Essen, Germany, who used "the cartilage palisade technique" for the reconstruction of the TM and the auditory canal wall [15] [16]. The mechanical characteristics of cartilage offer the advantage of high resistance to retraction and re-perforation. Cartilage has a constant shape, firmer than fascia and also lacks fibrous tissue, so that the post-operative dimensions remain the same and it is also nourished by diffusion and shows great adaptation with tympanic membrane [1].

2. Objective

The work was planned to evaluate the results of cartilage graft in the surgical treatment of chronic suppurative otitis media.

3. Material & Methods

The present study "Role of Cartilage as a Graft Material for Tympanic Membrane and in Middle Ear Reconstruction" was conducted in the Department of Otorhinolaryngology and Head & Neck Surgery of JLN Medical College & Hospital, Ajmer from August 2011 to December 2013.

Study design: prospective study.

Study population: inclusion criteria:

1) Tubotympanic type of CSOM in the quiescent stage that included occasional wet ears.

2) Patients of active CSOM, tubotympanic type not improving with conservative treatment that included persistent wet ears.

3) Patients with retraction pocket and conductive hearing loss.

4) Patients of CSOM atticoantral type where cartilage would be kept for ossiculoplasty and mastoid cavity reconstruction.

Exclusion criteria:

1) Patients of tubotympanic CSOM having septic foci in nose and throat. Such patients were considered after elimination of the septic foci medically and/or surgically.

2) Patients of atticoantral CSOM where cartilage was not used for reconstruction after mastoidectomy.

Sample size: 100.

All patients had undergone thorough history taking and complete ear, nose and throat (ENT) examination including tuning fork tests. A battery of investigations including routine blood investigations, urine examination, X-ray mastoid (lateral oblique view), X-ray chest (posteroanterior view), electrocardiogram, audiometry, tuning fork tests and examination under microscope was done in all patients. Pus for culture and sensitivity, tympanometry, High Resolution Computed Tomography (HRCT) scan temporal bone were done in some cases. Preanaesthetic check up was done and after anaesthetic fitness patients were posted for surgery.

Anaesthesia: general/local.

Technique of surgery:

The surgical areas were cleaned with povidine iodine 0.5% and 70% methylated spirit. 2% lidocaine with 1:200,000 adrenaline solution was infiltrated locally.

Post-aural Wilde's incision was made in majority of the patients. Posterior tympanomeatal flap was elevated up to the fibrous annulus which was detached from the bony annulus and positioned anteriorly thus exposing the middle ear. Status of the middle ear structures was then assessed to decide the type of tympanoplasty and size and shape of cartilage graft required. Conchal or tragal cartilage used as autograft. Mastoidectomy either cortical or canal wall down mastoidectomy was done as per the requirement. Then ossicular chain was checked.

If the ossicular chain was intact than type I tympanoplasty via underlay technique was done using cartilage of 1 mm thickness made by cartilage slicer. If there was necrosis of the incus, than cartilage was reshaped and kept over stapes head and malleus in type II tympanoplasty. In patients with cholesteatoma, canal wall down mastoidectomy was done and cartilage was used for reconstruction. Gel foam was kept in middle ear to stabilize the graft in position. The posterior tympanomeatal flap was then repositioned back and canal wall filled with gel foam.

Closure was done in two layers (subcutaneous and skin). Mastoid dressing was given for 7 days. Total suture removal was done at 7 postoperative day. Patients were given antibiotic cover for 3 weeks.

Follow up was done at 1 month, 6 weeks and 3 months. At each follow up the complaints of the patients were noted. Microscopic examination was done to see the condition of the canal and the graft. Pure tone audiometry was done at 3rd month of follow up. Graft uptake was considered as successful if there was no residual perforation on follow up at 3 months. Hearing results were compared using the guidelines recommended by Committee on Hearing and Equilibrium of the American Academy of Otolaryngology-Head and Neck Surgery for the evaluation of results for conductive hearing loss [17]. This includes reporting of the mean, standard deviation and range of the postoperative air bone gap. Statistical analysis of these results was done by using paired "t" test.

4. Results

54 patients were residing in rural communities while the rest 46 belonged to urban areas. Out of the 100 studied cases 54 subjects were operated on the right ear while 46 were operated on left ear.

The age of the patients included in the study ranged from 14 years to 52 years with mean age of presentation of 27.8 ± 10.8 years. The commonest age group was 21 - 30 years having 38 patients followed by <20 years age group having 28 patients, 41 - 50 years age group having 10 patients, >50 years age group having 4 patients. In the current study, there were 54 males (54%) and 46 females (46%). Slight male preponderance was recorded (**Table 1**).

The commonest complaint of patients was ear discharge, seen in 100% of the patients including occasional or persistent wet ears. Second common presenting complaint was hearing impairment which was seen in 88% of patients. There was associated earache in 24% patients and 4% of patients had tinnitus and vertigo each in the present study.

Pre-operative hearing assessment was done using pure tone audiometry. Out of the 100 studied cases, 42 patients had air conduction level between 21 to 30 decibels. 20 patients had air conduction level between 41 - 50 decibels followed by 31 - 40 decibels in 14 patients and 12 patients had air conduction level above 50 decibels. 12 subjects had air conduction level below or equal to 20 decibels.

In present study, out of 100 patients, 66 patients had bone conduction level between 5 to 10 dB and 18 patients had air conduction level ≤ 5 dB. 12 patients had bone conduction level between 11 to 15 dB followed by 2 patients 16 to 20 dB and 2 above 20 dB.

Table 1. Age and sex distribution of patients.

Age group	Number of patients		Percentage	
	Male	Female	Male	Female
<20	15	13	15%	13%
21 - 30	20	18	20%	18%
31 - 40	10	10	10%	10%
41 - 50	6	4	6%	4%
>50	3	1	3%	1%

In present study most of the patients (48) had air bone gap between 16 to 25 decibels. 30 patients had air bone gap between 60 - 40 decibels and 14 patients had ≤15 decibels.

Pre-operatively mean air conduction was 35 dB with standard deviation of 12 dB. Mean bone conduction was 8.76 with standard deviation of 3.8 dB and mean air bone gap was 26.4 dB with standard deviation of 10 dB (**Table 2**).

This table shows that most common intra-operative finding was central perforation which was seen 46% patients. Most commonly involved ossicle was incus, involved in 62% patients followed by stapes in 36% patients. Malleus was involved only in 4% patients (**Table 3**).

In the present study, type I tympanoplasty was carried out in 36 cases. Type II tympanoplasty was performed in 28 patients and type III tympanoplasty in 36 patients. Mastoidectomy was performed in 76 patients. Mastoidectomy was done in cases of tympanic membrane (TM) retraction, cholesteatoma and granulations. 40 patients underwent modified intact canal wall mastoidectomy, out of which type II tympanoplasty was done in 28 and type I in rest 12 cases. In 36 cases canal wall down mastoidectomy with type III tympanoplasty was done.

Successful graft uptake was achieved in 90% of the 100 operated ears. In 10% residual perforation was seen at the end of 3 months study period.

Post-operatively out of 100 studied cases, 44 patients had air conduction level below or equal to 20 decibels. 22 patients had air conduction level between 21 - 30 decibels and 18 patients had between 41 - 50 decibels followed by 16 patients between 31 - 40 decibels.

Out of 100 patients, 66 patients had bone conduction level between 6 to 10 dB. 16 patients had bone conduction level ≤ 5 dB and 10 patients had between 11 to 15 dB. 6 patients had bone conduction level between 16 - 20 dB and only 2 patients had more than 20 dB.

Post-operative hearing assessment was done using the same parameters as those used for preoperative hearing assessment. Post-operatively 56 patients had air bone gap ≤ 15 dB and 30 patients had between 26 - 40 dB followed by 14 patients between 16 - 25 dB. The AB Gap in 10 cases of graft failure was >25 dB.

Post-operatively mean air conduction was 27.4 dB with standard deviation of 11.5 dB. Mean bone conduction was 9.26 with standard deviation of 4.03 dB and mean air bone gap was 18 dB with standard deviation of 9 dB (**Table 4**).

On comparison of pre-operative and post-operative hearing results there was a mean improvement in air conduction threshold by 7.6 dB. On applying "t" test it showed that this difference was highly significant (*P* value = 0.0017) thus verifying the efficacy of cartilage graft in restoring the distorted sound conduction mechanism of

Table 2. Pre-operative audiometric evaluation.

Type of hearing loss	Range (in dB)	Mean (in dB)	SD (in dB)
Air conduction	15 - 60	35	12
Bone conduction	5 - 25	8.76	3.8
Air bone gap	5 - 44	26.4	10

Table 3. Intra-operative findings.

Intra operative findings	No. of patients	Percentage
Central perforation	46	46%
Marginal	30	30%
Posterosuperior retraction	22	22%
Cholesteatoma	36	36%
Plastered tympanic membrane	6	6%
Tympanosclerotic plaque	10	10%
Malleus necrosed	4	4 %
Incus necrosed	62	62%
Stapes erosion	36	36%

the ear. However, as can be expected there was no significant change in bone conduction thresholds (P value = 0.52). On analysing the audiometric parameter of air-bone gap by the same paired "t" test there was again significant improvement in air-bone gap (8.4 dB) after surgery (P value = 0.00003) (**Table 5**).

5. Discussion

Cartilage is a reliable graft for tympanic membrane reconstruction as it is nourished by diffusion and becomes well incorporated in the tympanic membrane [1].

The demographic and clinical data was collected which included age, sex, rural/urban population, diagnosis (chronic suppurative otitis media with or without cholesteatoma), prior otologic surgery, details of surgical technique, intra-operative findings (middle ear mucosa status, ossicular chain status, and reconstruction), post-operative findings (graft incorporation), hearing and duration of follow-up. The main outcome measures were both anatomical and functional in form of graft incorporation and postoperative hearing function.

In the present study, successful graft uptake was achieved in 90 ears (90%) of the 100 ears operated. In 10 ears (10%) residual perforation was seen at the end of the study period. These results are comparable to the study by Sapci T *et al*. [18] in which 92% successful closure of tympanic membrane was achieved using tragal cartilage graft.

Results of tympanic membrane closure achieved by cartilage graft are comparable to those achieved by different workers for temporalis fascia graft-Dabholkar JP *et al*. [19] (84% graft uptake), Ozbek C *et al*. [20] (70.2%), Sirena E *et al*. [21] (80%), Yetiser S *et al*. [22] (95%).

Results of graft uptake in the present study are more or less better than those which have been achieved by the use of other graft materials like tragal perichondrium-Dabholkar JP *et al*. [19] (80% success rate), skin graft by Wright WK [23] (74% success) and tympanic membrane homograft by Marquet JFE [24] (80% success rate).

The thickness of cartilage creates stiffness that is more resistant than the fascia to the anatomic deformities caused by negative middle ear pressure thus improving the long term integrity of the graft.

In present study, the mean air conduction preoperatively was 35 decibels which improved to 27.4 decibels post-operatively. The mean pre-operative bone conduction was 8.76 decibels as compared to mean postoperative bone conduction of 9.26 decibels. The mean air bone gap pre-operative was 26.4 decibels which was reduced to 18 decibels post-operatively thus giving improvement in hearing of 8.4 decibels.

These results are comparable to the study done by Mahadevaiah A *et al*. [25] in which they achieved difference of mean pre- and post-surgery air bone gap of 13 decibels.

Factors which predicted the success rate of the middle ear reconstruction include occasionally/persistently wet ear, ossicular status, mobility/fixity of ossicular chain, pathology including cholesteatoma/granulations, type of surgery performed and nutritional status, smoking that definitely have role in healing.

There was no immediate postoperative or long term complications of surgery except for 10 cases in which there was failure of graft uptake.

A potential drawback of cartilage graft was the graft opacity, as it may be more difficult to detect eventual residual/recurrent cholesteatoma.

Table 4. Post-operative audiometric evaluation.

Type of hearing loss	Range (in dB)	Mean (in dB)	SD (in dB)
Air conduction	10 - 48	27.4	11.5
Bone conduction	5 - 25	9.26	4.03
Air bone gap	4 - 38	18	9

Table 5. Comparison of pre- and post-operative hearing results.

Hearing results	Pre-operative (mean ± S.D.)	Post-operative (mean ± S.D.)	P value
Air conduction	35 ± 12	27.4 ± 11.5	0.0017
Bone conduction	8.76 ± 3.8	9.26 ± 4.03	0.5248
A-B gap	26.4 ± 10	18 ± 9	0.00003

6. Conclusions

The cartilage graft is a very effective option for the repair of the conducting mechanism of the ear with good take-up rates, less chances of rejection or extrusion and very few significant complications.

- There was a 7.6-dB improvement in mean air conduction threshold post-operatively which was statistically significant (P value 0.0017).
- There was no significant improvement in the bone conduction threshold. This was as per expectations as the surgery was aimed to reconstruct the conduction mechanism only.
- A mean closure of average air bone gap of 8.4 dB was noted. This is also statistically significant (P value 0.00003) as derived by applying the paired "t" test.
- Cartilage is an effective autologous graft for the reconstruction of the conduction mechanism of ear. Thus we conclude that cartilage is an effective graft material for middle ear reconstruction.
- The results of cartilage in middle ear reconstruction are comparable to that of other graft materials as reported in literature.

Conflict of Interest

None.

References

[1]   Levinson, R.M. (1987) Cartilage-Perichondrial Composite Graft Tympanoplasty in the Treatment of Posterior Marginal and Attic Retraction Pockets. *Laryngoscope*, **97**, 1069-1074.
      http://dx.doi.org/10.1288/00005537-198709000-00013

[2]   Buckingham, R.A. (1992) Fascia and Perichondrium Atrophy in Tympanoplasty and Recurrent Middle Ear Atelectasis. *Annals of Otology, Rhinology Laryngology*, **101**, 755-758. http://dx.doi.org/10.1177/000348949210100907

[3]   Milewski, C. (1993) Composite Graft Tympanoplasty in the Treatment of Ears with Advanced Middle Ear Pathology. *Laryngoscope*, **103**, 1352-1356. http://dx.doi.org/10.1288/00005537-199312000-00006

[4]   Committee on Conservation of Hearing of the American Academy of Ophthalmology and Otolaryngology (1964) Standard Classification for Surgery of Chronic Ear Disease. *Archives of Otolaryngology—Head and Neck Surgery*, **81**, 204-205.

[5]   Zollner, F. (1955) The Principles of Plastic Surgery of the Sound Conducting Apparatus. *Journal of Laryngology and Otology*, **69**, 637-652. http://dx.doi.org/10.1017/S0022215100051240

[6]   Wullstein, H.L. (1952) Functional Operation in the Middle Ear with Split Thickness Skin Graft. *Archives of Otorhinolaryngology*, **161**, 422-436. http://dx.doi.org/10.1007/BF02129204

[7]   Heermann, H. (1960) Tympanic Membrane Plastic Repair with Temporalis Fascia. *Hals Nas Ohrenh*, **9**, 136-139.

[8]   Salen, B. (1968) Tympanic Membrane Grafts of Full Thickness Skin, Fascia and Cartilage with Its Perichondrium, an Experimental and Clinical Investigation. *Acta Oto-Laryngologica*, **244**, 5-73.

[9]   Bocca, E., Cis, C. and Zernotti, E. (1959) L'impiego di lembi liberi di periostio nella tympanoplastica. *Archivio Italiano di Otologia, Rinologia e Laringologia. Supplemento*, **40**, 205.

[10] Tabb, H.G. (1960) Closure of Perforation of the Tympanic Membrane by Vein Grafts: A Preliminary Report of 20 Cases. *Laryngoscope*, **70**, 271-274. http://dx.doi.org/10.1288/00005537-196003000-00004

[11] Albrite, J.P. and Leigh, B.G. (1966) Dural Homograft (Alloplastic) Myringoplasty. *The Laryngoscope*, **76**, 1687-1693. http://dx.doi.org/10.1288/00005537-196610000-00006

[12] Jansen, C. (1963) Cartilage-Tympanoplasty. *The Laryngoscope*, **73**, 1288-1302. http://dx.doi.org/10.1288/00005537-196310000-00006

[13] Salen, B. (1963) Myringoplasty Using Septum Cartilage. *Acta Otolaryngologica*, **57**, 82-91.

[14] Utech, H. (1959) Ueber diagnostische und therapeutische Moeglichkeiten der Tympanotomie bei Schalleitungsstoerungen. *Zeitschrift für Laryngologie, Rhinologie, Otologie und ihre Grenzgebiete*, **38**, 212-221.

[15] Heermann, J. (1978) Auricular Cartilage Palisade Tympano-, Epitympano-, Antrum- and Mastoid-Plastics. *Clinical Otolaryngology & Allied Sciences*, **3**, 443-446. http://dx.doi.org/10.1111/j.1365-2273.1978.tb00726.x

[16] Heermann, J. (1992) Autograft Tragal and Conchal Palisade Cartilage and Perichondrium in Tympanomastoid Reconstruction. *Ear, Nose & Throat Journal*, **71**, 344-349.

[17] Guidelines of the Committee on the Hearing and Equilibrium (1995) Committee in Hearing and Evaluation of Results

of Treatment of Conductive Hearing Loss. *Otolaryngology—Head and Neck Surgery*, **106**, 865-867.

[18] Sapci, T., Almac, S., Usta, C., Karavas, A., Mercangoz, C. and Evimik, M.F. (2006) Comparison between Tympano-plasties with Cartilage Perichondrium Composite Graft and Temporal Fascia Graft in Terms of Hearing Levels and Healing. *Kulak Burun Boğaz İhtisas Dergisi*, **16**, 255-260.

[19] Dabholkar, J.P., Vora, K. and Sikdar, A. (2007) Comparative Study of Underlay Tympanoplasty with Temporalis Fascia and Tragal Perichondrium. *Indian Journal of Otolaryngology and Head & Neck Surgery*, **59**, 116-119.
http://dx.doi.org/10.1007/s12070-007-0035-0

[20] Ozbek, C., Cifta, O., Tuna, E.E., Yazkan, O. and Ozdem, C. (2008) A Comparison of Cartilage Palisades and Fascia in Type I Tympanoplasty in Children: Anatomic and Functional Results. *Otology & Neurotology*, **29**, 679-683.
http://dx.doi.org/10.1097/MAO.0b013e31817dad57

[21] Sirena, E., Carvalho, B., Buschle, M. and Mocellin, M. (2010) Timpanoplastia Myringoplasty Type 1 and in Residency Surgical Results and Audiometric. *International Archives of Otorhinolaryngology*, **14**, 60-65.

[22] Yetiser, S. and Hidin, Y. (2009) Temporalis Fascia and Cartilage Perichondrium Composite Shield Graft for Recon-struction for Tympanic Membrane. *The Annals of Otology, Rhinology, and Laryngology*, **118**, 570-574.

[23] Wright, W.K. (1956) Repair of Chronic Central Perforation of Tympanic Membrane by Skin Grafting. *The Laryngo-scope*, **66**, 1464-1487. http://dx.doi.org/10.1002/lary.5540661104

[24] Marquet, J.F.E. (1968) Myringoplasty by Eardrum Transplantation. *The Laryngoscope*, **78**, 1329-1336.
http://dx.doi.org/10.1288/00005537-196808000-00006

[25] Mahadeviah, A. and Parikh, B. (2008) Modified Intact Canal Wall Mastoidectomy: Long Term Hearing Results in Hearing and Healing. *Indian Journal of Otolaryngology and Head & Neck Surgery*, **60**, 317-323.
http://dx.doi.org/10.1007/s12070-008-0109-7

10

Clinical and Histological Patterns of Oropharyngeal Tumors in Selected Health Institutions in North Western Nigeria

Kufre Robert Iseh*, Mohammed Abdullahi, Daniel Jiya Aliyu, Stanley Amutta, Stephen Semen Yikawe, Joseph Hassan Solomon

Department of ENT, Usmanu Danfodiyo University Teaching Hospital, Sokoto, Nigeria
Email: *frobih@yahoo.com

Abstract

Background: Tumors of the oropharynx affect a common pathway for deglutition, respiration and speech and therefore pose a challenge to both the patient and clinician. This paper attempts to present clinical and histologic patterns, and therapeutic challenges of oropharyngeal tumors from three selected health facilities in North Western Nigeria. Materials and Methods: The medical records of patients seen in the Usmanu Danfodiyo University Teaching Hospital, Sokoto, Federal Medical Centre Birnin Kebbi and Shepherd Specialist Hospital, Sokoto with oropharyngeal tumors over a fourteen-year period were reviewed (January 2000 to December 2013). Results: A total of 36 patients were seen. Twenty (56%) were males and 16 (44%) were females, making the male:female ratio, 1.3:1, (P value of 0.004 for the null hypothesis). The age range was 3 to 80 years, with a mean age of 45.5 years. Majority of patients were in their 5th decade of life (33%). Nineteen (53%) patients presented with dysphagia, 11 (28%) with mass in the mouth (soft palate), 7 (17%) with neck swelling, while 3 patients (7%) presented with upper airway obstruction. Twenty-six patients (72%) presented at an advanced stage. Squamous cell carcinoma accounted for 31% of the cases, followed by lymphoma 14%, adenoid cystic carcinoma 8%, pleomorphic adenoma 5%, mucoepidermoid carcinoma 5%, peripheral nerve sheath tumour 3%, alveolar rhabdomyosarcoma (3%), tuberculoma (3%) and inflammatory polyp (3%). Surgery was carried out in 31 cases (86.1%) for the purpose of obtaining biopsy and removal of tumour, followed by chemotherapy (5.5%) and radiotherapy (5.5%) where histologic diagnosis was malignant. Five (13.9%) did not consent for any intervention. Conclusion: Oropharyngeal tumours are varied in presentation. Squamous cell carcinoma (31%) was the commonest histologic type followed by lymphoma (14%) and adencystic carcinoma (8%). About 72% of the cases were in advanced stages (T4). More than half of the tumours (53%) were of soft palate origin.

*Corresponding author.

Keywords

Oropharyngeal Tumour, Squamous Cell Carcinoma, Lymphoma, North Western Nigeria

1. Introduction

Tumours of the oropharynx affect a common pathway for deglutition, respiration, and speech and therefore pose a challenge to both the patient and clinician when these functions are compromised [1]. Because the oropharynx is hidden, tumours growing in this region appear to have an insidious onset, with patients presenting at an advanced stage [2]-[4]. The oropharynx is a musculofascial tube which extends from the level of the hard palate above to the hyoid bone below. It is divided into the following sub-sites for therapeutic and diagnostic purposes; soft palate, tonsillar fossa (lateral wall), base of the tongue, and posterior pharyngeal wall [2] [5].

Histologically, the oropharynx contains squamous epithelium, lymphoid tissues and minor salivary glands. Tumours of the oropharynx could arise from any of these tissues, and could be either benign or malignant, but majority of epithelial tumours are squamous cell carcinomas [1] [2] [5]-[8]. The amount of lymphoid tissue in the oropharynx is high and this could explain the higher incidence of oropharyngeal lymphoma compared to other sites in the body [1] [2].

Benign lesions are usually slow growing until obstructive features manifest and are more commonly located on the soft palate; while for the malignant lesions, the lateral oropharyngeal wall is the sub site more commonly affected [1] [2] [5] [9]. Cancers of the base of the tongue are difficult to detect because of its location and relative absence of pain fibres, hence patients with base of the tongue tumours present at an advanced stage [1] [2] [5]. Common clinical features include the following: dysphagia, difficulty in breathing, throat pain, feeling of throat mass, voice changes, oral bleeding, ear pain, and neck mass [1] [3]. Therefore, the oropharynx should be evaluated in cases of respiratory distress, stridor, voice changes, or dysphagia.

This paper attempts to present clinical and histologic patterns, and therapeutic challenges of oropharyngeal tumours from three selected health facilities in north western Nigeria.

2. Materials and Methods

This is a retrospective study of all patients that presented to ENT Departments of Usmanu Danfodio University Teaching Hospital Sokoto, Federal Medical Centre Birnin Kebbi, and Out-Patient Unit of Shepherd Specialist Hospital, Sokoto with oropharyngeal tumours, over a fourteen-year period (January 2000 to December 2013).

Patients who had oropharyngeal tumors were recruited for the study. Medical records of patients were reviewed, relevant data extracted (such as bio data, clinical presentation, treatment modalities) and analysed using Statistical Package for Social Sciences (SPSS) version 20. Patients with incomplete clinical information were excluded from the study.

3. Results

A total number of 36 patients were seen. Twenty (56%) were males and 16 (44%) were females, with a male to female ratio of 1.3:1, (P value of 0.004 for the null hypothesis). The age range was 3 to 80 years, with a mean age of 45.5 years. Majority of patients [12 (33%)] were in their 5th decade of life.

Nineteen (53%) patients presented with dysphagia, 11 (31%) with mass in the mouth, 7 (19%) with neck swelling, 3 patients (8%) presented with upper airway obstruction necessitating emergency tracheostomy while some presented with a combination of above symptoms. Twenty-six patients (72%) presented at an advanced stage. Five patients (13.9%) had a history of cigarette smoking but history of alcohol consumption was not identified among the patients.

Nineteen (53%) tumours involved the soft palate alone, 1 (3%) was limited to the tonsils. Sixteen (44%) of the tumours involved the entire oropharynx. Twenty-two (61%) were malignant tumors while 5 (14%) were benign. Histology results for 4 cases could not be traced (**Figure 1**).

Squamous cell carcinoma accounted for 11 (31%) of cases, lymphoma 5 (14%), adenoid cystic carcinoma 3 (8%), pleomorphic adenoma 2 (5%), mucoepidermoid carcinoma 2 (5%), alveolar rhabdomyosarcoma 1 (3%),

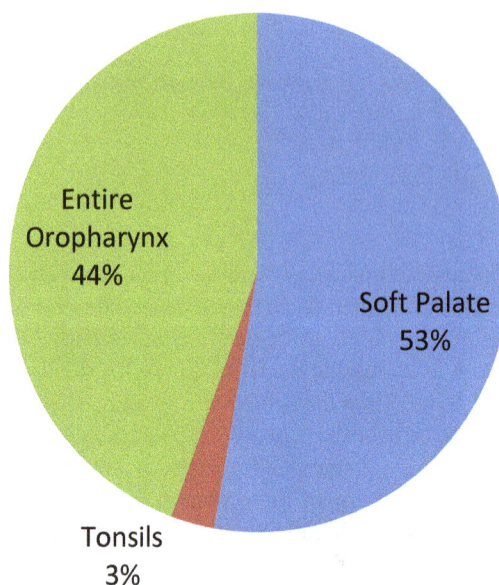

Figure 1. Site of oropharynx affected by the tumor.

tuberculoma 1 (3%), benign peripheral nerve sheath tumour 1 (3%), and inflammatory polyp 1 (3%).

Surgery was carried out on 31 (86.1%) cases for the purpose of obtaining biopsy and debulking of tumour, followed by chemotherapy (5.5%) and radiotherapy (5.5%) where histologic diagnosis was malignant. Five (13.9%) did not consent to any form of intervention.

4. Discussion

Oropharyngeal tumours account for 10% - 12% of all malignancies of the upper aerodigestive tract worldwide [1]. It accounted for 3.8% of all head and neck cancers seen in Sokoto, Nigeria [10], and 0.4% of all neoplasms seen in Ibadan, Nigeria [11].

Studies on the head and neck cancers showed that the median age of diagnosis is in a patient's early 60s, with a male predominance [12]. However, for oropharyngeal malignancies especially for squamous cell carcinoma, it is diagnosed predominantly in patients over the age of 45 years. Over the past two decades, diagnosis had been made in patient less than 45 years especially with implication of HPV type 16 [13] [14]. In our study, majority of the patients were between the ages of 40 - 49 years which agrees with the similar study done in Maiduguri, North eastern part of Nigeria [6] (**Figure 2**). Precise reasons for Involvement of younger age group with Oropharyngeal cancer are not well defined as in studies from the western countries [15] [16]. Proposed mechanism may be related to poor nutritional status involving the deficiency of vitamin A, chronic irritant and poor dental hygiene may be more relevant in our environment coupled with low socioeconomic status, ignorance and bad culture like chewing herbal medicine, kola nuts, tobacco and drinking highly concentrated gin. In a recent study by Iseh *et al.* in the same region the analysis of frequency of food intake amongst head and neck cancer patients demonstrated low consumption of vegetables, selenium, lycopene and pytochemicals rich food which are consistent with increased risk of cancer [17]. In that study low income, large family size, ignorance and low literacy rate were identified as poor prognostic factors affecting their financial capabilities in accessing a balanced diet thereby predisposing to poor health status and head and neck cancer [17]. Males were more commonly affected with a male:female ratio of 1.3:1, this agrees with other studies [6] [18] [19] this difference between males and females was however not statistically significant (P value of 0.004 for the null hypothesis) in this study.

There are well documented etiologies of the oropharyngeal cancers in literatures [6] [20]-[22]. However, smoking could only be implicated in only 5 (13.9%) in our study. This finding may be due to the limitations of a retrospective study where the surgeon(s) who first came in contact with the patient(s) may not have taken the appropriate histories such as the predisposing factors and others. Therefore, a prospective study which may involve the role of human papillomavirus in the pathogenesis of head and neck cancer in our local environment is much desired as this may help in the prevention protocols of oropharyngeal squamous cell carcinoma.

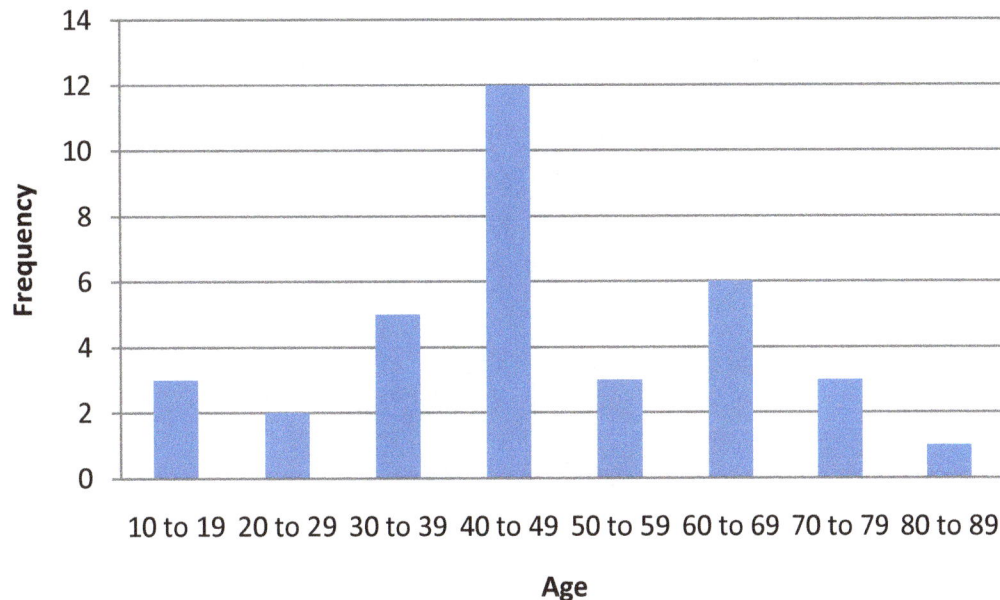

Figure 2. Age distribution.

Benign tumors occur more frequently in the oral cavity than the oropharynx [1]. This could explain our findings in the present study were only 14% are benign tumors. For malignant tumors of the oropharynx, our present study showed that squamous cell carcinoma was the commonest which agrees with studies in both local and the western countries [1] [2] [5] [7] [8] [18].

Generally in Sub-Saharan Africa, cancer presentation is usually in advanced stage [6]. Seventy-two percent of our patients had advanced tumor with various clinical presentations: dysphagia (53%), mass in the mouth (soft palate) (31%), cervical mass (19%) and difficulty in breathing (8%) which necessitated tracheostomy. The late presentation can be attributed to ignorance and the use of traditional medications taken before seeking medical help [23]. Our finding in this study is similar to the studies carried out in Jos and Maiduguri, both in Nigeria [23] (**Figure 3** and **Figure 4**).

Surgery was carried out on 86.1% of patients, with only 5.5% of them having chemo radiation. With most of our patients presenting at an advanced stage, it is expected that most of them will have undergone post operative chemo radiation as is the practice worldwide [1], but it wasn't so in this study. This is due to poverty, ignorance and in those who presented before 2010, reluctance to travel over 400 km to get radiotherapy. Other factors that may be responsible for this poor health seeking behaviour in our environment may be; cultural beliefs, scepticism about orthodox medicine, exploitation by quacks, large family size and conflict of interest, so it's not surprising that 9 patients did not consent for any form of treatment but signed and left against medical advice. This may also be the reason for poor follow up among our patients as most of them did not come for follow up after surgery, resulting in low rate of post operative chemo-radiation.

Public enlightment for the community and continuous medical education for Health workers is needed, to enable persons with features of early lesion to be referred to an otolaryngologist for further evaluation and care, and to discourage harmful traditional practices and beliefs. Appropriate legislation through advocacy should also be put in place to enable indigent patients access to medical care at affordable cost.

5. Conclusion

Oropharyngeal tumors in this study were malignant (61%) and benign (14%). Squamous cell carcinoma (31%), followed by lymphoma (14%) was the commonest histologic types seen, with majority of patients (72%) presenting at an advanced stage of the disease with multiple symptoms, some life threatening requiring urgent airway surgical intervention. However, some patients were not too keen on continuing with other modalities of treatment because of poverty and ignorance, accounting for a low number of patients having post operative radiotherapy and chemotherapy. More is needed on advocacy and public enlightment in this regard.

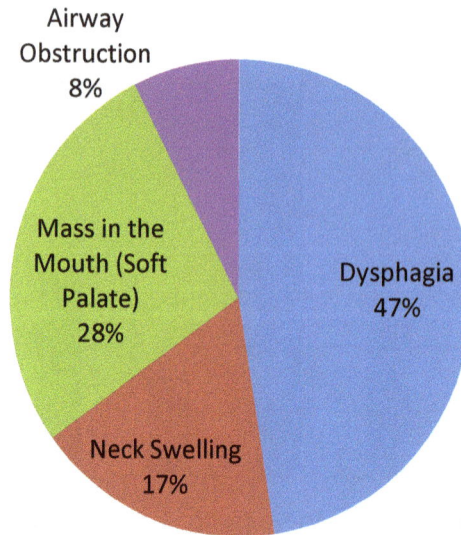

Figure 3. Clinical features.

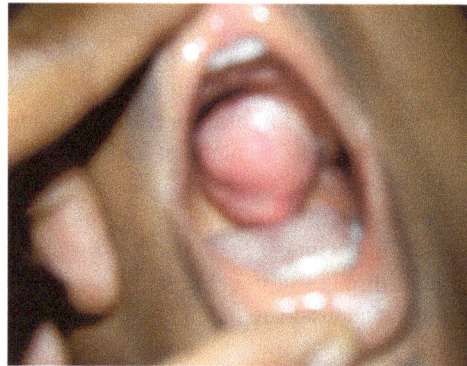

Figure 4. Patient with soft palatal mass.

Competing Interest

The authors declare that they have no competing interest.

Author's Contribution

K. R. Iseh, conceived and designed the study and drafted the manuscript. M. Abdullahi, S B Amutta & D. J. Aliyu participated in coordinating the study and drafting the manuscript. S. S. Yikawe & J. H. Solomon drafted the manuscript and performed statistical analysis. All authors read and approved the final manuscript.

References

[1]   Bradley, J.P. (2008) Oropharyngeal Tumours. In Gleeson, M., Browning, G.C. and Burton, M.J., *et al.*, Eds., *Scott-Brown's Otorhinolaryngology, Head and Neck Surgery*, 7th Edition, Hodder Arnold, London, 2577-2593. http://dx.doi.org/10.1201/b15118-212

[2]   Gassner, G.H. and Sabri, A.N. (2005) Oropharyngeal Malignancy. In Cummings, C.W., Flint, P.W., Lund, V.J., *et al.*, Eds., *Cummings Otolaryngology Head & Neck Surgery*, 4th Edition, Elsevier Mosby, Amsterdam, 1717-1754.

[3]   Pitchers, M. and Marthin, C. (2006) Delay in Referral of Oropharyngeal Squamous Cell Carcinoma to Secondary Care Correlates with a More Advanced Stage at Presentation, and Is Associated with Poor Survival. *British Journal of Cancer*, **94**, 955-958. http://dx.doi.org/10.1038/sj.bjc.6603044

[4]   Dhooge, I.J. and Albers, F.W. (1996) Clinical Characteristics and Diagnostic Delay of Head and Neck Cancer: Results from a Prospective Study in Belgium. *European Journal of Surgical Oncology*, **22**, 354-358.

http://dx.doi.org/10.1016/S0748-7983(96)90220-6

[5]   Homer, J. and Rees, G. (2012) Pharynx: Oropharynx. In Watkinson, J.C. and Gilbert, R.W., Eds., *Stell & Maran's Textbook of Head and Neck Surgery and Oncology*, 5th Edition, Hodder Arnold, London, 612-617. http://dx.doi.org/10.1201/b13389-37

[6]   Garandawa, H.I., Abdullahi, I., Haruna, A.N., Sandabe, M.B. and Samdi, M.T. (2012) Oropharyngeal Cancers in Maiduguri, Nigeria: A Ten Year Review of Clinical Profile. *Online Journal of Medicine and Medical Science Research*, 1, 116-121.

[7]   Otoh, E.C., Johnson, N.W. and Danfillo, I.S. (2004) Primary Head and Neck Cancers in North Eastern Nigeria. *West African Journal of Medicine*, 23, 305-313.

[8]   Lilly-Tariah, O.B., Nwana, E.J.C. and Okeowo, P.A. (2000) Cancers of the Ear, Nose and Throat. *Nigerian Journal of Surgical Sciences*, 10, 52-56.

[9]   Ologe, F.E., Adeniji, K.A. and Segun-Busari, S. (2005) Clinicopathological Study of Head and Neck Cancers in Ilorin, Nigeria. *Tropical Doctor*, 35, 2-4. http://dx.doi.org/10.1258/0049475053001949

[10]   Iseh, K.R. and Malami, S.A. (2006) Pattern of Head and Neck Cancer in Sokoto. *Nigerian Journal of Otorhinolaryngology*, 3, 77-83.

[11]   Abiose, B.O., Ogunniyi, J. and Oyejide, O. (1991) Oral Soft Tissue Malignancies in Ibadan, Nigeria. *African Journal of Medicine Medical Sciences*, 20, 107-113.

[12]   Parkin, D.M., Bray, F., Ferlay, J. and Pisani, P. (2005) Global Cancer Statistic. *CA: A Cancer Journal for Clinicians*, 55, 74-108. http://dx.doi.org/10.3322/canjclin.55.2.74

[13]   Gillison, L.M., Koch, M.W., Capone, B.R., Spafford, M., Westra, H.W. and Wu, L. (2000) Evidence of Causal Association between Human Papillomavirus and a Subset of Head and Neck Cancer. *Journal of the National Cancer Institute*, 92, 709-720. http://dx.doi.org/10.1093/jnci/92.9.709

[14]   Gillison, M.L. (2007) Current Topics in the Epidemiology of Oral Cavity and Oropharyngeal Cancers. *Head & Neck*, 29, 779-792. http://dx.doi.org/10.1002/hed.20573

[15]   D'Souza, G., Kreimer, A.R., Viscidi, R., Pawlita, M., Fakhry, C., Koch, W.M., *et al.* (2007) Case-Control Study of Human Papillomavirus and Oropharyngeal Cancer. *New England Journal of Medicine*, 356, 1944-1956. http://dx.doi.org/10.1056/NEJMoa065497

[16]   McKaig, R.G., Baric, R.S. and Olshan, A.F. (1998) Human Papillomavirus and Head and Neck Cancer: Epidemiology and Molecular Biology. *Head and Neck*, 20, 250-265. http://dx.doi.org/10.1002/(SICI)1097-0347(199805)20:3<250::AID-HED11>3.0.CO;2-O

[17]   Iseh, K.R., Essien, E. and Bilbis, L.S. (2013) Demographic Characteristics and Food Consumption Pattern of Head and Neck Cancer Patients in a Tertiary Health Institution North West Nigeria. *Pakistan Journal of Nutrition*, 12, 897-902. http://dx.doi.org/10.3923/pjn.2013.897.902

[18]   Silas, O.A. and Adoga, A.A. (2012) Histopathologic Patterns of Malignant Tumours of the Oropharynx of the Jos University Teaching Hospital. *Journal of Clinical Pathology and Forensic Medicine*, 3, 9-11.

[19]   Psyrri, A., Prezas, L. and Burtness, B. (2008) Oropharyngeal Cancer. *Clinical Advances in Hematology and Oncology*, 6, 604-612.

[20]   Blot, W.J., McLaughlin, J.K., Winn, D.M., Austin, D.F., Greenberg, R.S., Preston-Martin, S., *et al.* (1988) Smoking and Drinking in Relation to Oral and Pharyngeal Cancer. *Cancer Research*, 48, 3282-3287.

[21]   Brugere, J., Guenel, P., Leclerc, A. and Rodriguez, J. (1986) Differential Effect of Tobacco and Alcohol in Cancer of the Larynx, Pharynx and Mouth. *Cancer*, 57, 391-395. http://dx.doi.org/10.1002/1097-0142(19860115)57:2<391::AID-CNCR2820570235>3.0.CO;2-Q

[22]   Talamini, R., Favero, A., Franceschi, S., La Vecchia, C., Levi, F. and Conti, E. (1998) Cancer of the Oral Cavity and Pharynx in Nonsmokers Who Drink Alcohol and in Nondrinkers Who Smoke Tobacco. *Journal of the National Cancer Institute*, 90, 1901-1903. http://dx.doi.org/10.1093/jnci/90.24.1901

[23]   Adoga, A.A., Nimkur, T.L. and Silas, O.A. (2011) Clinicopathological Profile of Malignant Tumors of the Oropharynx at the Jos University Teaching Hospital, Jos, Nigeria. *Journal of Medicine in the Tropics*, 13, 36-40. http://dx.doi.org/10.4314/jmt.v13i1.69331

11

Triple-c Cartilage Tympanoplasty: Case Series

Kartik Parelkar, Smita Nagle, Mohan Jagade, Vandana Thorawade, Poonam Khairnar, Anoop Attakil, Madhavi Pandare, Rajanala Nataraj, Reshma Hanwate, Rajesh Kar

Department of ENT, Grant Govt Medical College & Sir J J Group of Hospitals, Mumbai, India
Email: kartikparelkar@ymail.com

Abstract

The triple-c cartilage tympanoplasty *i.e.* (composite chondroperichondrial clip) technique was devised by Fernandes in 2003. Objectives: The objective of our case series was to assess the success rate and efficacy of the triple-c cartilage tympanoplasty by transcanal approach. Study Design: A retrospective analysis of patients subjected to the technique was conducted. Methods: 20 cases who met the inclusion criteria were assessed by otomicroscopy and pure tone audiometry before and 2 months after the surgery. Results: All patients had complete take-up of the graft and a hearing improvement which was statistically significant. Conclusions: Thus the triple-c technique provides an effective method of closing nonmarginal perforations of the tympanic membrane.

Keywords

Triple-c, Cartilage, Tympanoplasty

1. Introduction

Ideal graft material for tympanoplasty has always been a dilema. Heerman was the first to consider temporalis fascia as a grafting material. Storrs successfully employed it thereafter [1]. The concept of grafting tragal cartilage and perichondrium was introduced by Good hill [1].

Tragal cartilage with perichondrium (**Figure 1**) fulfills all the required qualities of an ideal graft material namely low rejection rate, sufficient quantity, good tensile strength, conductive properties similar to that of tympanic membrane and easy availability.

Fernandes from Newcastle, Australia published the technique of composite chondroperichondrial clip tympanoplasty using the tragal cartilage [2].

In this technique the cartilage-perichondrium graft is both an onlay and underlay graft similar to the butterfly

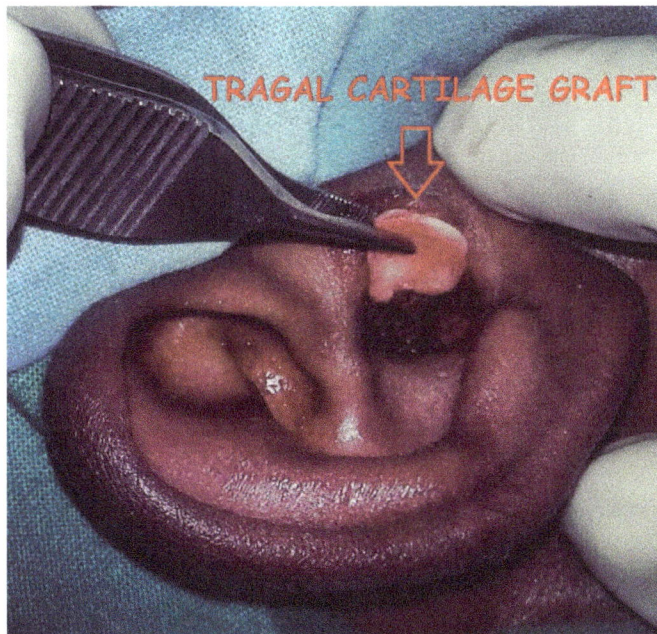

Figure 1. Tragal cartilage with perichondrium being harvested.

technique without its disadvantages. Many cases with small harmless perforations of the ear drum are operated by retroauricular approach using fascia due to the cartilage and onlay phobia. In these cases the triple-c cartilage tympanoplasty by transcanal approach would be a splendid and minimally invasive solution.

The triple-c technique is fairly simple, sutureless and effective method [3] of type-1 tympanoplasty with good patient compliance and reduced hospital stay in our experience as discussed below.

2. Methodology

20 cases in the age group of 12 to 50 years with small to moderate sized perforations and a dry ear (for at least 6 months) were selected. Patients with marginal perforations were excluded.

These patients had a hearing loss no greater than 40 db at any frequency on preoperative pure tone audiometry.

All 20 cases underwent meticulous preoperative assessment which included otomicroscopy, pure tone audiometry and routine workup.

Eustachian tube patency was tested by valsalva and methylene blue dye test.

The ossicular status and mobility were assessed by endoscopy through the moderate perforations specially in patients having hearing loss on the higher side.

The graft take-up and the hearing were assessed 2 months postoperatively (**Figure 2**) with otomicroscopy and pure tone audiometry respectively.

3. Technique

1) Transcanal method was used and tragal cartilage with perichondrium on both sides harvested.

2) The perichondrium from the medial side of the graft was removed while that from the lateral side of the graft raised 1 - 2 mm from all around the margins (**Figure 3**).

3) The fashioned graft was then slipped through the perforation in a similar way as the lens in its capsule in ophthalmology and dialled in place using a pick.

4) The perichondrium was then gently pulled out from the perforation and spread over the denuded margins in an overlay fashion (**Figure 4**).

Thus making the cartilage proper as an underlay graft and perichondrium an onlay one, clipping the freshened margins of the perforation.

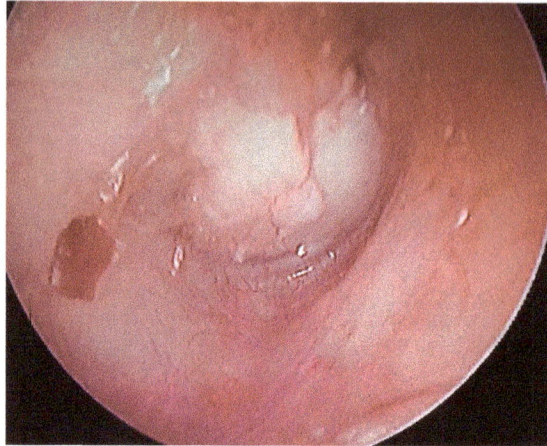

Figure 2. 2 months postoperatively showing take-up of the graft.

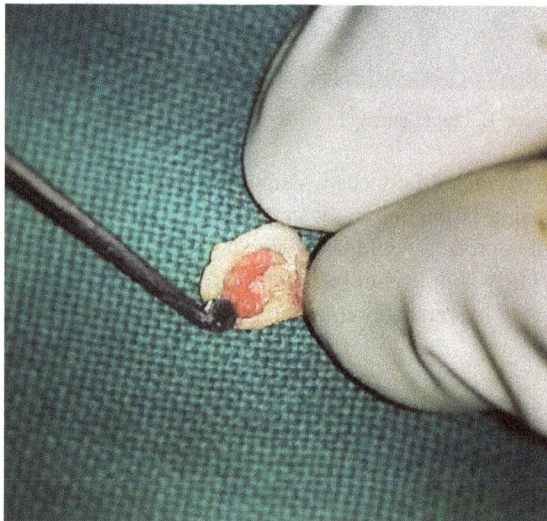

Figure 3. Perichondrium from lateral side raised all along the margins of the cartilage.

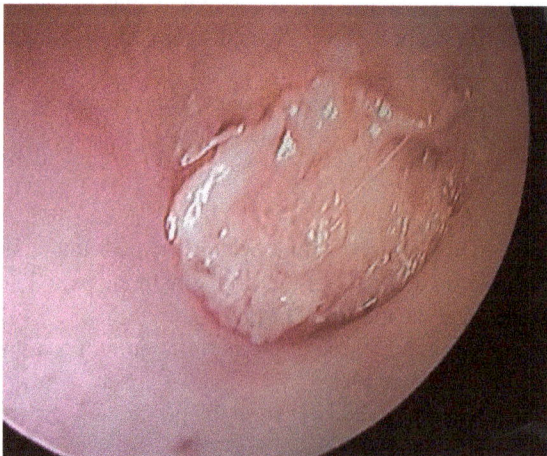

Figure 4. Perichondrium spread in overlay fashion and the cartilage proper placed as an underlay graft.

4. Results

The following table shows the hearing improvement 2 months post-operatively in our case series.

Sr. no.	Pre-operative hearing loss (db)	Post-operative hearing loss (db)	Difference	Deviation	Square of deviation
1.	45	30	−15	2.35	5.52
2.	45	25	−20	−2.65	7.02
3.	40	23	−17	0.35	0.12
4.	40	20	−20	−2.65	7.02
5.	40	20	−20	−2.65	7.02
6.	40	20	−20	−2.65	7.02
7.	40	20	−20	−2.65	7.02
8.	40	25	−15	2.35	5.52
9.	45	25	−20	−2.65	7.02
10.	35	20	−15	2.35	5.52
11.	40	25	−15	2.35	5.52
12.	40	25	−15	2.35	5.52
13.	40	25	−15	2.35	5.52
14.	40	20	−20	−2.65	7.02
15.	35	20	−15	2.35	5.52
16.	45	25	−20	−2.65	7.02
17.	40	20	−20	−2.65	7.02
18.	40	25	−15	2.35	5.52
19.	40	25	−15	2.35	5.52
20.	40	25	−15	2.35	5.52

Difference Scores Calculations: T-value calculation: $t = (M − \mu)/S_M = (−17.35 − 0)/0.56 = 31.06$; Mean: −17.35; $\mu = 0$; $S^2 = SS/df = 118.55/(20 − 1) = 6.24$; $S_M^2 = S^2/N = 6.24/20 = 0.31$; $S_M = \sqrt{S_M^2} = \sqrt{0.31} = 0.56$; The value of t is −31.062793. The value of p is <0.00001. The result is significant at $p \leq 0.05$.

5. Discussion

Tympanic membrane perforations significantly impair the quality of life for millions of patients [4].

Though temporalis fascia is the most commonly used graft material it should be noted that cartilage contributes minimally to an inflammatory tissue reaction and is well incorporated with tympanic membrane layers; it also provides firm support to prevent retraction. The main advantage of the cartilage graft has been thought to be its very low metabolic rate. It receives its nutrients by diffusion, is easy to work with because it is pliable, and it can resist deformation from pressure variations [5].

The perceived disadvantage of the cartilage graft is that it creates an opaque tympanic membrane, which could potentially hide a residual cholesteatoma [6].

Mirko Tos described 23 known cartilage tympanoplasty methods to reconstruct the eardrum and proposed a classification into six main groups [7]. The triple-c and the butterfly technique belong to group-F as per this classification.

Eavey was the first to describe the butterfly cartilage inlay grafting technique. The edges of the cartilage perichondrial composite graft curve out like butterfly wings when the edge is split [8]. Though an attractive technique there maybe problems with epithelisation of the graft and accumulation of keratin under the wing of the cartilage causing displacement of the graft similar to a grommet. In the triple-c technique we did not face such issues.

When partial thickness cartilage with perichondrium on the lateral aspect alone is fashioned, there is curling of the cartilage possibly due to the pull by the perichondrium, this can be addressed to a certain amount by the triple-c technique as here the perichondrium is raised all along the margins of the cartilage.

There is very limited data regarding curling of the cartilage, four incisions of the perichondrium "the anticurling incisions" have been described by Mirko Tos but a systematic study is still required to validate them.

Using a normal tympanic membrane as a reference, Zahnert et al. noted that a cartilage plate with a thickness of less than 0.5 mm gave the least acoustic transfer loss [9]. Though recent studies show no difference in hearing results between the full thickness and partial thickness grafts.

Also histomorphological studies of cartilage grafts (Hitari, 2006) have shown that there is wide replacement of the chondrocytes by fibrous tissue and loss of lipid vacuoles over time which makes the cartilage graft more homogenous in nature. This transfers the acoustic energy better than normal cartilage.

In 2004, Gierek et al. [10] performed 112 cases with cartilage and 30 cases with temporalis fascia. They observed that there was no significant hearing difference between the two groups. Couloinger et al. [11] observed 59 cartilage graft tympanoplasties and 20 temporalis fascia graft tympanoplasties in 2005 and they reported no postoperative hearing difference between the two groups.

Hence even though temporalis fascia is the current choice, cartilage grafts with minimally invasive techniques such as the triple-c technique may replace fascia for small to moderate sized non-marginal perforations.

Also in near future endoscopic approach for this technique will be in vogue. Otoendoscopy gives the surgeon a panoramic view and helps in visualization of many hidden areas of the middle ear [12], it may modify this novel technique even further.

6. Conclusions

In our experience the composite chondroperichondrial "clip" tympanoplasty using the tragal cartilage and transcanal approach has the following advantages:
- Minimally invasive
- Sutureless
- Reduced operative time
- Excellent hearing improvement
- Assurance of graft take-up
- Better patient compliance and reduced hospital stay

Though a highly efficacious technique, comparative studies between the triple-c and the butterfly technique are necessary. Also long term follow-up of cases managed with this technique and studies regarding the fate of cartilage graft would help us understand cartilage tympanoplasty in greater depths.

References

[1]   Glasscock, M.E. and Shambaugh, G.E. Surgery of the Ear 5th Edition Pathology and Clinical Course of Inflammatory Disease of the Middle Ear. Vol. 21, 428-429.

[2]   Fernandes, S.V. (2003) Composite Chondroperichondrial Clip Tympanoplasty: The Triple-C Technique. Otolaryngology—Head and Neck Surgery: Official Journal of American Academy of Otolaryngology-Head and Neck Surgery, 128, 267-267. http://dx.doi.org/10.1067/mhn.2003.88

[3]   Ahmed, S., Raza, N., Ullah, S. and Shabbir, A. (2013) Chondroperichondrial Clip Myringoplasty: A New Technique for Closure of Tympanic Membrane Perforations. The Journal of Laryngology & Otology, 127, 562-567. http://dx.doi.org/10.1017/S0022215113000595

[4]   Rahman, A. (2007) Healing of Tympanic Membrane Perforation: An Experimental Study. Karolinska Institute and University Hospital, Stockhole.

[5]   Yung, M. (2008) Cartilage Tympanoplasty: Literature Review. The Journal of Laryngology & Otology, 122, 663-672.

[6]   Ghanem, M.A., Monroy, A., Alizadeh, F.S., Nicolau, Y. and Eavey, R.D. (2006) Butterfly Cartilage Graft Inlay Tympanoplasty for Large Perforations. Laryngoscope, 116, 1813-1816. http://dx.doi.org/10.1097/01.mlg.0000231742.11048.ed

[7]   Tos, M. (2009) Cartilage Tympanoplasty: Classifications of Methods—Techniques—Results. Edition I, Thieme.

[8]   Eavey, R.D. (1998) Inlay Tympanoplasty: Cartilage Butterfly Technique. Laryngoscope, 108, 657-661. http://dx.doi.org/10.1097/00005537-199805000-00006

[9]   Zahnert, T., Huttenbrink, K.-B., Murbe, D. and Bornitz, M. (2000) Experimental Investigations of the Use of Cartilage in Tympanic Membrane Reconstruction. *American Journal of Otolaryngology*, **21**, 322-328.
http://dx.doi.org/10.1016/S0196-0709(00)80039-3

[10] Gierek, T., Slaska-Kaspera, A., Majzel, K. and Klimczak-Gotqb, L. (2004) Results of Myringoplasty and Type I Tympanoplasty with the Use of Fascia, Cartilage and Perichondrium Grafts. *Otolaryngologia Polska*, **3**, 529-533. (In Polish)

[11] Couloigner, V., Baculard, F., El Bakkouri, W., Viala, P., Francois, M., Narcy, P., *et al.* (2005) Inlay Butterfly Cartilage Tympanoplasty in Children. *Ontology Neurotology*, **26**, 247-251.
http://dx.doi.org/10.1097/00129492-200503000-00020

[12] Harugop, A.S., Mudhol, R.S. and Godhi, R.A. (2008) A Comparative Study of Endoscope Assisted Myringoplasty and Microscope Assisted Myringoplasty. *Indian Journal of Otolaryngology and Head Neck Surgery*, **60**, 299-302.
http://dx.doi.org/10.1007/s12070-008-0099-5

12

Transmucosal Bleomycin for Tongue Lymphatic Malformations

Eric W. Cerrati[1], Teresa M. O. March[2]*, David Binetter[2], Yelena Bernstein[2], Milton Waner[2]

[1]Department of Otolaryngology, New York University, New York, USA
[2]Vascular Birthmark Institute of New York, Lenox Hill and Manhattan Eye, Ear and Throat Hospitals, New York, USA
Email: *to@vbiny.org

Abstract

Purpose: Bleomycin is an antibiotic medication that inhibits the synthesis of DNA, RNA, and proteins and is now used in a variety of medical conditions including vascular anomalies. The aim of this study was to evaluate the clinical efficacy of transmucosal intralesional injection of bleomycin in the management of tongue lymphatic malformations. Method: A single institutional case series was presented on patients with recalcitrant lymphatic malformations of the tongue who were treated with bleomycin. Age at the time of injection, gender, number of treatments, amount of bleomycin injected per session, post-injection complications, pre- and post-injection symptoms, and anatomic extent of the lymphatic malformation were all recorded and analyzed. Results: Five patients received transmucosal bleomycin and were followed over a 10-month period. The patients included 4 females and 1 male, aged from 3.25 to 36 years (average 13.52 years). Four patients had one treatment while 1 required two treatments. A total of 1 to 6 units were injected per session. Overall reduction in size of the lymphatic malformation and improvement in all symptoms were observed in the patients by day 14. Average follow-up was 9 to 12 months. Conclusion: Intralesional injection of bleomycin is an effective treatment modality in patients with lymphatic malformations of the tongue.

Keywords

Bleomycin, Sclerotherapy, Lymphatic Malformation, Tongue

1. Introduction

Vascular malformations manifest as either high-flow lesions (arteriovenous malformations and fistulae) or low-

---
*Corresponding author.

flow lesions (venous, lymphatic, capillary, or mixed malformations) [1]-[3]. Lymphatic malformations (LMs) are composed of dilated lymphatic vessels with inappropriate drainage patterns and are lined with endothelial cells. They are estimated to occur in 0.5% of the general population and commonly result in a painless focal mass (macrocystic) or diffuse tissue swelling or overgrowth (microcystic) [2]. While these lesions can occur anywhere on the body, they show a predilection for the cervicofacial region and from a recent review of the anatomic distribution of airway LMs, the most common locations are the oral cavity (75%), oropharynx (35%), and the parapharyngeal space (30%) [4]. LMs involving the tongue tend to be microcystic and poorly defined giving the characteristic granular appearance over the lingual dorsum. Treatment for lymphatic malformations of the tongue is guided by the degree of involvement and the condition of the surrounding structures. Grading systems have been proposed to help standardize treatment; however, these have not been universally accepted. In general, isolated superficial LMs or those confined to only a portion of the tongue allow surgical resection to be an effective treatment. For more advanced LMs, surgical resection alone is inadequate and is often performed in conjunction with other modalities such as laser therapy, radiofrequency ablation, and sclerotherapy.

Currently in non-oral cavity LMs, direct puncture sclerotherapy is used both as an adjunct and as an alternative to surgery [1] [2]. The sclerosants are injected directly into the malformation, causing endothelial damage, inflammation, thrombosis, fibrosis, and eventual destruction of the lesion. The advantages of sclerotherapy include rapid recovery, no incisions, and a low risk of nerve injury and infection [1]. Several different sclerosants have been described in the treatment of LMs. Of these, the most common are sodium tetradecyl sulfate (STS), OK-432, and doxycline [2]. Unfortunately, most of the sclerosants described in the literature produce a significant amount of postoperative swelling limiting their use when treating airway LMs [1] [2].

Bleomycin, an antibiotic with cytotoxic antitumor properties via the inhibition of DNA, RNA, and protein synthesis, has been used in a variety of medical conditions including in a role as a sclerosant. It is favored by some clinicians because of its clinical efficacy combined with a low incidence of significant postoperative edema [5]-[7]. Bleomycin's use has yet to be applied to oral cavity lymphatic malformations.

2. Case Report

A case series of 5 patients with lymphatic malformations of the oral tongue treated with transmucosal bleomycin sclerotherapy between June 2013 and March 2014 is presented. The target lesions were identified preoperatively with computed tomography (CT) and magnetic resonance imaging (MRI). The following inclusion criteria were met by all of the patients: presence of an extensive lymphatic malformation involving the majority (>75%) of the anterior tongue; prior treatment consisting of partial CO_2 laser ablations; recalcitrant disease with chronic hemorrhagic vesicles, malodor, pain, and swelling; and pre- and post-operative photographs for assessment and comparison. The outcome measures were overall tongue size, number of vesicles, presence of leakage from the vesicles and interval time between treatments.

If and when these patients developed lymphangitis or acute inflammation involving the malformation, treatment consisted of high dose corticosteroids and antibiotics. We recorded the age at the time of the injection, gender, number of treatments, amount of bleomycin injected per session (0.5 mg/kg was the maximum dose per session), postinjection complications, pre-/post-injection symptoms and anatomic extent of the LM.

All procedures were performed in the operating room under general anesthesia. A Denhardt mouth gag was used to provide adequate exposure along either a towel clamp on the distal tongue or a Weider retractor to hold the tongue to one side. A 1-cc syringe with a 25-gauge needle was used. The total amount of bleomycin available per session was 0.5 mg per kilogram with a maximum of 15 mg per session. The needle was advanced across the region of the malformation and filled the malformation with the sclerosant in a retrograde fashion while gradually withdrawing the needle.

The five patients were followed for a period of 9 to 12 months (mean of 10.8) and consisted of four females and one male with ages ranging from 3.25 to 36 years (average 13.52 years). Four of the patients required only one treatment while one required a total of two. A total of 1 to 6 units were injected per session, depending on the patient's weight (**Table 1**).

All of the patients developed early reactive swelling; however, no airway interventions were necessary. Due to this finding, the injections were limited to the anterior 1/2 - 2/3 of the tongue. In 2 patients, oral corticosteroids were prescribed after 3 - 4 days as the pain from the swelling was affecting their oral intake. At the two-week follow-up appointment, the swelling was noted to be completely resolved and the overall size of the

Table 1. Patient data.

Patient (age in years, gender)	Location of LM	# of treatments	Bleomycin amount (units)
36F	Anterior tongue, floor of mouth	1	6.0
3M	Anterior tongue, floor of mouth	1	1.8
7M	Anterior tongue	1	1.7
9F	Anterior tongue	2	6.0
10F	Anterior tongue	1	1.0

tongue was reduced. At the end of the follow-up, the patients reported an overall reduction in tongue size, decreased number of vesicles and increased length of interval time between treatments. The patients also reported an improvement in their quality of life given the effectiveness their improvement in speech and reduction/elimination of hemorrhage, malodor, pain, and swelling.

3. Discussion

The treatment for extensive lymphatic malformations of the tongue involves any combination of sclerotherapy, laser therapy, and surgery. Unfortunately, there is no conclusive evidence demonstrating which sclerosant is the best. So far in the literature and with our experience, Bleomycin is the ideal sclerosant for airway lesions because of its effectiveness along with its minimal postoperative swelling [1].

The other sclerotherapy agents such as STS, doxycycline, ethanol and OK-432 have shown varying degrees of effectiveness with significant risk factors. For example, ethanol, though inexpensive and very effective, is associated with nerve injury, skin necrosis and systemic effects such as cardiopulmonary collapse. OK-432, an agent once described as being the most widely used sclerosant for LMs, reported a regression of disease in 96% of patients. Its side effects include swelling, erythema, pain and a low-grade fever for up to 5 days post-injection [2]. Doxycycline has been shown to result in an 83% mean reduction in lesion size and is deemed more effective in treating microcystic LMs than OK-432. Again, its side effects include pain and significant swelling, which limits its application in airway lesions [3].

Bleomycin was first introduced as a sclerosant in 1977 by Yura *et al*. It is an antibiotic with cytotoxic antitumoral properties [6]. The agent's low tendency to induce post-injection swelling makes it a preferred sclerosant for airway lesions, especially in patients without tracheotomy at the time of intervention [1] [6] [7]. Our experience has demonstrated a reactive swelling when used specifically in the tongue, which has limited our application of bleomycin to the anterior tongue. This swelling, which was not observed in the supraglottic area specifically, may be secondary to the increased lymphatics and vasculature of the tongue itself [1]. The most worrisome side effect of bleomycin is pulmonary fibrosis. While this complication been documented in the oncology literature as a dose-dependent response to those who receive the drug systemically, it has never been reported in reference to its use as a sclerosant [8] [9]. The cumulative dose that is associated with the increased risk of pulmonary fibrosis is 450 mg [1]. When used in sclerotherapy, not only is bleomycin not absorbed into the bloodstream but the maximum amount per session is only 15 mg (0.5 mg/kg/session), making it extremely unlikely to even approach the high cumulative dose of 450 mg [1] [9].

The more common side effect is hyperpigmentation, which is reported to occur in 8% - 38% of patients. This finding does not seem to be dose dependent as it has been reported to occur with doses as low as 5 mg. The mechanism of action is unknown; however, histologic studies have shown that bleomycin reduces the epidermal turnover resulting in a prolonged contact between melanocytes and keratinocytes [10]. Local skin irritation after bleomycin results in hyperemia and increased concentration of bleomycin to the area. We, therefore, take the following measures in an effort to reduce the risk of hyperpigmentation: leave all tape including that placed around intravenous lines and EKG leads on the patient until after 72 hours, and advise against scratching the skin. Fortunately, the hyperpigmentation is usually reversible with cessation of the drug but can take up to 6 months to resolve.

Although our case series has only 5 patients, bleomycin has shown promising results in the oral tongue. Once the cohort of patients is increased and the results can be collected on an objective scale, a direct comparison can be made of the different (**Figure 1** and **Figure 2**) treatments such as other sclerosants. Bleomycin has been

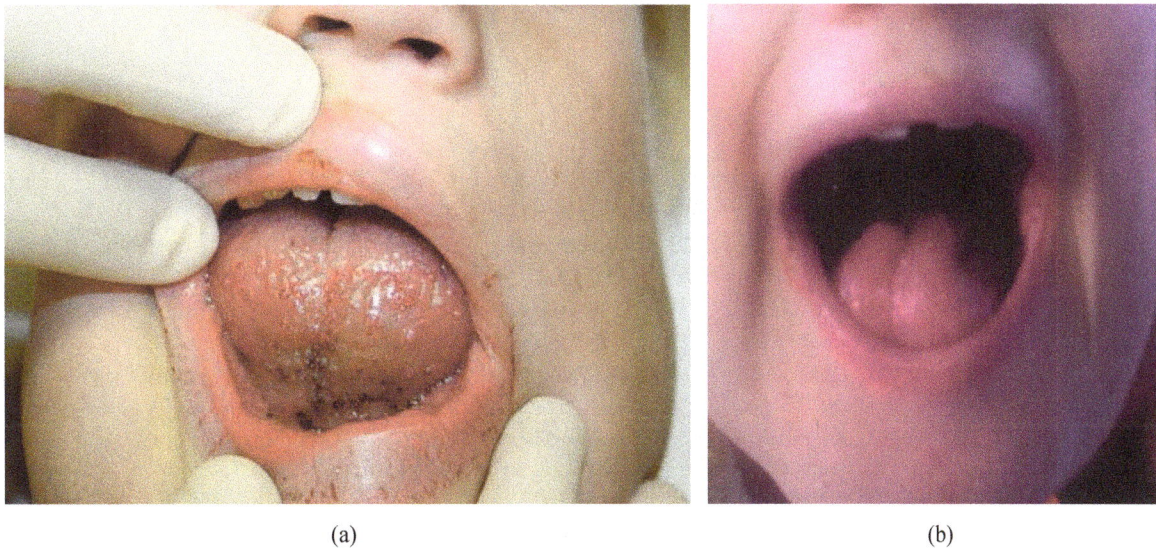

Figure 1. 10-year-old male with a persistently enlarged tongue despite multiple resections (a); One unit of bleomycin was injected and the follow-up photo was taken 4.5 months later (b).

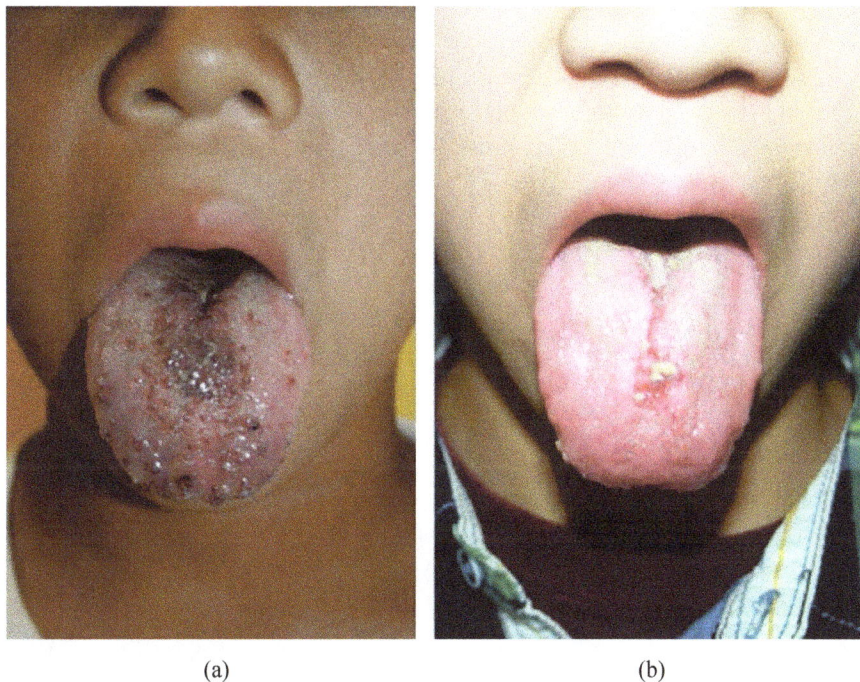

Figure 2. 7-year-old male demonstrating the classic changes of the tongue after a bleomycin injection (a); At the routine follow-up, the tongue size is reduced and the mucosa has returned to the usual appearance (b).

extremely effective in treating laryngeal LMs and this new application in the tongue will likely be equally successful.

4. Conclusion

Intralesional injection of bleomycin is an effective modality of treatment for patients with lymphatic malformations of the tongue. Bleomycin is shown to be an effective sclerosant with a low risk profile. All of the patients in this series were extremely satisfied with the results and no complications or side effects of bleomycin were reported.

Conflict of Interest

None.

References

[1]   Oomen, K.P., Paramasivam, S., Waner, M., *et al.* Endoscopic Transmucosal Direct Puncture Sclerotherapy for Management of Airway Vascular Malformations. Pending Publication.

[2]   Gurgacz, S., Zamora, L. and Scott, A. (2014) Percutaneous Sclerotherapy for Vascular Malformations: A Systemic Review. *Annals of Vascular Surgery*, **28**, 1335-1349. http://dx.doi.org/10.1016/j.avsg.2014.01.008

[3]   Burrows, P.E., Mitri, R.K., Alomari, A., *et al.* (2008) Percutaneous Sclerotherapy of Lymphatic Malformations with Doxycycline. *Lymphatic Research and Biology*, **6**, 209-216. http://dx.doi.org/10.1089/lrb.2008.1004

[4]   O, T.M., Rickert, S.M., Diallo, A.M., *et al.* (2013) Lymphatic Malformations of the Airway. *Otolaryngology—Head and Neck Surgery*, **149**, 156-160. http://dx.doi.org/10.1177/0194599813485065

[5]   Wiegand, S., Eivazi, B., Zimmermann, A., *et al.* (2009) Microcystic Lymphatic Malformations of the Tongue: Diagnosis, Classification, and Treatment. *Archives of Otolaryngology—Head and Neck Surgery*, **135**, 976-983. http://dx.doi.org/10.1001/archoto.2009.131

[6]   Bai, Y., Jia, J., Huang, X.X., *et al.* (2009) Sclerotherapy of Microcystic Lymphatic Malformations in Oral and Facial Regions. *Journal of Oral and Maxillofacial Surgery*, **67**, 251-256. http://dx.doi.org/10.1016/j.joms.2008.06.046

[7]   Mathur, N.N., Rana, I., Bothra, R., *et al.* (2005) Bleomycin Sclerotherapy in Congenital Lymphatic and Vascular Malformations of Head and Neck. *International Journal of Pediatric Otorhinolaryngology*, **69**, 75-80. http://dx.doi.org/10.1016/j.ijporl.2004.08.008

[8]   Jules-Elysee, K. and White, D.A. (1990) Bleomycin-Induced Pulmonary Toxicity. *Clinics in Chest Medicine*, **11**, 1-20.

[9]   Ionescu, G., Mabeta, P., Dippenaar, N., *et al.* (2008) Bleomycin Plasma Spill-Over Levels in Pediatric Patients Undergoing Intralesional Injection for the Treatment of Hemangiomas. *South African Medical Journal*, **98**, 539-540.

[10] Khenaizan, S. and Al-Berouti, B. (2011) Flagellate Pigmentation: A Unique Adverse Side Effect of Bleomycin Therapy. *European Journal of Dermatology*, **21**, 146.

13

A Rare Case of Nasal Glial Heterotopia Presenting as Sphenochoanal Polyp*

Pavol Surda, Jonathan Hobson

Ear, Nose and Throat Department, Warrington and Halton Hospitals, Warrington, UK
Email: pavol.surda@gmail.com

Abstract

Objective: This paper reports a rare case of nasal glial heterotopia presenting as sphenochoanal polyp. So far, literature has revealed only few cases. Case Report: A 55-year-old woman presented with a 2-month history of left sided nasal obstruction. Rigid endoscopy showed greyish left nasal polyp and anterior discharge. Subsequently, CT scan of the sinuses revealed sphenochoanal polyp filling the left nasal cavity, without signs of expansion, or destruction and no obvious connection with intracranial tissue. Mass was removed endoscopically and histology confirmed glial nature of the mass. Conclusion: Any mass arising from sphenoid sinus should be carefully evaluated on CT scan for existence of fibrous stalk, or connection with brain tissue and needs to be considered in the differential diagnosis of the sphenochoanal mass. Complete surgical excision is the treatment of choice, which is curative.

Keywords

Heterotopic Glial Heterotopia, Sphenoid Sinus, Nasal Cavity, Sphenochoanal Polyp

1. Introduction

Nasal Glial Heterotopias (NGH) are congenital tumours of the midline frontonasal space arising from a normal neurectodermal tissue entrapped during the closure of the anterior neuropore. NGH, or differentiated neural tissue outside the cranial vault is uncommon, and these anomalies most commonly occur in the nasal cavity [1] [2]. However, heterotopic brain tissue has also less commonly been reported to occur in other sites, such as the pharynx, lung, orbits, palate, tongue, cheek, lip, and neck [3]. The reported incidence is 1 in every 20,000 to 40,000 births. The most common congenital nasal masses are nasal dermal sinus cysts, nasal encephaloceles, and NGH. These masses appear to share a similar embryogenic origin. They occur when the neuroectodermal and ecto-

---

*The paper was presented as poster at the congress of European Rhinologic Society in Amsterdam 2015.

dermal tissues fail to separate during the development of the nose. NGH might link the intracranial dura mater through the foramen cecum and evidence of this connection is observed in about 15% of histopathological studies and referred as a "fibrous stalk" [4].

The extranasal form (60%) is superficially located, and expands into the subcutaneous space [4]. Intranasal NGH, the topic in this case report, account for 30% of all NGH seen at birth and are frequently revealed by respiratory distress in the early life. Majority of intranasal form involves the cribriform plate. NGH presenting as sphenochoanal mass are rare. Mixed form (10%) associates both extranasal and intranasal extensions [5].

Histologically, they are composed of astrocytes and neuroglial fibers intermixed with a fibrovascular connective tissue stroma. Occasionally, rare neurons and/or ependymal cystic structures may be present as well. These cells were S-100 protein and glial fibrillary acid protein (GFAP) positive, confirming their glial nature [6].

Unilateral lesion occupying sphenoid sinus is uncommon. Etiology may be inflammatory (including chronic invasive fungal sinusitis), a benign neoplasm (e.g. inverted papilloma, hemangioma, angiofibroma), malignant neoplasm, congenital tumor (encephalocele), an internal carotid artery aneurysm, a pituitary adenoma or an ectopic pituitary [7].

CT and MR imaging are useful in the evaluation of masses involving the skull base. CT provides information about the adjacent osseous structures while MR imaging, because of its improved soft-tissue resolution, helps to characterize the soft-tissue abnormality. Angiofibromas and hemangiomas are vascular tumors that enhance avidly after contrast administration and may show an abundance of flow voids on MR images. Nasopharyngeal carcinoma involving sphenoid sinus will show replacement of fat in this location and, if extensive, may result in expansion of the sinus.

Complete surgical excision is the treatment of choice. In the early management of NG, bifrontal craniotomy has been recommended [5] [8]. Improvements in technology, surgical technique, and medical environment result in introducing a single staged endoscopic endonasal procedure in the treatment of NGH [9].

The objective of this paper is to raise awareness of this rare congenital tumour, which should take part in differential diagnosis of all unilateral solitary sphenoidal lesions.

2. Case Report

We report the case of 55-year-old woman with Turner's syndrome, who presented with left sided sphenochoanal polyp causing nasal obstruction over 2 months. There has been an associated mucoid discharge, but no epistaxis, facial pain and cranial nerves were intact. Physical examination revealed a greyish nasal polyp and anterior discharge. There was no history of hoarseness, dysphagia, dyspnea, fever, weight loss, or any systemic or local complaints. Besides Turner's syndrome, the patient experienced common childhood diseases, diabetes II type and hypertension. She was never hospitalized before due to these minor ailments nor had she undergone any kind of surgeries. There was no relevant past allergy or drug history. Family history was negative. The results of complete blood count, white blood cell count, serum biochemistry and chest X-ray were normal. CT scan of the sinuses revealed sphenochoanal polyp filling left nasal cavity, without signs of expansion, or destruction (**Figure 1**). The osteomeatal complex was normal.

Patient underwent endoscopic endonasal removal of the polyp. Under general anesthesia we first examined nasal cavity. We identified greyish nasal polyp in left middle meatus arising from sphenoid sinus. There were no signs of abnormal mass pulsatility. Polypectomy was then progressively achieved with help of microdebrider and meticulous bipolar haemostasis to keep the operative field free of bleeding. We firstly removed the nasal portion and subsequently opened sphenoid sinus and completely removed the rest of the polyp. A fibrous stalk wasn't identified and there was no perioperative CSF leak. The histology of this polyp was confirmed following immuno-staining as containing heterotopic glial tissue (**Figure 2**).

At the post-op review, patient mentioned one episode of clear fluid leaking from her left nostril, which made impression of CSF leak. On examination with 30 degree rigid nasendoscopy the sphenoidotomy was nice and clear, there was no obvious fluid leakage or pooling and no recurrence of her polyps. Postoperative CT scan revealed a defect in the inferomedial aspect of the left temporal fossa communicating with the left sphenoid sinus and positive beta-2 transferrin test. Subsequently, we referred patient for further surgical CSF leak management to ENT department in Crewe Hospital, which was successfully achieved. In the 10 months follow-up period patient remained disease free with no signs of CSF leak.

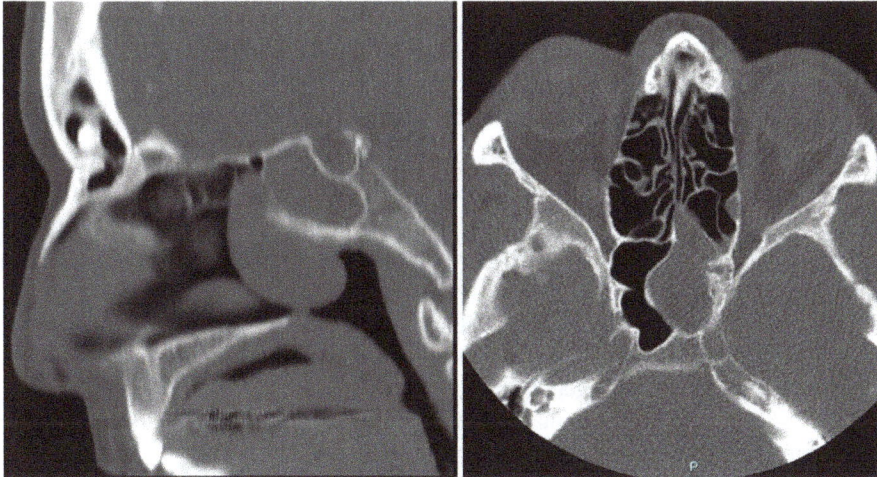

Figure 1. A 55-year-old woman with NGH in the sphenoid sinus: Axial and Sagittal CT scan shows a well-demarcated soft-tissue mass, which is extending into nasal cavity/post-nasal space.

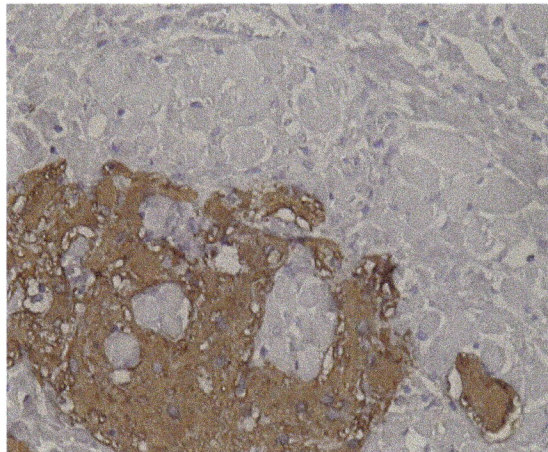

Figure 2. Immunohistochemical detection of glial fibrillary acidic protein.

3. Discussion

NGH of the spehonoidal sinus is a rare disease. The biggest challenge in the diagnostic process is the differentiation between encephalocele, which typically presents with marked connection between the mass and the intracranial tissue. However, NGH might link the intracranial dura mater through the foramen cecum. Evidence of this connection is observed in about 15% while still showing no communication with the brain parenchyma. Histopathological studies refer this connection as a "fibrous stalk". Clinically encephaloceles might present preoperatively with meningitis.

NGH are on T1-weighted images hypointense to isointense to gray matter. On T2-weighted images, T2 hyperintensity caused by gliosis is often observed within the mass. Dysplastic tissue does not typically enhance. The two entities may be distinguished from one another in that encephaloceles usually retain a visible connection with the brain [10] [11]. Rahbar *et al.*, discussed this pathological finding, emphasizing difficulties in diagnosis, and concluded that gliomas should be distinguished from encephalocele only after clinicopathological correlation [12]. CT is useful for identifying small bone defects at the skull base, whereas MR imaging, with its multiplanar capabilities, is excellent for identifying communication with the adjacent brain.

Histologically, NGH and encephaloceles are characterized by varying proportions of neurons and glia, with three cases also showing gemistocytic astrocytes. There are varying degrees of fibrosis, frequently associated with inflammation (40% of cases). Calcifications and ependymal-type cystic degeneration was also occasionally seen. Mason's trichrome stain combined with S-100 protein and glial fibrillary acidic protein can be most help-ful in accentuating the neural tissue in the background fibrosis. Neuron specific enolase may be used if the other stains fail. It should be noted that there are no significant histologic differences between lesions with and with-out demonstrable CNS connection. Therefore, the accurate diagnosis of heterotopia versus encephalocele re-quires knowledge of the patient's radiographic and/or operative findings [6].

4. Conclusions

- Any mass arising from sphenoid sinus should be carefully evaluated on CT scan for existence of fibrous stalk, or connection with brain tissue.
- The diagnosis is usually uncertain until the final pathological report.
- Surgeons have to always perioperatively examine sphenoid sinus for any signs of CSF leak. CSF leak may be closed endoscopically in the first stage, or in the second stage in case of small defect.
- If the diagnosis of NGH was confirmed and there was no evident perioperative CSF leak, during the follow-up we should perform regular nasal endoscopy of sphenoid sinus.
- If CSF leak is not clearly present, we can measure beta-trace and beta-2 transferrin present in nasal fluid/blood. If CSF leak is not clear, intrathecal fluorescein is very helpful.
- Incidence of perioperative CSF leak is 66% [9].

Conflict of Interest

We have got no conflicts of interest to disclose.

References

[1]   Ducic, Y. (1999) Nasal Gliomas. *Journal of Otolaryngology*, **28**, 285-287.

[2]   Uemura, T., Yoshikawa, A., Onizuka, T. and Hayashi, T. (1999) Heterotopic Nasopharyngeal Brain Tissue Associated with Cleft Palate. *Cleft Palate-Craniofacial Journal*, **36**, 248-251.
       http://dx.doi.org/10.1597/1545-1569(1999)036<0248:HNBTAW>2.3.CO;2

[3]   Hendrickson, M., Faye-Petersen, O. and Johnson, D.G. (1990) Cystic and Solid Heterotopic Brain in the Face and Neck: A Review and Report of an Unusual Case. *Journal of Pediatric Surgery*, **25**, 766-768.
       http://dx.doi.org/10.1016/S0022-3468(05)80015-6

[4]   Thomson, H.G., Al-Qattan, M.M. and Becker, L.E. (1995) Nasal Glioma: Is Dermis Involvement Significant? *Annals of Plastic Surgery*, **34**, 168-172. http://dx.doi.org/10.1097/00000637-199502000-00009

[5]   Walker Jr., E.A. and Resler, D.R. (1963) Nasal Glioma. *Laryngoscope*, **73**, 93-107.
       http://dx.doi.org/10.1288/00005537-196301000-00008

[6]   Penner, C.R. and Thompson, L. (2003) Nasal Glial Heterotopia: A Clinicopathologic and Immunophenotypic Analysis of 10 Cases with a Review of the Literature. *Annals of Diagnostic Pathology*, **7**, 354-359.
       http://dx.doi.org/10.1016/j.anndiagpath.2003.09.010

[7]   Sethi, D.S., Lau, D.P.C., Linchon, W.J. and Chong, V. (1998) Isolated Sphenoethmoid Recess Polyps. *Journal of La-ryngology Otology*, **112**, 660-663. http://dx.doi.org/10.1017/S0022215100141386

[8]   Hughes, G.B., Sharpino, G., Hunt, W. and Tucker, H.M. (1980) Management of the Congenital Midline Nasal Mass: A Review. *Head and Neck Surgery*, **2**, 222-233. http://dx.doi.org/10.1002/hed.2890020308

[9]   Bonne, N.X., Zago, S., Hosana, G., Vinchon, M., Van den Abbeele, T. and Fayoux, P. (2012) Endonasal Endoscopic Approach for Removal of Intranasal Nasal Glial Heterotopias. *Rhinology*, **50**, 211-217.

[10]   Fuse, T., Aoyagi, M., Ota, N., Koike, Y. and Yuda, F. (1992) Heterotopic Brain Tissue of the Soft Palate. *ORL Journal for Oto-Rhino-Laryngology and Its Related Specialties*, **54**, 54-56. http://dx.doi.org/10.1159/000276260

[11]   Grossman, R.I. and Yousem, D. (1994) Neuroradiology: The Requisites. Mosby, St. Louis.

[12]   Rahbar, R., Resto, V.A. and Robson, C.D. (2003) Nasal Glioma and Encephalocele: Diagnosis and Management. *La-ryngoscope*, **113**, 2069-2077. http://dx.doi.org/10.1097/00005537-200312000-00003

14

Atypical Gunshot Injury to the Ear: A Case Report

Sai Spoorthi Nayak, Ehrlson De Sousa, Saumyata Neeraj

Department of ENT, Goa Medical College, Goa, India
Email: Saumyata16@gmail.com

Abstract

Bullet injuries to head and neck are usually associated with high mortality and morbidity due to a number of vital structures lying in close proximity. We present a rare case of air-gun injury with an unusual entry wound. The pellet having a simple trajectory was lodged into middle ear avoiding all important structures.

Keywords

Bullet, Perforated Tympanic Membrane, Metallic Foreign Body

1. Introduction

Bullet injuries are a very rare occurrence in a peace loving state as ours. Civilian firearms in Goa are either accidental or suicidal and very rarely homicidal. Penetrating injuries to the middle ear are usually caused by ear buds, Q-tips, pencils, hairpins, etc., which have very localized injury and predictable path. However, penetrating bullet injury to the ear with virtually no entry wound is in itself a rare occurrence. A very unique case of penetrating bullet injury came walking to our casualty with as minimal damage to the ear as one could possibly imagine.

In the event of any trauma to face, our innate sense of protection is directed towards the eyes and face. We instinctively turn away from any approaching insult exposing one of our ears to projectiles, blows, blasts, etc. The pinna and temporal bone encase and deflect injury from deeper middle ear and inner ear structures. But once the pinna and external auditory canal are by passed, the fragile tympanic membrane and subsequently the middle ear are readily damaged.

2. Case Report

A 23 years old male presented to our casualty with history of accidental gun-shot to the right ear by an unknown person. The patient presented with earache and bleeding from right ear and sudden conductive hearing loss of around 40 dB (**Figure 1**).

On examination, there was only a minor abrasion on the right pinna in the cymba concha with pooling of blood in external auditory canal; obscuring the view of tympanic membrane. However no entry wound was visible. Facial nerve functions were normal.

HRCT temporal bone revealed multiple artefacts with streaking in the external auditory canal and middle ear going upto the Eustachian tube. The ossicles appeared intact. The facial nerve canal, inner ear and carotid canal were spared (**Figure 2** and **Figure 3**).

The patient was taken up for exploratory tympanotomy under local anaesthesia. Examination under microscope revealed traumatic perforation of the tympanic membrane through which the bullet was seen lodged in the middle ear. The skin of the external auditory canal was avulsed. Bullet fragments were seen to be lodged in the roof of external auditory canal. Mucosa of the middle ear was also found to be avulsed. The entire bullet was found to be in the anterior mesotympanum with no damage to the ossicles whatsoever (**Figure 4**).

The bullet fragments were removed and the tympanic membrane was reconstructed using the patient's own temporalis fascia.

The patient was hospitalized for about a week for intravenous antibiotics and discharged on 7th post-operative day after suture removal. He was followed up every week for 3 months. Post-operative hearing documented on audiogram on 3rd post-operative month was recorded as normal (**Figure 5**).

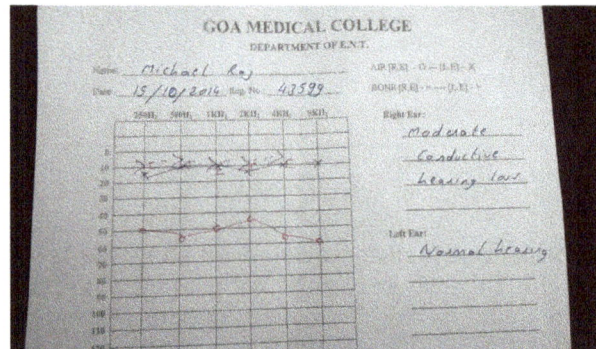

Figure 1. Pure tone audiometry (preoperative findings).

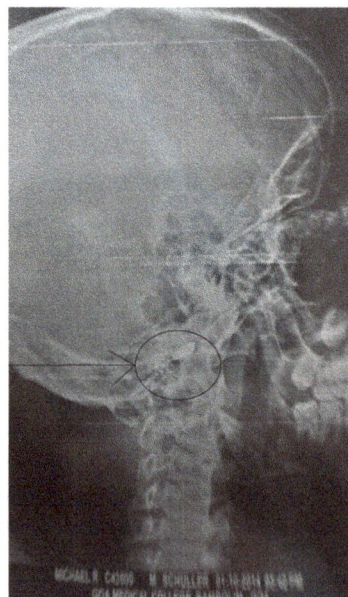

Figure 2. X-ray mastoid showing foreign body anterior to external acoustic meatus.

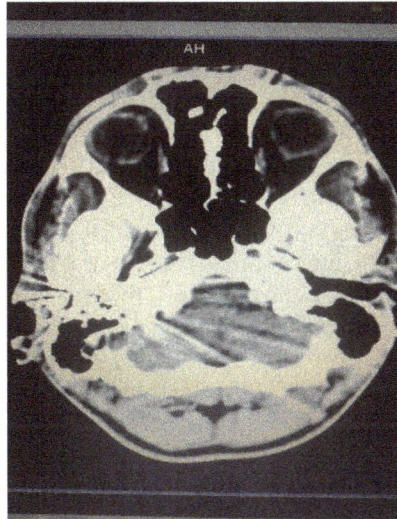

Figure 3. HRCT temporal bone showing multiple artefacts with streaking in the external auditory canal and middle ear.

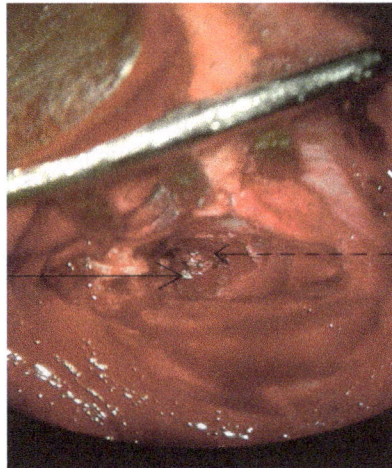

Figure 4. Showing metallic foreign body (bullet) in middle ear through ruptured tympanic membrane following posterior meatotomy. Dotted arrow showing ruptured tympanic membrane and solid arrow showing metallic foreign body (bullet).

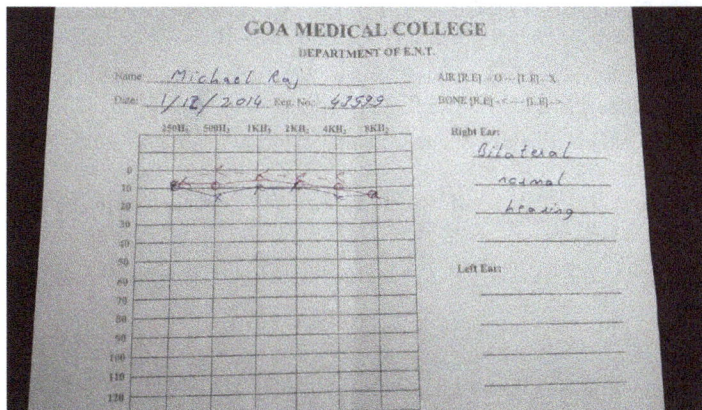

Figure 5. Pure tone audiometry (post operative findings).

3. Discussion

Bullet wound could be ricocheting shots or grazing ones. While some shots leave bullets lodged in the body, others have an exit wound. The location of an entrance wound and the projectile path are the most important factors in causing significant injury or death following shooting [1]. The extent of tissue damage is influenced by the type of bullet, its velocity and mass as well as the physical characteristics of tissues [2]. Gun-shot injuries are characterized by irregular path as well as localised destruction of bones and tissues [1].

Penetrating injuries to the middle ear could be due to misguided cotton tip, hairpin, key or pencil/pen. Blast injuries are also counted under penetrating injuries. However penetrating bullet injuries through the external auditory canal are considered among the rarest of the rare cases. Injuries caused by the afore mentioned objects are usually localized and often have a predictable path as compared to the bullet injuries which don't [3].

Handguns and shotguns are generally low velocity (<1000 frequency/second), unless fired at close range. Rifles usually project high velocity missiles (>2000 frequency/second). Skin is penetrated by a projectile at the rate about 163 frequency/second while bone requires 213 frequency/second to fracture [3]. The bullet which was found in our case measured 0.177 caliber (4.5 mm).

Whatever the case, the presentation is almost similar viz-pain, conductive hearing loss, sensorineural hearing loss, vertigo, tinnitus, rarely dysguesia/facial palsy. Delayed effects like infections, otorrhoea and tertiary cholesteatoma may also result [3].

Upto 88% of traumatic tympanic membrane perforations heal spontaneously within 3 - 10 months. The rate of spontaneous healing is inversely proportional to the size of perforation. Perforations that do not heal spontaneously within this time may require tympanoplasty to reduce the risk of chronic infection or cholesteatoma. In Kronenburg and colleagues series, the risk of post injury cholesteatoma was limited to patients whose perforation did not heal in 10 months [4].

Our main objective in the particular case was to remove the foreign body, reconstruct the middle ear, achieve fairly normal hearing and prevent tertiary choleasteatoma formation.

In this particular case, as the bullet entered through the external auditory canal and was lodged in the middle ear extra complications of bullet path and cavity did not come into play. The fragile tympanic membrane was damaged. This being a low velocity missile, the bullet had lost a significant amount of velocity by the time it entered the middle ear. The firing range is assumed to be long as the patient claimed to have not seen the assailant. Even though the patient's hearing returned back to normal, the patient has to be followed up indefinitely for the fear of cholesteatoma formation.

4. Conclusion

Penetrating bullet injury to the ear with virtually no entry wound is a rare occurrence. Even though we removed the foreign body and achieved an intact ear drum and a normal hearing post operatively, the patient has to be followed up indefinitely for the fear of tertiary cholesteatoma formation.

References

[1]   Reiss, M., Reiss, G. and Pilling, E. (1998) Gunshot Injuries in Head and Neck Area. Basic Principles, Diagnosis and Management. *Schweizerische Rundschav fur Medizin Praxis*, **87**, 832-838.

[2]   Maiden, N. (2009) Ballistics Review: Mechanisms of Bullet Wound Trauma. *Forensic Science, Medicine, and Pathology*, **5**, 204-209. http://dx.doi.org/10.1007/s12024-009-9096-6

[3]   Willings, D.B. and Pacher, M.D.N. (2009) Trauma to Middle Ear, Inner Ear and Temporal Bone. Ballingers Otorhinolaryngology. *Head and Neck Surgery*, **1**.

[4]   Kronenberg, J., Ben-Shoshan, J. and Wolf, M. (1993) Perforated Tympanic Membrane after Blast Injury. *American Journal of Otolaryngology*, **14**, 92-94.

15

Head and Neck Primary Mucosal Melanoma: Report of 17 Cases

Btissaam Belhoucha[1], Zahra Essaadi[2], Youssef Rochdi[1], Hassan Nouri[1], Lahcen Aderdour[1], Mona Khouchani[2], Abdelaziz Raji[1]

[1]Department of ENT, CHU Med VI, Marrakech, Morocco
[2]Department of Oncology and Radiotherapy, CHU Med VI, Marrakech, Morocco
Email: btissambelhoucha@gmail.com

Abstract

Introduction: Mucosal melanoma (MM) is a rare disease, accounting for 1.7% - 3% of all melanomas and 8% of all head and neck melanomas. It's a rare cancer with a very poor prognosis. Materials and Methods: We retrospectively reviewed the records of 17 patients with primary mucosal melanomas of the head and neck who were diagnosed between January 2007 and December 2012. Results: Our patient population included 9 women and 8 men. The age ranged from 61 to 75 years. The primary site of disease was in the sinonasal cavity for 12 patients (70%) and oral cavity for 5 patients. Treatment modalities for mucosal melanoma include surgical resection with or without neck dissection, immunochemotherapy, and radiation therapy (RT). 15 patients had attempted curative resections. Two patients received palliative radiation therapy as the primary treatment and chemotherapy as the adjuvant treatment. Discussion: Primary mucosal melanoma is a rare cancer and represents only 1.7% - 3% of all primary melanomas [1]-[3]. Mucosal melanoma must always be considered for multimodality therapy: surgical excision, medical oncology, and radiation therapy. Despite its radioresistant nature of tumor, the role of radiation therapy following surgical intervention has typically been advocated.

Keywords

Malignant Melanoma, Oral Mucosa, Sinonasal Cavity, Radiation Therapy, Prognosis

1. Introduction

Mucosal melanoma is a rare disease, accounting for 1.7% - 3% of all melanomas and 8% of all head and neck melanomas. It's a rare cancer with a very poor prognosis. Oral mucosal melanoma typically presents earlier than sinonasal mucosal melanoma. Head and neck melanoma also tends to affect a slightly older aged group than melanomas in other sites; it includes a mean age of 60 - 69 years and equal male/female preponderance. It involves in decreasing order of frequency, the sinonasal cavity (50%), oral cavity (45%), and other sites (5%) such as pharynx, larynx, and upper esophagus [1] [4] [5].

There is typically decreased nodal metastasis in comparison to cutaneous melanoma. The prognosis for a patient with mucosal melanoma is dismal, with a 5-year survival rate of 5% to 17% [1] [4] [5]. The purpose of this article is to discuss the optimal treatment and outcomes for head and neck mucosal melanoma.

2. Materiels and Methods

We retrospectively reviewed the records of 17 patients with primary mucosal melanomas of the head and neck who were diagnosed and prospectively followed up at the department of ENT surgery and the department of oncology between January 2007 and December 2012. We have exclude from the study Patients with cutaneous melanomas, including cutaneous melanomas encroaching on the sinonasal area, patients with associated pathology that may influence the overall survival of our patients (kidney, lung or heart disease) and lost sight patients. Limitations of our study include its retrospective nature and its limited patient numbers.

Patient and disease characteristics included age, gender, race, and primary site of disease, disease stage, and treatment received have been reviewed.

3. Results

Sinonasal mucosal melanoma was defined as a pathological diagnosis of malignant melanoma arising on the mucosa of the oral cavity, nasal cavity, nasopharynx, or sinuses, according to the final pathological report. In all cases the diagnosis of mucosal melanoma was established after standard microscopic and immunohistochemical examinations (positivity for HMB-45 and S-100 protein) of incisional biopsy specimens. Thorough history taking and physical examination ruled out the possibility of occult melanotic lesions elsewhere in the body, to finally declare the lesions "primary."

Disease was almost equally common in men and women; our patient population included 9 women and 8 men. The age ranged from 61 to 75 years, with median age of 67, 83 years for patient with sinonasal melanoma and 70, 40 years for patient with patient with oral cavity melanoma.

The primary site of disease was in the sinonasal cavity for 12 patients (70%) and oral cavity for 5 patients (30%). Patients' most common complaints included epistaxis (10 patients: 58%), facial pressure (5 patients: 30%) and nasal obstruction (6 patients: 35%). Most frequently sino nasal tumors were in the maxillary sinus (6 patients), nasal cavity (3 patients) and nasal septum (2 patients) (**Figure 1** and **Figure 2**).

Symptoms of oral melanomas vary and include a bleeding lump (3 patients) and pain (1 patient); 4 patients had a history of a continuously growing exophytic hyperplastic mass of a dark color (**Figure 3**).

Mucosal melanoma of oral cavity was most frequent on the hard palate (2 patients) and less frequently in the buccal mucosa (1 patient), mandibular gingiva (1 patient) and alveolar ridge (1 patient).

The median duration of symptoms before presenting to an otolaryngologist was 2 months (range 1 month to 04 months). All patients with oral mucosal melanoma (5 pattients) present with neck metastasis while only 2 patients of sinonasal melanoma present initially with neck involvement (**Figure 4**).

The tumors were stratified according to UICC (Union Internationale Contre le Cancer) staging [5] [6]: stage I, confined to the primary site (10 patients); stage II, positive cervical lymph nodes (05 patients); and stage III, distant metastases (02 patients). Of these patients, the liver and the lung were the most common locations.

According to TNM classification , The sinonasal tumors were stratified T3N0M0 in three cases, T4N2M0 in two cases, T1N0M0 in six cases and T4N3M+ in one case; The oral tumors were stratified T1N1M0 in two cases; T1N2M0 in one case, T4N2M0 in one case and T4N3M+ in one case.

Treatment modalities for mucosal melanoma include surgical resection with or without neck dissection, immunochemotherapy, and radiation therapy (RT). The type of surgery varied, based on anatomic location. 15 patients had attempted curative resections. Additionally, control of neck disease was achieved with the help of a modified radical neck dissection in the patient who presented with neck lymph node involvement (6 patients). Of the 15 patients who underwent upfront surgical resection, surgical margins were negative in 12 patients and positive in three patients. No patient underwent lymphoscintigraphy and sentinel node mapping.

All patients received postoperative RT to the involved sites of disease. The median radiation dose delivered

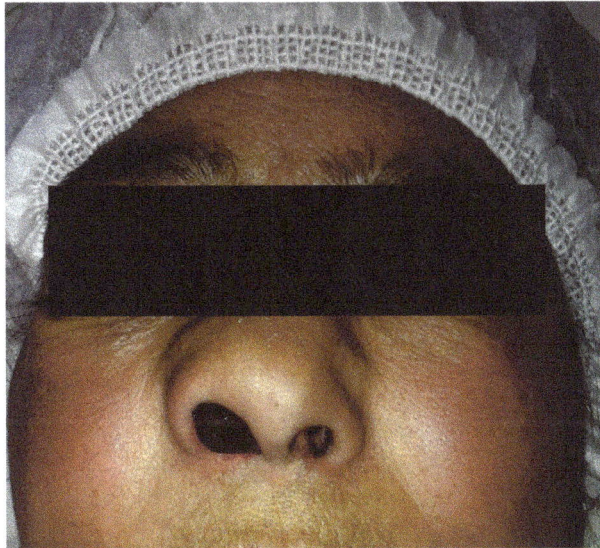

Figure 1. Photograph of A patient showing a black polypoidal mass in the left nasal cavity.

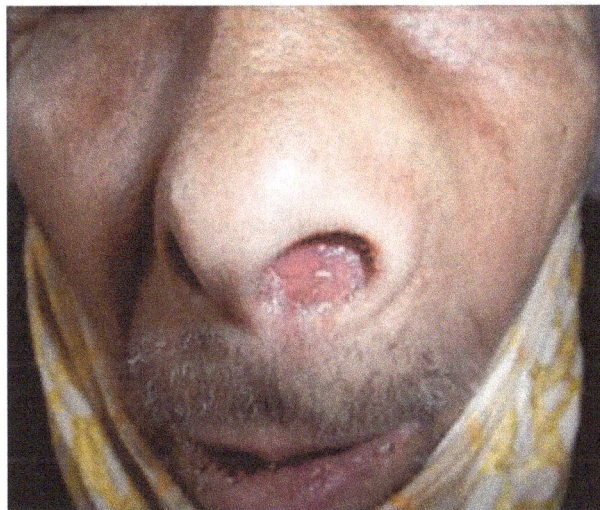

Figure 2. Not pigmented, melanoma involving the nasal cavity.

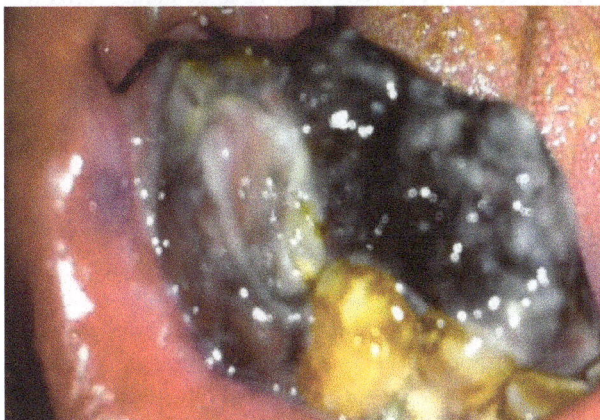

Figure 3. Macroscopic appearance of the oral tumor.

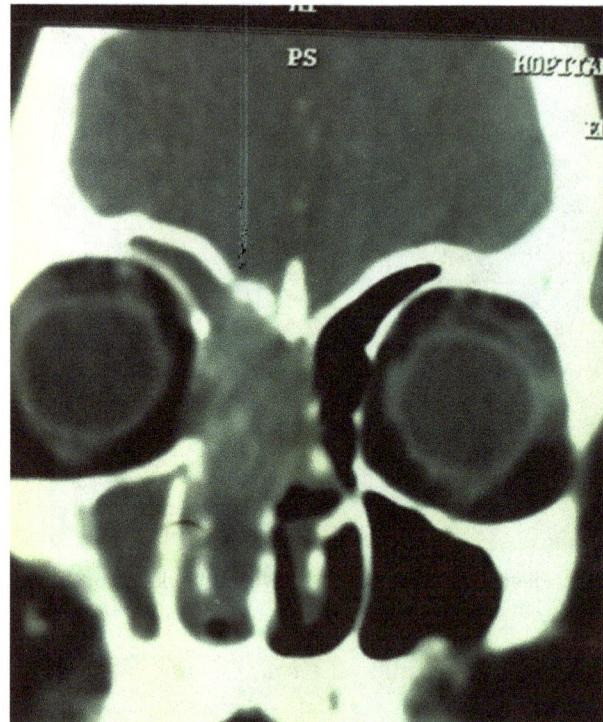

Figure 4. CT scan of paranasal sinuses, coronal view showing an extensive mass involving nasal cavity with signs of bony destruction.

was ranged from 30 to 70 Gy, These patients typically received a total of 10 fractions over 2 to 4 weeks to the involved sites of disease. Immunochemotherapy was administered in an adjuvant fashion to surgery in all patients, the protocol included DTC (dimethyltriazeno-imidazole-carboxamide), ACNU (nimustine hydrochloride), and VCR (vincristine), which is also known as the DAV protocol. Using this aggressive approach; a combination of surgery, RT, and/or systemic therapy; we had just 3 patients recurred at follow-up. Of these patients, two patients recurred locally and one distantly. Two patients received palliative radiation therapy as the primary treatment and immunochemotherapy as the adjuvant treatment. Eventually, these patients developed liver and pulmonary metastases.

All patients were followed in regular intervals by clinical, endoscopic and radiological examination. A MRI control was made in the 6th and 12th month follow-up. The local control rates vary from approximately 50% to 70% at 5 years.

Although the majority of recurrences are observed within 15 to 29 months after treatment.

Overall survival (OS) was defined as the time from surgery/biopsy to death from any cause, with surviving patients censored at date of last follow-up. Surgery with adjuvant medical treatment seems to be effective for local control of the disease. Survival ranged between 5 to >61 months (patient alive at 61 months), In comparison with other studies, our patients, who received a combination of surgery radiotherapy and immunochemotherapy had the longest survival (**Table 1** and **Table 2**).

4. Discussion

Primary mucosal melanomas represent only 1.7% - 3% of all primary melanomas [1]-[3]. The most frequent head and neck site of occurrence of mucosal melanoma is the conjunctiva, followed by the upper respiratory tract and the oral cavity [6]. The majority of the upper respiratory tract arises from the nasal cavity (80%) and the rest from the sinuses (20%). Common sites in order include the nasal septum, lateral nasal wall, turbinates, and nasal vestibule [3] [4] [6]. The maxillary sinus was the most commonly involved site among the paranasal sinuses accounting for 6% of all mucosal melanoma followed by the ethmoid, frontal, and sphenoid sinus cavities [3] [4]. In this study, we found that the maxillary sinus was the most commun site of the sino nasal melanoma.

Table 1. Clinical and treatment data of the patients with sinonasal melanoma.

Age gender	Symptome	Primary site	Classification		Primary treatment	Adjuvant treatment	Lymph node	Evolution
			Ballantyne	TNM				
61 female	Epistaxis nasalobstruction	Maxillary sinus	I	T3	Surgery (paralateronasal)	Immunochemotherapy radiation		Alive at 11 months
65 female	Epistaxis facial pressure	Maxillary sinus	II	T4	Surgery (paralateronasal)	Immunochemotherapy radiation	N+	Death at 10 months
67 female	nasalobstruction	Nasal cavity	I	T1	Surgery endonasal	Immunochemotherapy radiation		Alive at 61 months
W < 68 female	Epistaxis nasalobstruction	Septum	I	T1	Surgery (paralateronasal)	Immunochemotherapy radiation		Alive at 42 months
68 female	epistaxis	Nasal cacity (cornet inf)	I	T1	Surgery endonasal	Immunochemotherapy radiation		Alive at 18 months
72 female	epistaxis facial pressure	Maxillary sinus	III	T4	Surgery (paralateronasal)	Immunochemotherapy radiation	M+	Death at 07 months
75 female	Epistaxis nasalobstruction	Nasoethmoidal	I	T3	Surgery (paralateronasal)	Immunochemotherapy radiation		Alive at 16 months
61 male	epistaxis facial pressure	Maxillary sinus	II	T4	Surgery (paralateronasal)	Immunochemotherapy radiation	N+	Death at 6 months
67 male	facial pressure	Maxillary sinus	I	T3	Surgery (paralateronasal)	Immunochemotherapy radiation		Death at 9 months
68 male	epistaxis facial pressure	Maxillary sinus	I	T1	Surgery (paralateronasal)	Immunochemotherapy radiation		Alive at 51 months
71 male	Epistaxis nasalobstruction	Nasal cavity	I	T1	Surgery endonasal	Immunochemotherapy radiation		Alive at 31 months
73 male	Epistaxis nasalobstruction	Nasal septum	I	T1	Surgery (paralateronasal)	Immunochemotherapy radiation		Alive at 30 months

Table 2. Clinical and treatment data of the patient with oral melanoma.

Age gender	Symptome	Primary site	Classification		Primary treatment	Adjuvant treatment	Lymph node	Evolution
			Ballantyne	TNM				
68 male	Gingivorragia bleeding lump cervical node	Hard palate	II	T1	Wide local excision	Immunochemotherapy radiation	N+	Alive at 42 months
71 male	Facial pain gingivorragia	Hard palate	II	T4	-	Immunochemotherapy radiation	N+	Death at 09 months
73 male	Gingivorragia pigmented lesion	Mandibular gingiva	I	T1	Alveolectomy	Immunochemotherapy radiation	N+	Alive at 22 months
68 female	Bleeding lump	Buccal mucosa	III	T4	-	Immunochemotherapy radiation	N+ M+	Death at 05 months
72 female	Bleeding lump	Alveolar ridge	II	T1	Alveolectomy	Immunochemotherapy radiation	N+	Alive at 28 months

Oral mucosa is the second most common site of head and neck mucosal melanoma, representing 0.2% to 8% of all melanomas and 0.5% of all oral malignancies [1] [6], with nearly 70% arising in the upper alveolus and hard palate [3]. We found similar results in accordance with the literature. Oropharyngeal and laryngeal mucosal melanomas are exceedingly rare and only mentioned in case reports [1] [4] [6].

Generally, oral cavity melanoma appears to occur at a younger age than sinonasal mucosal melanoma [4]. Such a difference was not found in our study.

Sinonasal mucosal melanoma has typical presentations of epistaxis, nasal obstruction, facial deformity and facial pain. Typically, sinonasal mucosal melanoma presents as an expansive mass encroaching on several sub-sites of the paranasal sinuses, orbit, or cranial fossa and more than likely not pigmented [3] [4]. Symptoms of oral melanomas vary and include a bleeding lump and, rarely, pain. The diagnosis is often unfortunately delayed until symptoms resulting from ulceration, growth, or bleeding are noted [1] [2] [6].

Oral lesions are often flat and pigmented. These patients are often asymptomatic at time of presentation, and by this time, significant vertical invasion of the tumor cells into the underlying tissues has already occurred [1] [2] [6].

Unlike their skin counterparts, mucosal melanomas cannot be classified into the cutaneus melanomas categories due to different clinical and histologic characteristics. Patients may be staged according to the American Joint Committee on Cancer staging system. Alternatively, tumors may be stratified as follows according to UICC (Union Internationale Contre le Cancer) staging: stage I, confined to the primary site; stage II, positive cervical lymph nodes; and stage III, distant metastases [5] [6].

Mucosal melanoma must always be considered for multimodality therapy: surgical excision, medical oncology, and radiation therapy [5] [6]. 25% of patients with oral mucosal melanoma present with neck metastasis while only 6% of sinonasal melanoma patient present initially with neck involvement [3] [4]. In this paper, 5/5 patients with oral melanoma had cervical lymph nodes in time of presentation and just 2/12 patients with sinonasal had cervical lymph nodes (**Figure 5**).

Sentinel Lymph Node Biopsy in the Head and Neck. The widespread use of sentinel lymph node (SLN) biopsy in the management of head and neck melanoma has been limited by several concerns. One is that the lymphatic drainage in the head and neck region is complex, with multiple primary channels and the potential for multiple SLN sites.

Secondarily excision of these nodes can be technically challenging as small distances between sentinel nodes make detection and isolation difficult. Furthermore, approximately 25% - 30% of the sentinel nodes is found within the parotid gland, and concern of facial nerve injury has led many surgeons to advocate superficial parotidectomy over SLN biopsy.

And lastly, the cooperation of experienced pathologists and nuclear medicine staff are essential to the success of the procedure. But it still remains an area for future evaluation [1] [4] [7] [8].

For oral mucosal melanoma, the topic of prophylactic neck dissections has been debated more due to the greater frequency of regional metastasis upon initial presentation. The rate of regional recurrence in oral mucosal melanomas is much greater, estimated around 70% [2] [5] [6]. Prophylactic neck dissections in treatment of sinonasal mucosal melanoma are not advocated.

Metastatic disease should be evaluated for at onset including CT Chest and PET/CT.

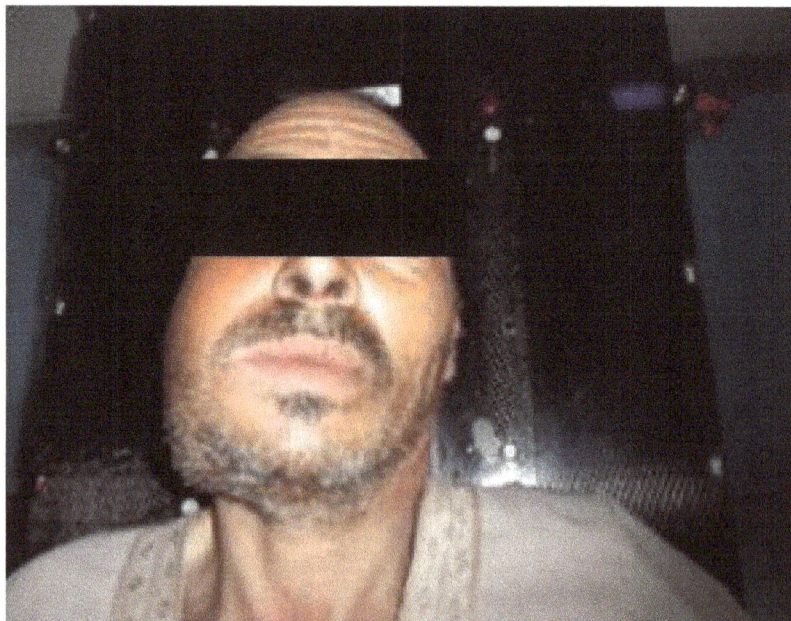

Figure 5. Patient with oral melanoma and nodal involvement.

Unlike cutaneous melanoma, the common sites of distant metastasis are the lungs (33%) and brain (14%), with multiple sites being involved in 33% of cases in the literature [3]-[5]. In this study we found that two patients had a distant metastasis, at initial presentation, in multiple sites; lung and liver: (1 patients), brain and liver (1 patient).

Despite its radioresistant nature of tumor, the role of radiation therapy following surgical intervention has typically been advocated. However, the topic of primary radiation therapy has been debated. Gaze *et al.* demonstrated complete clinical response in 8/13 patients with primary radiation therapy alone [9]. Remainder of studies advocate radiotherapy for inoperable tumors or recurrence.

Post-operative radiation therapy has shown to improve local control in several retrospective series. Benlyazid *et al.* demonstrated greater improved local control (62% vs 26%) in patients treated surgery and radiation therapy versus those with surgery alone [10]. Similarly, Owens *et al.* found similar benefit with 83% vs 55% in comparing those patient receiving surgery with post-operative radiation therapy and those receiving surgery alone [11].

The authors of a series from the University of Florida agree that surgery with postoperative RT should be used in nearly all cases of head and neck mucosal melanomas. However, they also suggest that elective nodal irradiation should be used to address subclinical regional disease [12]. In this study we have use an aggressive approach: a combination of surgery, RT, and immunochemotherapy, and we found that Surgery with adjuvant medical treatment seems to be effective for local control of the disease. Survival ranged between 05 to >61 months (alive at 61 months), In comparison with other studies, our patients had the longest survival. Although this is a very small sample of patients; this result is in accordance with the treatment recommended by many authors. More studies are needed to determine treatment modalities, prophylactic neck dissection, adjuvant treatment, the prognostic value of tumor thickness and invasion of mucosal melanoma. This would also help to establish a clinically useful classification of mucosal melanomas and thus to improve therapy.

The final area of treatment lies with immunochemotherapy. KIT gene has been identified in nearly 15% - 30% of mucosal melanoma cases. Some preliminary studies have even suggested that treatment with a KIT inhibitor may lead one further year of survival.

The domain of medical oncology and genetic research may provide further clues, especially in light of preliminary benefits noted of KIT inhibitors [13]-[15].

5. Conclusion

The occurrence of primary mucosal melanoma is very rare. It is most frequently present in the nose and/or sinuses, followed by the oral cavity and nasopharynx. Head and neck melanoma is a complex disease especially in its treatment considerations. The prognosis remains poor despite adequate locoregional control of the disease. The generally advanced stage of the tumor at initial diagnosis leads to a poorer survival because of their development in hidden and clinically silent areas. As in any other cancer, the best opportunity for cure lies in early and aggressive treatment. Further research in the use of adjuvant therapy (chemotherapy, immunotherapy, biological therapy) will be necessary to improve the outcome of patients with mucosal melanoma.

Conflict of Interest

None.

References

[1] Shashanka, R. and Smitha, B.R. (2012) Head and Neck Melanoma. *International Scholarly Research Network ISRN Surgery*, **2012**, Article ID: 948302.

[2] Greenberg, M.S. and Glick, K.M. (2008) Pigmented Lesions of the Oral Mucosa. In: *Burket's Oral Medicine*, 11th Edition, BC Decker, Hamilton, 586.

[3] Narasimhan, K., *et al.* (2009) Sinonasal Mucosal Melanoma: A 13-Year Experience at a Single Institution. *Skull Base*, **19**, 255-262. http://dx.doi.org/10.1055/s-0028-1115321

[4] Rapidis, A., Apostolidis, C., Vilos, G. and Valsamis, S. (2003) Primary Malignant Melanoma of the Oral Mucosa. *Journal of Oral and Maxillofacial Surgery*, **61**, 1132-1139. http://dx.doi.org/10.1016/S0278-2391(03)00670-0

[5] Gavriel, H., McArthur, G., Sizeland, A. and Henderson, M. (2011) Review: Mucosal Melanoma of the Head and Neck. *Melanoma Research*, **21**, 257-266. http://dx.doi.org/10.1097/CMR.0b013e3283470ffd

[6]   Chang, A., Karnell, L. and Menck, H. (1998) The National Cancer Data Base Report on Cutaneous and Noncutaneous Melanoma: A Summary of 84,836 Cases from the Past Decade. The American College of Surgeons Commission on Cancer and the American Cancer Society. *Cancer*, **83**, 1664-1678.
      http://dx.doi.org/10.1002/(SICI)1097-0142(19981015)83:8<1664::AID-CNCR23>3.0.CO;2-G

[7]   Jethanamest, D., Vila, P.M., Sikora, S.G. and Morris, L.G.T. (2011) Predictors of Survival in Mucosal Melanoma of the Head and Neck. *Annals of Surgical Oncology*, **18**, 2748-2756. http://dx.doi.org/10.1245/s10434-011-1685-4

[8]   Leong, S.P., Accortt, N.A., Essner, R., Ross, M., Gershenwald, J.E., Pockaj, B., *et al.* (2006) Impact of Sentinel Node Status and Other Risk Factors on the Clinical Outcome of Head and Neck Melanoma Patients. *Archives of Otolaryngology—Head Neck Surgery*, **132**, 370-373. http://dx.doi.org/10.1001/archotol.132.4.370

[9]   Gaze, M.N., Kerr, G.R. and Smyth, J.F. (1990) Mucosal Melanomas of the Head and Neck: The Scottish Experience. The Scottish Melanoma Group. *Clinical Oncology* (*Royal College of Radiologists*), **2**, 277-283.
      http://dx.doi.org/10.1016/S0936-6555(05)80955-0

[10] Benlyazid, A., Thariat, J., Temam, S., Malard, O., Florescu, C., Choussy, O., *et al.* (2010) Postoperative Radiotherapy in Head and Neck Mucosal Melanoma: A GETTEC Study. *Archives of Otolaryngology—Head Neck Surgery*, **136**, 1219-1225. http://dx.doi.org/10.1001/archoto.2010.217

[11] Owens, J.M., Roberts, D.B. and Myers, J.N. (2003) The Role of Postoperative Adjuvant Radiation Therapy in the Treatment of Mucosal Melanomas of the Head and Neck Region. *Archives of Otolaryngology—Head Neck Surgery*, **129**, 864-868. http://dx.doi.org/10.1001/archotol.129.8.864

[12] Wagner, M., Morris, C.G., Werning, J.W. and Mendenhall, W.M. (2008) Mucosal Melanoma of the Head and Neck. *American Journal of Clinical Oncology*, **31**, 43-48. http://dx.doi.org/10.1097/COC.0b013e318134ee88

[13] Hodi, F.S., Friedlander, P., Corless, C.L., Heinrich, M.C., Mac Rae, S., Kruse, A., *et al.* (2008) Major Response to Imatinib Mesylate in KIT-Mutated Melanoma. *Journal of Clinical Oncology*, **26**, 2046-2051.
      http://dx.doi.org/10.1200/JCO.2007.14.0707

[14] Quintás-Cardama, A., Lazar, A.J., Woodman, S.E., Kim, K., Ross, M. and Hwu, P. (2008) Complete Response of Stage IV Anal Mucosal Melanoma Expressing KIT Val560Asp to the Multikinase Inhibitor Sorafenib. *Nature Clinical Practice Oncology*, **5**, 737-740. http://dx.doi.org/10.1038/ncponc1251

[15] Handolias, D., Salemi, R., Murray, W., Tan, A., Liu, W., Viros, A., *et al.* (2010) Mutations in KIT Occur at Low Frequency in Melanomas Arising from Anatomical Sites Associated with Chronic and Intermittent Sun Exposure. *Pigment Cell Melanoma Research*, **23**, 210-215. http://dx.doi.org/10.1111/j.1755-148X.2010.00671.x

16

Long Term Outcomes of Cross-Hatching Eustachian Tuboplasty

Carlos Yanez, Sandra Velázquez, Nallely Mora

American British Medical Center, Mexico City, Mexico
Email: carlosyanez_md@yahoo.com

Abstract

Objective: To review the long term outcomes of cross-hatching Eustachian Tuboplasty (ChEt) in patients with chronic obstructive Eustachian tube dysfunction (COETD), as well as assess the clinical factors associated with surgical success. Study Design: Retrospective case series review. Setting: Tertiary healthcare institution. Methods: This is a retrospective review of non-revision ChET for COETD. Follow-up period was 5 years. The inclusion criteria were persistent otitis media with effusion, conductive hearing loss of 5 or more years, and constant COETD related-symptoms. The curvature of the posterior cushion was modified using an argon laser to alter the spring of the cartilage alleviating the obstructed valve's aperture. Several clinical factors were reviewed in relation to the successful opening of Eustachian tube valve. Results: One hundred and twenty patients, 72 males/48 females, average age 42.4 + 2 years old, met study inclusion criteria. COETD patients/ obstructive causes were: Posterior cushion hypertrophy, 68 (56.6%); Tensor Veli and Levator Veli Palatini muscles hypertrophy, 15 (12.5%); Remarkable mucosal hypertrophic disease, 37 (30.8%). Total of ET tubes was 198. Bilateral 143 (72.2%), 55 unilateral (27.7%) ET valve was seen more open postoperatively on simple endoscopy (SE) and slow motion video analysis (SMVEA). There were no complications. Mean pure tone average improved by 20 dB postoperatively; P = 0.015. Mean immitance changes in tympanometric measurements improved postoperatively at least 0.10 mmhos in 91% of the patients (P = 0.010). Resolution of symptoms was considered a successful outcome. Failure correlated with the severity of disease. Conclusion: High rates of improvement (96%) were achieved. ChEt is a promising technique for the treatment of COETD.

Keywords

Obstructive Eustachian Tube Dysfunction, Eustachian Tuboplasty

1. Introduction

Chronic obstructive Eustachian tube dysfunction (COETD) is a common disorder causing repeated visits to the doctor's office and substantial medical expenses. The most common symptoms are autophony, hypoacusia, tinnitus and fullness of the ear. When medical treatment fails, surgery should be considered an option. Tympanostomy tube placement is the common procedure. Multiple insertions of ventilating tubes are required if refractory otitis media persists. Numerous surgical procedures have been proposed for correcting COETD. Hopf *et al.* [1] proposed that intraluminal surgery improves Eustachian tube dysfunction using laser techniques. Kujawski [2] [3] performed the first in 1997 using a CO_2 laser focused on the cartilaginous portion and reported that 81% of his 38 patients were symptom-free after 36 months of follow-up. Poe, Metson and Kujawski [4] describe their preliminary results on Laser Eustachian Tuboplasty on 2003. We [5] described the laser-assisted cross-hatching Eustachian Tuboplasty (ChEt) and reported the preliminary results in 25 patients including a 15-month follow-up. Overall results showed that 92% were free of middle ear effusion with symptoms improving. Nowadays, laser-assisted ChEt is being considered a minimally invasive surgical modality for COETD, although further studies are required for determining whether it is alternative to COETD, instead of repeated tympanostomy tube placement in selected patients. We also developed a Eustachian tube dysfunction numerical staging, as well as results reporting system that better assists in the analysis of Eustachian tube surgery [6]. We present here the outcomes of ET surgery in our personal clinical patient series.

2. Materials and Methods

This is a retrospective case series review carried out at the Sinus Surgery Center, inside a Tertiary Care Hospital, the American British Cowdray Medical Center, located in Mexico City, where 120 consecutive patients with COETD were diagnosed between February 2001 and June 2008. Patients were classified according to the Yanez Classification System [6], surgically treated with ChET and followed for 5 years postoperatively. The inclusion criteria were persistent otitis media with effusion, with a history of multiple tympanostomy tube insertions; conductive hearing loss of 5 or more years, and constant COETD related-symptoms. Age and gender were equally distributed. Exclusion criteria were allergic rhinitis, laryngopharyngeal reflux and other type of otologic or nasal surgery. We included 72 males and 48 females, mean age 42.4 ± 2 years, the youngest being 4 and the oldest 60 years old. They served as their own controls. All patients provided informed consent for the surgical procedure and the study was reviewed and approved by the Ethics Committee of the Sinus Surgery Center.

For the classification system, patients were studied as following:

1) Axial and coronal computer tomography scans of the ear were taken for measuring the width of the bony portion of the Eustachian tube (ET) and the cartilaginous portion morphology, studied while the patients performed the Valsalva maneuver, as well as identifying the internal carotid artery and the relationship with the ET. The radiological pathology of the cartilaginous portion of the ET was classified based on mucosal intraluminal swelling as normal, or swollen/opacified; done by a Radiologist that doesn't know the patients.

2) Preoperative symptoms (earache, hearing loss, ear fullness, tinnitus, autophony and vertigo) were recorded using a 3-point scale (0 = absent; 1 = mild; 2 = moderate; 3 = severe symptom).

3) All patients underwent a trans-nasal endoscopic slow motion video analysis (SMVEA) of their Eustachian tubes, done with a 30° view angle using a rigid Hopkins rod endoscope measuring 4.0 mm or 2.7 mm diameter, (Karl Storz, Tuttinghem, Germany), recorded and analyzed on a S-VHS/SR-VCR in normal time, in slow motion and single frame viewing at 30 frames per second. Examinations were performed while the patient was awake and administered topical anesthesia by placing two or three cotton swabs soaked in a 2% Pontocaine solution and left for 5 to 7 minutes in the inferior meatus. The endoscopes were directed into the pharyngeal orifice while the patient remained sitting and rested his/her head in the chair's headrest. The entire nose was first inspected and the 30° angle view was directed laterally. The ET medial structures and valve were examined. Subjects were asked to repeat the letter K, to swallow and to yawn for better viewing of the palate, medial cartilaginous lamina, tensor veli palatine muscle (TVPM), levatorveli palatine muscle (LVPM), sphenopharyngeousmuscle (SphM) and record valve dynamics in both normal and forced motion modes. **Figure 1** shows the phases of valve dilation in a normal Eustachian tube valve.

4) All patients underwent auditory battery tests (pure tone audiometry, tympanometry, Eustachian tube—tympanometric tests).

5) Patients were classified following the staging system used to identify the extent of the surgical procedure required for every patient.

SLOW MOTION VIDEO ENDOSCOPY PHASES OF VALVE DILATION

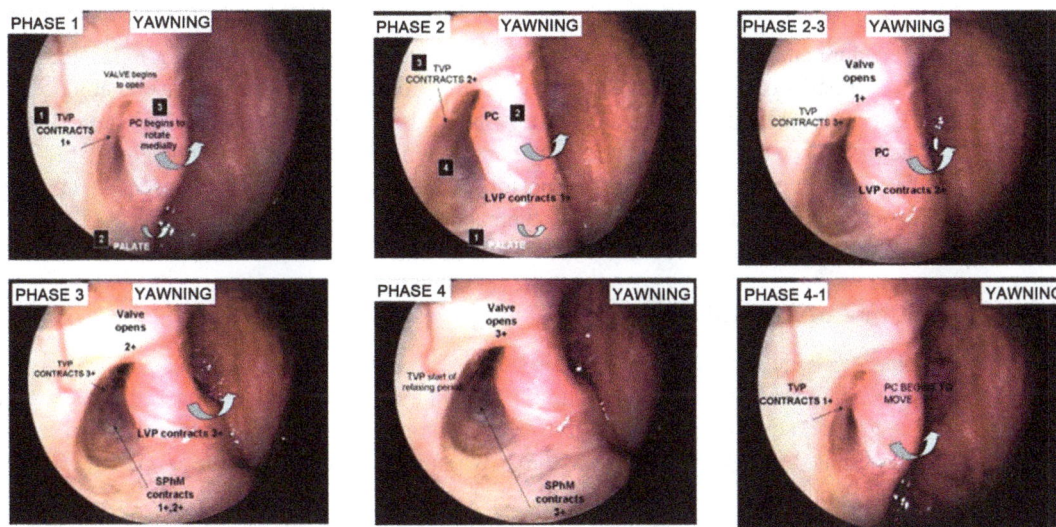

Figure 1. Slow-motion video-endoscopic analysis. We can see the phases of valve dilation that are useful to classify the Eustachian tube dysfunction.

2.1. Laser Eustachian Tuboplasty Procedure—Cross-Hatching

All patients were operated under general anesthesia by the senior author of this article. The ChEt procedure included a bilateral diagnostic nasal endoscopy carried out under general anesthesia. Special attention was paid to examining the ET valve, TVPM, LVPM and SphM areas. Mucosal contact areas, polypoid or granulomatous tissue were studied in detail. Anatomical variations, such as altered cartilaginous spring of the posterior cushion, abnormally wide or thick posterior cushion, valve morphology, pronounced superior direction of the lumen and valve or absence of the posterior cushion cartilaginous super-structure (congenital or iatrogenic) were also noted and recorded. Obstructive and/or hypertrophic areas of the tube were confirmed by instrument palpation and direct visualization and its direct impact to the valve area was recorded. A tonsil mouth gag was inserted and the mouth opened.

Instruments were placed in a combined fashion using both the endonasal and oral route. An auto-static holder for the endoscopes (Microfrance, Medtronic-Xomed, Jacksonville, Fla.) was mounted on the table and adjusted to the endoscope, facilitating a four-handed technique. No lidocaine and epinephrine injections were administered. The orifice of the tube was visualized with a 30° angled view endoscope (4 mm in diameter) and the medial cartilaginous lamina and valve palpated with a curved ball tipped instrument. After identifying these structures, a KTP 532 nm fiber-delivered laser (Laserscope, San Jose, California, USA) was then introduced through the nose into the nasopharynx and positioned toward the diseased area of the mucosa to be ablated in the medial cartilaginous lamina within the posterior cushion. An endostat single-use fiberoptichandpiece designed for handheld surgery on very small delicate structures was used housing a 0.6 mm fiber. The settings were 2 - 4 watts continuously. Laser ablation of the mucosa was begun over the medial edge of the posterior cushion where a mucosal defect was created starting in the center ablating most mucosa on the anterior surface of the posterior cushion. Laser ablation of the submucosal tissue and perichondrium was also accomplished until the cartilaginous superstructure of the posterior cushion was identified and discovered creating a defect from the proximal to distal portion into the tubal lumen to a point 3 - 4 mm from the functional valve. The valve area was not touched with the laser. Mild, moderate and severe obstructive conditions were treated differently.

The shape and size of the area to be ablated was assessed preoperatively depending on the stage of COETD. In all cases, ChEt was applied to the ET cartilage frame as proposed by the authors. Half or full thickness incisions were made on the concave side of the cartilaginous superstructure of the posterior cushion and extended as close as possible toward the valve area. The opposite mucoperichondrium was not reached. This resulted in a far more effective release of inherent interlocked forces in the cartilage and more reliable long term straightening favoring better TVPM mobility.

No ET packing or stents were used at the end of the procedure. Care was taken not to injure the mucosa of the anterior edge of the ET to avoid scar band formation. Patients were discharged from the hospital on the same day of the surgical procedure and were instructed to gently blow their noses and use hypertonic saline solution for rinsing their noses. All patients received postoperative nasal steroids and oral dexametasone at a dose of 40 mg daily for 5 days. Both were started on day 2 and were suspended on day 8, postoperatively. Immediate post-operative control visits took place two and four weeks later and long term follow-up was done in all 120 patients at a year, two, and five years, postoperatively. In the postoperative visits we made the 3-point scale symptom recording tool, auditory battery tests (tone audiometry, tympanometry, ET—tympanometric tests) the SMVEA and compared to the preoperative data.

2.2. Statistical Method of Analysis

All patient data and findings were recorded. The data was transferred into a microcomputer and analyzed using the StatPac statistical software program (Bloomington, MN). Symptom scores were estimated for every preoperative, those at one and four weeks, one, two and five years postoperative symptoms and analyzed using the Wilcoxon's test with one-tailed interpretation. Wilcoxon's two-tailed test was used for analyzing the pre and postoperative simple endoscopic findings and slow-motion endoscopic analysis data and also when correlations of ET patency on pre and postoperative differences in symptoms and findings were tested. In cases of bilateral symptoms, only the worst ET was used in the analyses.

3. Results

Analysis of data obtained from preoperative CT scans of the ear showed the following: normal shape and width (1.3 mm - 3.5 mm) of the bony portion of the ET in all 120 patients (100%). No bony dehiscence were recognized in the carotid canal and no opacification was seen in the bony portion. The intraluminal ET mucosa was preoperatively classified as seen on CT scans as normal in 2% of the patients and hypertrophic in 98%.

According to the Yañez and Mora Classification System [6] we found 8 patients (7%) with Stage 0 COETD (score < 13) 14 patients (12%) with Stage 1 COETD with a score < 22 indicating mild COETD. 28 patients (23%) had Stage 2 (score < 34) indicating moderate COETD. 70 patients (58%) had Stage 3 disease (score < 39) indicating severe COETD. **Table 1** shows the classification system corresponding to the surgical plan on each patient.

Comparing the data of slow motion video endoscopic analysis, before surgery half of the patients had moderate impairment of valve aperture, and the other half between mild and severe impairment. Mobility of the medial aspect of the ET seen during SMVEA improved notoriously the first year in 87% of the cases (105 patients) with good valve dilation. Fifteen patients (13%) had a moderate improvement in ET mobility. At five years postoperatively, 118 of the 120 patients had normal middle ears and their tympanic membranes looked well and also demonstrate a good valve dilation on SMVEA (**Figure 2**). One patient had another episode of middle ear effusion in one ear and required a third tympanostomy tube placement. A titanium middle ear grommet was inserted for permanent ventilation.

Table 1. Stages of chronic obstructive Eustachian tube disease and laser ablation extension.

Disease stage	Extension of laser ablation in the Eustachian tube
1	Ablation of the mucosa overlying the leading edge of the lateral cartilaginous lamina and the posterior cushion. Oval shaped ablation defect is centered over this cartilage. Perichondrium is not ablated.
2	Mucosa and submucosal tissue (perichondrium) overlying the leading edge of the lateral cartilaginous lamina and the posterior cushion oval shaped ablation defect is centered over this cartilage only. No ablation is carried out distally to the Eustachian tube valve.
3	Mucosa, submucosal, perichondrium and cartilage are thinned. Effort is made to weaken the spring of the cartilage. Oval shaped ablation defect is centered over this cartilage only. Medium thickness cross-hatching of the PC tissue ablation is extended distally to within 4 - 5 mm of the Eustachian tube valve.
4	Mucosa, submucosal, perichondrium and cartilage are thinned. Effort is made to weaken the spring of the cartilage. Oval shaped ablation defect is centered over this cartilage and extended distally to within 4 - 5 mm to adjacent structures. Full thickness cross-hatching of the posterior cushion.

SLOW MOTION VIDEO ENDOSCOPY BEFORE SURGERY

17%

34%

49%

n=120

■ MILD ▨ MODERATE ■ SEVERE

SLOW MOTION VIDEO ENDOSCOPY ANALYSIS AT 1 YEAR POSTOPERATIVELY

14%

86%

■ Good Valve Dilation ▨ Moderate Valve Dilation

SLOW MOTION VIDEO ENDOSCOPY ANALYSIS AT 5 YEAR POSTOPERATIVELY

2%

98%

▨ Good Valve Dilation ■ Moderate Valve Dilation

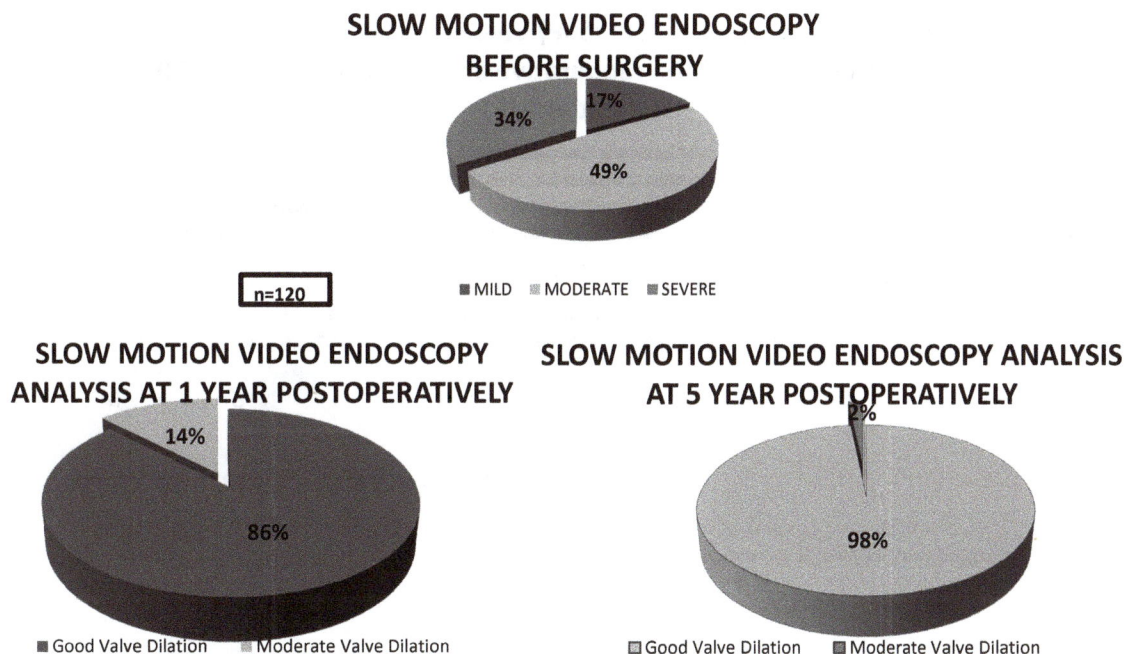

Figure 2. Before surgery 49% had moderate valve impairment. After the first year 87% of patients had good valve dilation, at the end of the study 98% reach good valve dilation. Slow motion video endoscopy analysis before surgery, 1 year and 5 years after the procedure. n = number of patients.

Intraoperative anatomical variations of the ET most commonly found included severely malformed posterior cushion cartilage in 28 patients (23.33%) with severe obstruction of the functional valve area. Obstructive hypertrophy of the TVPM, LVPM and SphM areas was seen in 35 patients (29.16%). Remarkable mucosal hypertrophic disease of the PC was seen in 31 patients (25.83%), and in 16 patients (13.33%) recorded in the vicinity of the functional valve area. Severe scarring tissue completely occluding the proximal tubal lumen and partially obscuring the PC was seen in one patient (0.83%) the remaining 9 had polypoid obstruction

Ninety three patients (77.5%) were seen after a week. The rest (27 patients) 22.5% were unable to return for their postoperative visit because they lived distant from the city. These patients did not refer any complaints when spoken to on the telephone. One hundred and twelve patients (93.3%) did go to the 1st year postoperative visit and 120 patients (100%) did go to the 2nd, and 5th year follow-up examination.

3.1. Pre and Postoperative Symptoms

A symptom severity product (SSP) value was estimated for the 3-point scale symptom preoperatively, at one, two and five years postoperatively during follow-up and carefully compared. We observed how symptoms decrease during the follow up, being minimal at 5 years postoperatively (**Figure 3**).

3.2. Tympanometry Results

ET tympanometric tests were carried out in all patients at 1 year, 2nd and 5th year postoperative and compared to the preoperative data, we included 198 Eustachian tubes. Before Surgery we found 183 Type B Tympanometries, after the first year 176 were Type A curves and for the 5th year 185 were Type A curves (**Figure 4**).

4. Discussion

Cross-hatching Eustachian Tuboplasty is a relatively new procedure [5], careful patient selection criteria must be established. A lot has been written about Eustachian tube dysfunction and several procedures have been proposed in the last years [7]. A comparison of the studies assessing the efficacy of Eustachian tube surgery is often difficult due to the lack of a common staging system or a proper definition of COETD. There is a recent and promising classification proposed as a novel diagnostic tool [8], in this study, all eligible patients were studied

Symptom Severity Product (SSP) Values for Eustachian Tube Obstructive Dysfunction Preoperative and follow up data N=120 Patients

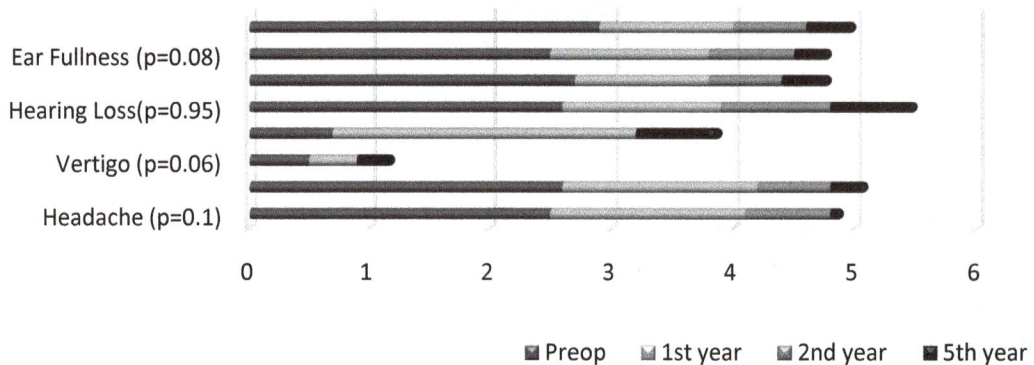

Figure 3. A symptom severity product (SSP) value was estimated for the 3-point scale. We can see that the symptoms trend to disappear at the end of the study.

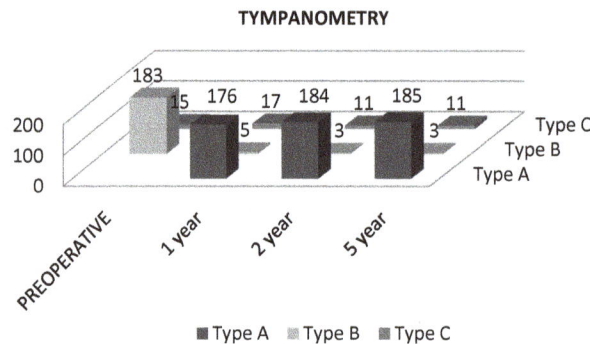

Figure 4. We include 198 Eustachian tubes. Preoperative there were 183 curve B Tympanometries, in the first year 176 were A and for the 5th year 185 were A curves.

using the classification system we proposed in 2008 [6].

The intraluminal ET mucosa on the CT scan was normal in 2% of the patients and hypertrophic in 98%, however, it is important to consider that often times X-rays, CT scans and other procedures produce considerably false negative results when edema, opacification and polyps occur and assessed in the ET lumen. CT scans are more useful when assessing the status of the isthmus and the bony ET portion.

Before surgery 93% of patients had Eustaquian tube disease, regarding our classification system, at the end of the study we reach 99% of patients without Eustachian tube dysfunction (Stage 0) the remaining 1% were patients that developed associate conditions (laryngo pharyngeal reflux, allergic rhinitis).

In the slow motion video endoscopy before surgery we found 49% of the patients with moderate impairment of valve aperture, and 51% between mild and severe impairment. At five years postoperatively, we can appreciate in 98% the improvement of valve dilation.

The improvement of symptoms was measured at 1, 2 and 5 years after surgery and compared with the preoperative data, having a 96% of patients without symptoms at the end of the study.

Although, the patient sample size is sufficient for drawing conclusions from the different outcomes in this report, large numbers of patients are still needed in more detailed studies in the near future. Correct diagnosis of COETD is of crucial importance in planning the surgical treatment of the chronic disease. Endoscopic methods have improved the diagnostic precision, the use of SMVEA is of the most important. In this study, SMVEA was the tool for reaching a detailed diagnosis of COETD and valve dilation capability.

The major drawback, in an attempt to quantify disease extension, is that repeated ET endoscopies for SMVEA may be considered painful or cause severe discomfort to patients. No other test for measuring ET function postoperatively is as reliable.

Additional useful information is obtained from the patient's history. In order to adequately choose the correct surgical approach, a staging system is helpful. Until now, there are no standardized criteria for the selection of cases that are appropriate for the ChEt procedure mainly because of differences in surgical techniques favored by each surgeon. According to our stage system, ChEt is recommended in COETD Stages 2, 3 and 4. However, a cautious interpretation of endoscopic findings is needed to compare the treatment results because of various extensions of the disease and surgical treatment. To clarify the indication of a ChEt approach in the future, the recurrence rate should be analyzed according to the stage of COETD. Therefore, preoperative staging is highly important. This will increase the choice of the adequate surgical ET tissue ablation extension and approach.

The Balloon dilatation of the Eustachian tube surgery [9] [10] is another technique for treating Eustachian tube dysfunction, it has been published a clear short term (6 months) benefit across all recorded outcome measures in a majority of cases, with symptom improvement in 67% of cases at 2 months.

We think we have to compare both techniques and large numbers of patients are still needed to reproduce results.

5. Conclusion

These outcome results suggest that ChEt is safe and efficacious in the treatment of COETD. Preoperative staging of COETD is useful for planning an appropriate surgical approach. The numerical score system used here can objectively quantify and provide a high level of agreement in the evaluation of COETD. We recommend it for reproducing it in ET surgery in large clinical studies. Further evaluation of longer term follow-up will be necessary to determine whether these patients achieve or continue to have good results.

References

[1]   Hopf, J., Linnarz, M., Gundlach, P., *et al.* (1991) Die Mikroendoskopie der eustachischen rohre und des mittelhres: Indikationen und klinischer einsatzpunkt. *Laryngorhinootologie*, **70**, 391-394. http://dx.doi.org/10.1055/s-2007-998060

[2]   Kujawski, O. (2000) Laser Eustachian Tuboplasty (LEPT): 4th European Congress of EUFOS. *Otolaryngology—Head and Neck Surgery*, **2**, 835-842.

[3]   Kujawski, O.B. and Poe, D.S. (2004) Laser Eustachian Tuboplasty. *Otology Neurotology*, **25**, 1-8. http://dx.doi.org/10.1097/00129492-200401000-00001

[4]   Poe, D.S., Metson, R.B. and Kujawski, O. (2003) Laser Eustachian Tuboplasty: A Preliminary Report. *Laryngoscope*, **113**, 583-591. http://dx.doi.org/10.1097/00005537-200304000-00001

[5]   Yañez, C. (2010) Cross-Hatching Technique for Eustachian Tuboplasty: Preliminary Report. *Otolaryngology—Head and Neck Surgery*, **142**, 688-693. http://dx.doi.org/10.1016/j.otohns.2009.12.046

[6]   Yañez, C. and Mora, N. (2008) Classification System for Results in Eustachian Tube Surgery. *Otolaryngology—Head and Neck Surgery*, **139**, P74. http://dx.doi.org/10.1016/j.otohns.2008.05.238

[7]   McCoul, E.D., Lucente, F.E. and Anand, V.K. (2011) Evolution of Eustachian Tube Surgery. *The Laryngoscope*, **121**, 661-666.

[8]   Schröder, S., Lehmann, M., Sauzet, O., Ebmeyer, J. and Sudhoff, H. (2014) A Novel Diagnostic Tool for Chronic Obstructive Eustachian Tube Dysfunction—The Eustachian Tube Score. *The Laryngoscope*. http://dx.doi.org/10.1002/lary.24922

[9]   Miller, B.J. and Elhassan, H.A. (2013) Balloon Dilatation of the Eustachian Tube: An Evidence Based Review of Case Series for Those Considering Its Use. *Clinical Otolaryngology*, **38**, 525-532. http://dx.doi.org/10.1111/coa.12195

[10] Poe, D.S., Silvola, J. and Pyykko, I. (2011) Balloon Dilation of the Cartilaginous Eustachian Tube. *Otolaryngology—Head and Neck Surgery*, **144**, 563-569. http://dx.doi.org/10.1177/0194599811399866

17

Nasal Schwannoma—A Case Report

A. Ravindran, A. Amirthagani, Prince Peterdhas, S. Nagarajan, P. Palanivel, Rekha Salini, A. S. Jagan

Department of Otorhonolaryngology, Thanjavur Madical College, Thanjavur, India
Email: amirent1976@gmail.com

Abstract

According to the literature, half of the schwannoma cases occur in the head and neck areas and only less than 4% occur in the sinonasal tract. In this case, a 50-year-old male patient, Mr. Jeyapal with a-year-long progressive left side nasal obstruction and purulent rhinorrhea, is presented [1]. The CT reveals a mass filling the left nasal cavity. During surgical intervention, the mass is found to originate from the medial side of the septum anteriorly and inferiorly. The pathological examination reveals capsulated tumor with palisading cellular arrangement and high cellular density [2]. The pathological findings and nervous origin of the tumor are discussed after an extensive review of the literature.

Keywords

Nasal Schwannoma, Chronic Nasal Obstruction, Nasal Polyp

1. Introduction

Half of the cases with schwannoma occur in the head and neck region, but less than 4% occur in the sinonasal area. This tumor is derived from the schwann cell, which can be found in many kinds of nerves, including cranial nerves (except olfactory and optic nerves), peripheral nerves, sympathetic and parasympathetic nerves. Clinically, these patients are indicated to have unilateral nasal obstruction, frequent epistaxis, anosmia, and painful sensation. The characteristics of the tumor are polyploid, slow-growing, and encapsulated. With nasal schwannoma, however, some special pathological findings are specific, which are not found in tumors from other regions.

2. Case Report

The patient was a 50-year-old male. He visited us because of a progressive left side nasal obstruction with intermittent purulent rhinorrhea for more than a year. No epistaxis, anosmia, or any other nasal symptom was mentioned. He denied any systemic disease and had never undergone any surgery. He was an agriculture coolie, smoked one pack of cigarettes per day and chewed betel nuts for over 10 years (**Figure 1**).

During his visit, under anterior rhinoscopy, a large polypoid mass was noted in his left nostril, which occupied the left nasal cavity and protruding out. Some yellowish mucopus was also found in the left nasal cavity. Posterior rhinoscopy revealed normal.

CT scan of the paranasal sinus showed a large soft tissue mass in the left nasal cavity with protrusion into the nasopharynx (**Figure 2**).

Patient underwent biopsy under local anaesthesia and it was reported as cellular schwanoma.

Lateral rhinotomy surgery was performed under general anesthesia with an impression of mass occupying nearly the entire left nasal cavity without much adhesion to nasal mucosa. Its insertion was at the vestibule left side. A deviated nasal septum, a laterally displaced left middle turbinate, and an atrophic inferior turbinate were found. These seemed to be secondary changes from the mass effect (**Figure 3**).

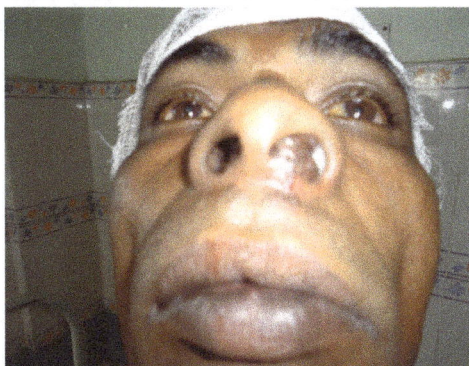

Figure 1. Clinical picture.

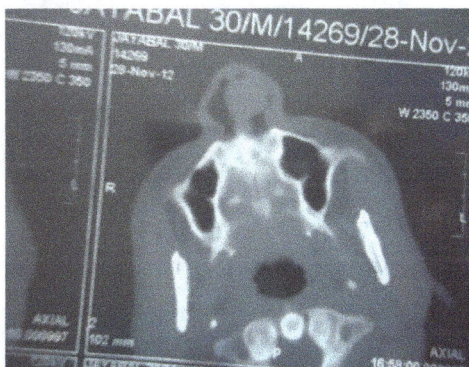

Figure 2. CT PNS axial cut.

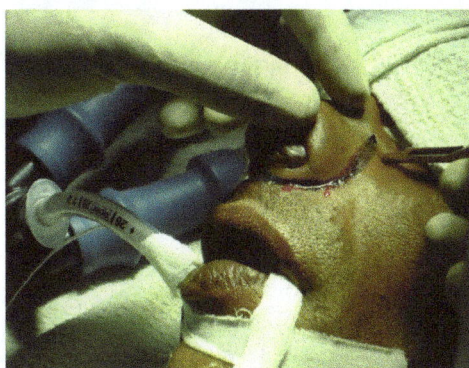

Figure 3. Lateral rhinotomy incision.

Lateral rhinotomy approach:

It was described by Moure in 1902. Incision starts under medial end of eyebrow, extending inferiorly, between medial canthus and nasal dorsum, along the deep nasal-cheek groove adjacent to nasal ala. To achieve en bloc resection, anterior nasal cavity entered through the inferior and anterior aspects of the medial wall of the maxilla. En bloc extirpation of the mass was possible because the tumour was occupying the anterior part of the nasal cavity. It was totally removed. The procedure was smooth and the patient's condition was uneventful (**Figure 4**).

The gross appearance of the specimen was yellowish white, soft, and polypoid (**Figure 5**).

Microscopically, a section showed a non-encapsulated hypercellular tumor composed of round to ovoid cells with palisading or fasicular arrangement in fibrillary background Verocay body-like structures were found in some sections Nuclear atypia was absent and the mitotic index was low (average of less than 1/10 HPF).

Immunohistochemically, the tumor cells were strongly and diffusely positive for vimentin and S-100 staining. Neuron specific enolase and smooth muscle actin stainings were focally positive. Cytokeratin, epithelial membrane antigen, and desmin staining were all negative. Therefore, benign nasal schwannoma was diagnosed.

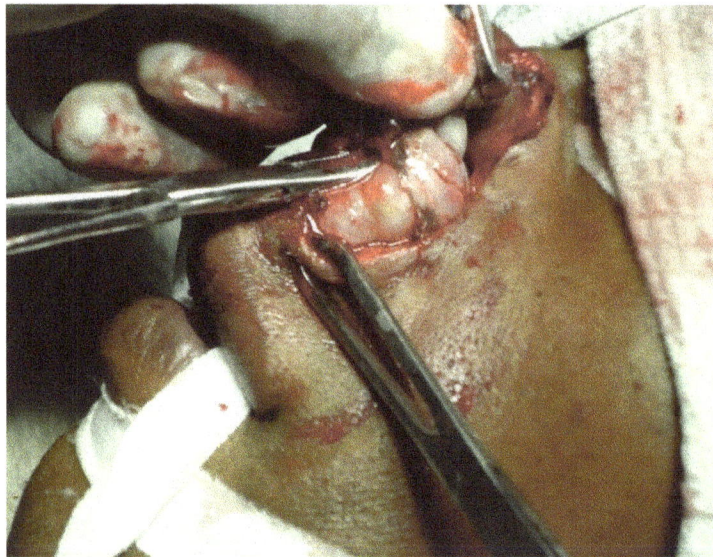

Figure 4. Intra operative picture showing the mass.

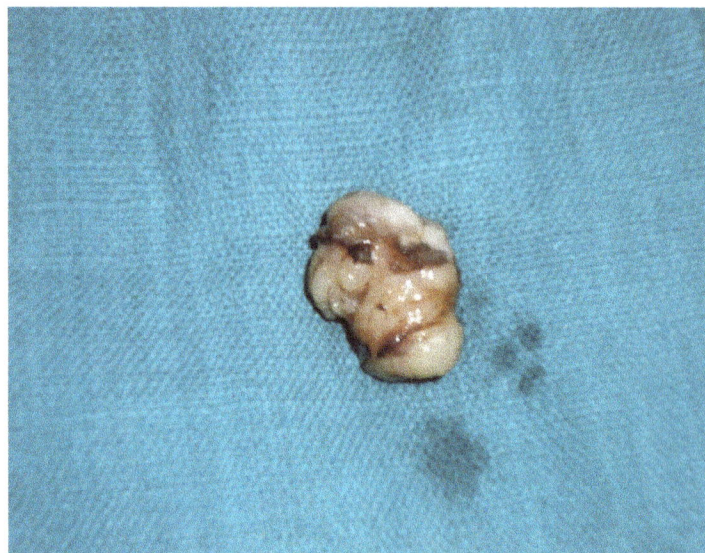

Figure 5. Exicised mass.

3. Discussion

Schwannoma is not a common tumor in the sinonasal tract. Only about 70 cases have been recorded in the literature [3]. A sinonasal schwannoma can be found in many sites, including the nasal septum, paranasal sinus, tip of the nose, turbinate, and nasopharynx [4]-[7]. The presenting symptoms of the tumor are always non-specific, depending on the site of the mass [8].

Generally, a unilateral nasal obstruction is the most common symptom, where patients usually feel a progressive unilateral nasal obstruction for a long period of time. Unilateral epistaxis is also a frequent complaint. Anosmia, painful sensation, and headache are noted because of the mass effect of the tumor [9].

Grossly, the schwannoma is usually reported to be an encapsulated mass with a smooth surface. Microscopically, Antoni A and Antoni B arrangements are diagnostic for this tumor [10]. Considering the neuro fibroma as the major differential diagnosis in this area, the typical pathological finding of proliferating spindle cells within wide-spreading keloid collagen bundles with branching vessels is not found in this case. According to one report [3], the pathological findings of schwannoma of the sinonasal tract are different from schwannomas in other regions. The differences include the loss of fibrous encapsulation and dominating hypercellularity. In this report, the pathological findings for our patient are compatible. No capsule was noted on the tumor surface. No typical Antoni B area was noted, and only interlacing weary cells with high density were found in all sections. These findings were compatible with the pathological findings of cellular schwannoma.

However, no typical fibrous capsule of cellular schwannoma was found, but a verocay body could be seen in some sections. These conflict the diagnostic criteria of cellular schwannoma [2].

On account of the hypercellular pattern of nasal schwannoma, it is always important to consider the possibility of malignancy. However, a scanty mitotic change in the average high power view may support the diagnosis of benign schwannoma. Cellular schwannoma also has a benign clinical course [2].

There was no malignant cell infiltration, which further confirmed the diagnosis of its benign nature.

Immunohistochemical stains are important in making these differentials diagnoses. Weary spindle cells are suggestive of nerve or muscle origin. Antibodies against vimentin, S-100, neuron specific enolase, smooth muscle actin, cytokeratin, epithelial membrane antigen and desmin were used. The tumor cells are strongly and diffusely positive for vimentin and S-100 stainings These are compatible with the diagnosis of either the typical or cellular schwannoma, but are not congruous with the differential diagnosis of juvenile angiofibroma, solitary fibrous tumor, hemangiopericytoma, fibroma, malignant peripheral nerve sheath tumor, or meningioma [2] [3]. Neuron specific enolase and smooth muscle actin stainings are focally positive, which revealed the possibility of a tumor of nerve or epithelial origin. However, antibodies against cytokeratin, epithelial membrane antigen, and desmin showed a negative result. Muscle origin is excluded after these stainings. These special staining patterns give a further confirmation of our diagnosis.

According to one report [3], schwannoma without a fibrous capsule has also been noted in gastric schwannoma. It is considered to be from the autonomic myenteric plexus because of the absence of a fibrous epineural sheath. Therefore, it is possible that the nasal schwannoma in our case is from autonomic nerve origin. Although the olfactory nerve is close to the location of the tumor, the lack of schwann cells in the olfactory nerve excludes this possibility.

In an overview of this case, we are reminded to include schwannoma in the clinical diagnosis when a patient presents with unilateral sinusitis and a large polyp. However, the extraordinary location, the lack of a fibrous capsule, and the presence of the Verocay body noted in this case are different from other reports [2]. Although a recurrence rate of 23% has been reported, nasal schwannoma usually has a benign clinical course [2]. Local wide excision of the tumor may be the first choice of management.

In our case, endoscopic sinus surgery was enough for removal of the tumor because of its definite origin. On account of its gigantic size and fragile consistency, en bloc resection is impossible. Complete removal is achieved by piecemeal resection. Nevertheless, considering the versatile entities of a unilateral polypoid mass, it is worthwhile to take a biopsy specimen before the operation for determining an appropriate surgical procedure. MRI evaluation before surgical exploration is recommended. Schwannoma presents as a solitary soft mass, with a high signal in the T2 weighted image in MRI. In some cases, the nerve is usually at the peripheral side of the mass [7]. These examinations promote better comprehension of the nature and the extent of the tumor. After clarification of the character and extent of the mass, endoscopic sinus surgery is enough for most benign lesions, otherwise, an external approach is the choice for unresolved cases. Finally, the findings in this case imply a possible relationship between the special pathological changes and the tumor origin, but the exact result needs further investigation.

4. Conclusion

Schwannoma is not a common tumor in the sinonasal tract. Only about 70 cases have been recorded in the literature. The presenting symptoms of the tumor are always non-specific, depending on the site of the mass. Microscopically, Antoni A and Antoni B arrangements are diagnostic for this tumor. MRI evaluation before surgical exploration is recommended. Local wide excision of the tumor may be the first choice of management.

References

[1]	Anonymous (1995) Case Records of the Massachusetts General Hospital. Weekly Clinicopathological Exercises Case 14-1995: A 12-Year-Old Boy with Progressive Nasal Obstruction. *New England Journal of Medicine*, **332**, 1285-1291. http://dx.doi.org/10.1056/NEJM199505113321908

[2]	Casadei, G.P., Scheithauer, B.W., Hirose, T., Manfrini, M., Van Houton, C. and Wood, M.B. (1995) Cellular Schwannoma. A Clinicopathologic, DNA Flow Cytometric, and Proliferation Marker Study of 70 Patients. *Cancer*, **75**, 1109-1119. http://dx.doi.org/10.1002/1097-0142(19950301)75:5<1109::AID-CNCR2820750510>3.0.CO;2-M

[3]	Hasegawa, S.L., Mentzel, T. and Fletcher, C.D.M. (1997) Schwannoma of the Sinonasal Tract and Nasopharynx. *Modern Pathology*, **10**, 777-784.

[4]	Kaufman, S.M. and Conard, L.P. (1976) Schwannoma Presenting as a Nasalpolyp. *Laryngoscope*, **86**, 595-597. http://dx.doi.org/10.1288/00005537-197604000-00017

[5]	Khalifa, M.C. and Bassyouni, A. (1981) Nasal Schwannoma. *Journal of Laryngology and Otology*, **95**, 503-507. http://dx.doi.org/10.1017/S0022215100091015

[6]	Leakos, M. and Brown, D.H. (1993) Schwannomas of the Nasal Cavity. *Journal of Otolaryngology*, **22**, 106-107.

[7]	Lemmerling, M., Moerman, M., Govaere, F., Prae, M., Kunnen, M. and Vermeersch, H. (1998) Schwannoma of the Tip of the Nose: MRI. *Neuroradiology*, **40**, 264-266. http://dx.doi.org/10.1007/s002340050582

[8]	Perzin, K.H., Panyu, H. and Wechter, S. (1982) Non-Epithelial Tumors of the Nasal Cavity, Paranasal Sinuses, and the Nasopharynx. A Clinicopathological Study, XII: Schwann Cell Tumors (Neurilemoma, Neurofibroma, Malignant Schwannoma). *Cancer*, **50**, 2193-2202. http://dx.doi.org/10.1002/1097-0142(19821115)50:10<2193::AID-CNCR2820501036>3.0.CO;2-0

[9]	Pasic, T.R. and Malielski, K. (1990) Nasal Schwannoma. *Otolaryngology—Head and Neck Surgery*, **103**, 943-946.

[10]	Verma, P.L. and Marwaha, A.R. (1970) Intranasalschwannoma. *Journal of Laryngology and Otology*, **84**, 1069-1071. http://dx.doi.org/10.1017/S002221510007287X

18

Histopathological Evidence for Irradiation Angiopathy in Head and Neck Cancer

Nobuhiro Uwa[1], Hiroyuki Hao[2], Yoshitane Tsukamoto[2], Tomonori Terada[1],
Kosuke Sagawa[1], Takeshi Mohri[1], Takashi Daimon[3], Hiroshi Doi[4], Yohei Sotsuka[5],
Guillaume van Eys[6], Marie-Luce Bochaton-Piallat[7], Seiichi Hirota[2], Masafumi Sakagami[1]

[1]Department of Otolaryngology, Hyogo College of Medicine, Nishinomiya, Japan
[2]Department of Surgical Pathology, Hyogo College of Medicine, Nishinomiya, Japan
[3]Department of Biostatistics, Hyogo College of Medicine, Nishinomiya, Japan
[4]Department of Radiology, Hyogo College of Medicine, Nishinomiya, Japan
[5]Department of Plastic Surgery, Hyogo College of Medicine, Nishinomiya, Japan
[6]Department of Genetics and Cell Biology, University of Maastricht, Maastricht, The Netherlands
[7]Department of Pathology and Immunology, University of Geneva-CMU, Geneva, Switzerland
Email: nobu-uwa@hyo-med.ac.jp

Abstract

Objective: To evaluate the incidence of cervical angiopathy caused by radiation therapy for head and neck cancer. Methods: Segments of 57 cervical arteries were obtained during surgery for head and neck malignant tumors and divided into two groups (irradiated group and non-irradiated group) based on the treatment prior to vascular resection. In order to evaluate vascular injury after radiation therapy, we examined the degree of medial atrophy, medial fibrosis, smooth muscle cell (SMC) differentiation in the media and intima, intimal hyperplasia and endothelial cell (EC) injury. Sections of arterial segments were stained with hematoxylin-eosin, Elastica van Gieson and Masson's trichrome, and immunohistochemistry for α-smooth muscle actin (α-SMA), smoothelin, S100A4 and CD31 in the resected vessels was conducted. Results: The median interval between the completion of radiation therapy and vascular resection was nine months. No significant differences were observed between the two groups in terms of medial atrophy, medial fibrosis and intimal hyperplasia. The ratio of the smoothelin-positive area per α-SMA-positive area in the media and the S100A4-positive proportion in the intima, indicating the degree of differentiation of the medial SMC and dedifferentiation of the intimal SMC, respectively, showed no significant differences, despite the tendency toward a lower smoothelin-positive area per α-SMA-positive area in the media of the irradiated arteries. The EC coverage revealed on CD31 immunohistochemistry was significantly decreased, with mural thrombus adhesion, in the irradiated group. Conclusions: The ECs of small arteries are damaged by irradiation. Although we did not confirm the statistical significance of medial SMC dedifferentiation, a decreased expression of smoothelin tended to be observed in the media of the irradiated arteries. Our findings provide histopathological evidence of irradiation angiopathy in head and neck cancer and may help to improve the surgical safety of microvascular anastomosis and determine the treatment strategy for head and neck tumors.

Keywords

Angiopathy, Endothlial Cell, Pathology, Radiation, Head and Neck

---

1. Introduction

Radiotherapy and/or chemoradiotherapy are often conducted as the initial treatment for head and neck cancer, with a focus on achieving functional preservation. However, in cases in which the tumors are not successfully treated with these approaches, the patient may be exposed to various postoperative complications after salvage surgery [1]. Moreover, in many cases of advanced head and neck cancer, microvascular free tissue transfer is essential for performing functional reconstruction after tumor resection. Although this technique is reliable for achieving head and neck reconstruction, with a success rate of 90% - 99% [2], necrosis of the transferred tissues, a severe complication of this procedure, may occur in cases involving occlusion of the anastomotic vessels. In the setting of microvascular anastomosis, the irradiated vessels reportedly display an increased incidence of thrombosis [3], whereas other reports have suggested that previous radiation therapy has no effect on the success rate for microvascular reconstruction [4] [5]. Therefore, the influence of radiotherapy on cervical vascular anastomosis has not yet been fully elucidated. In this study, immunohistochemistry for α-smooth muscle actin (α-SMA), smoothelin, S100A4 and CD31 was performed to evaluate the incidence of radiation angiopathy. It is known that α-SMA is widely expressed in vascular smooth muscle cells (SMCs) at various degrees of differentiation. On the other hand, smoothelin is expressed in a subset of differentiated SMCs [6], and S100A4 is expressed in dedifferentiated SMCs [7]. Additionally, CD31 is an established marker of vascular endothelial cells (ECs). For the purpose of improving the safety and clinical outcomes of treatment for head and neck cancer, we pathologically evaluated cervical vessels resected during head and neck surgery and examined the influence of irradiation on the cervical vessels.

2. Materials and Methods

2.1. Cases

Among cases of head and neck surgery performed at Hyogo College of Medicine in the period from May 2012 to August 2014, we resected recipient vessels for microvascular anastomosis or dissected segments of the vessels for malignant tumor resection in 62 cases. Of the 62 cases, we examined 57 cases (49 males, eight females; age range: 33 to 89 years old) for which accurate pathological findings were available. The primary tumor site was the hypopharynx in 18 cases, oral cavity in 13 cases, larynx in six cases, thyroid in five cases, esophagus in five cases, oropharynx in four cases, nasopharynx in two cases, nasal cavity in one case and sublingual gland in one case. Two cases of primary unknown neck cancer were included.

The vessels were thoroughly and carefully resected. The resected vessels were the superior thyroid artery in 32 cases, facial artery in 17 cases, lingual artery in four cases, transverse cervical artery in three cases and maxillary artery in one case. Of the 57 cases, the resected vessels in 11 cases were located within the irradiation field for previous radiotherapy. Based on the information for the anatomical sites and radiotherapy, the absorbed dose in the resected vessels was calculated and determined by both an otolaryngologist and radiation oncologist.

All patients provided their written informed consent. The ethics committee of our hospital granted approval for this study (approval number 1778).

2.2. Histological and Immunohistochemical Examinations

Segments of the cervical artery removed via surgery were fixed with 10% buffered formalin and embedded in paraffin. The specimens were cut into 3-μm-thick sections and stained with hematoxylin-eosin (HE), Elastica van Gieson (EVG) and Masson's trichrome (MT). The following mouse monoclonal antibodies were used for immunohistochemistry: anti-α-SMA (clone 1A4, DAKO, Glostrup, Denmark, 1:500 dilution), anti-smoothelin (clone R4A, produced by the Department of Genetics and Cell Biology, University of Maastricht, 1:10 dilution) [8], anti-S100A4 (clone 4B4 produced by the Department of Pathology and Immunology, University of Geneva, 1:20 dilution) [7] and anti-CD31 antibodies (clone JC70A, DAKO, 1:300 dilution). Heat-induced epitope retrieval was routinely performed. The sections were stained using an automated staining system (BOND-MAX-III, Leica Microsystems GmbH, Wetzlar, Germany). A morphometrical analysis was performed using the Image Analyze System equipped with a digital camera (Microscope System DP71. Olympus Co., Tokyo, Japan) and software program (Winroof, Mitani Co., Fukui, Japan) in each case.

The ratio of the medial thickness per total wall thickness on EVG and the blue-stained area on MT per medial area in each high-power field (×400) were evaluated as indicators of medial atrophy and medial fibrosis, respectively. The ratio of smoothelin-positive area per α-SMA positive area in the media was also calculated as an indicator of the medial SMC phenotype. In order to examine the degree of intimal hyperplasia of the cervical arteries, the ratio of the maximum intimal thickness per thickness of the underlying media was calculated using EVG. Immunohistochemistry for S100A4 was performed to detect the dedifferentiated SMC population in the intima. The highest S100A4 expression area per intimal area in each high-power field (×400) was calculated. Moreover, immunohistochemistry for CD31 was applied to evaluate the degree of luminal EC coverage. The EC coverage was classified into three grades: more than 2/3 of luminal EC coverage as Grade A, less than 1/3 as Grade C and between Grade A and Grade C as Grade B (**Figure 1**).

The histological and immunohistochemical examinations were conducted by a pathologist (H.H.) and otolaryngologist (N.U.) without any clinical information for the specimens.

2.3. Statistical Analysis

Continuous variables are summarized as the mean and standard deviation and categorical variables are expressed as frequencies with proportions. Continuous, unordered and ordered variables were compared using the t-test with Welch's correction, Fisher's exact test and the Mann-Whitney U test, respectively. All p values were two-sided, and a p value of <0.05 was considered to be statistically significant. The statistical analyses were performed using the R program (version 3.1.1).

3. Results

The 57 patients were divided into two groups, the irradiated (IR, n = 11) and non-irradiated (non-IR, n = 46) groups, according to the previous therapy prior to vessel resection. The absorbed dose in the resected vessels in the IR group was 50.3 to 72.9 Gy, with a mean dose of 61.8 Gy. Seven patients (63.6%) underwent radiotherapy with concurrent intravenous chemotherapy, whereas four patients (36.4%) received radiotherapy alone. The interval between the completion of radiotherapy and vascular resection was one to 108 months, with a median interval of nine months.

The clinical characteristics including atherosclerotic risk factors were compared between the IR and non-IR groups, and there were no significant differences between the two groups (**Table 1**).

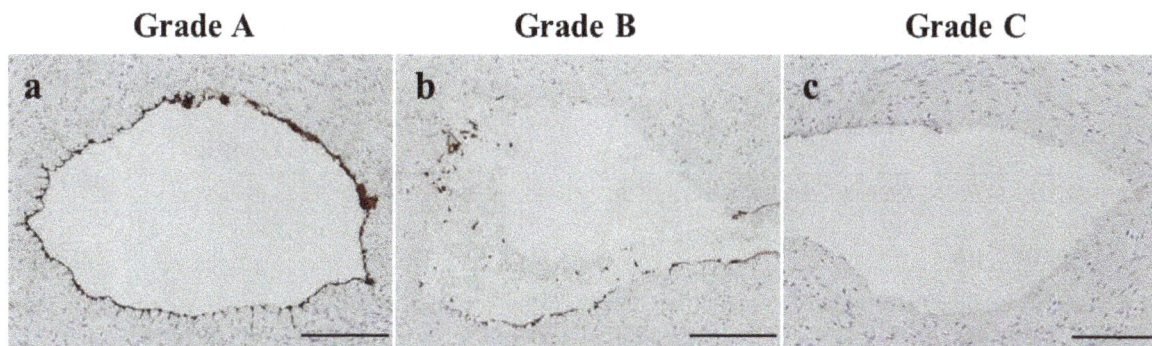

Figure 1. Classification of endothelial cell coverage using immunohistochemistry for CD31. The degree of endothelial cell coverage was classified into three grades: more than 2/3 of luminal endothelial cell coverage as Grade A (a), less than 1/3 as Grade C (c) and between Grade A and Grade C as Grade B (b). (a)-(c): Scale bar = 200 µm.

Although the IR group and non-IR group showed similar medial thickness and fibrosis proportion values (**Table 2**), a tendency toward a lower smoothelin-positive area per α-SMA-positive area in the media was observed in the IR group (**Table 2** and **Figure 2**). Few S100A4-positive cells were observed in the media of the IR group. The degree of intimal hyperplasia and S100A4-positive proportion in the intima showed no significant differences between the two groups (**Table 2**). Although more than 2/3 luminal EC coverage was observed in most cases in the non-IR group (44/46), specimens with less than 2/3 EC coverage were predominantly identified in the IR group (7/11, **Table 2**). A lack of EC coverage (**Figure 3(a)**) induced mural thrombus formation (**Figure 3(b)** and **Figure 3(c)**) in almost half of the IR group arteries (6/11, 54.5%). The thrombus consisted of various components, such as fibrin and platelet. There were no signs of artery occlusion due to thrombus formation in the specimens.

Table 1. Clinical characteristics of the 57 patients analyzed in this study.

		IR	Non-IR	p value
Gender	M	9 (81.8)	40 (87.0)	
	F	2 (18.2)	6 (13.0)	0.644
Age		66.09 ± 6.20	68.07 ± 12.59	0.459
Smoking history		10 (90.9)	33 (71.7)	0.261
Hypertension		7 (63.6)	17 (37.0)	0.173
Diabetes mellitus		2 (18.2)	10 (21.7)	1
Dyslipidemia		1 (9.1)	4 (8.7)	1
Renal failure		0 (0)	1 (2.2)	1
Intake of anticoagulant		1 (9.1)	4 (8.7)	1
Surgical history of vascular resection site		2 (18.2)	1 (2.2)	0.092

M: male, F: female, IR: irradiated. The proportion of patients in each group is shown in the brackets.

Table 2. Morphometrical analysis of the cervical arteries.

		IR	Non-IR	p value
Media				
Medial thickness/total wall thickness		0.76 ± 0.12	0.76 ± 0.15	0.964
Fibrosis proportion		54.4% ± 16.7%	54.9% ± 18.3%	0.943
Smoothelin-positive area/α-SMA-positive area		0.25 ± 0.22	0.37 ± 0.24	0.144
Intima				
Intimal thickness/medial thickness		0.34 ± 0.21	0.39 ± 0.43	0.572
S100A4-positive proportion		6.7% ± 7.1%	8.6% ± 7.7%	0.455
EC coverage	Grade A	4 (36.4)	44 (95.7)	
	Grade B	4 (36.4)	1 (2.2)	
	Grade C	3 (27.3)	1 (2.2)	p < 0.0001

IR: irradiated, α-SMA: α-smooth muscle actin, EC: endothelial cell. The proportion of patients in each group is shown in the brackets.

4. Discussion

A previous pathological study of radiation angiopathy using scanning electron microscopy demonstrated thickening of the vascular wall and intimal injury in irradiated arteries [9]. In addition, Schultze-Mosgau et al. [10] observed hyaline deposition and medial atrophy in patients who underwent radiotherapy with an absorbed dose of 60 - 70 Gy. Furthermore, irradiated mice gradually develop intimal thickness over time [11], and individuals treated with radiotherapy more than five years previously have a significantly higher rate of carotid artery stenosis

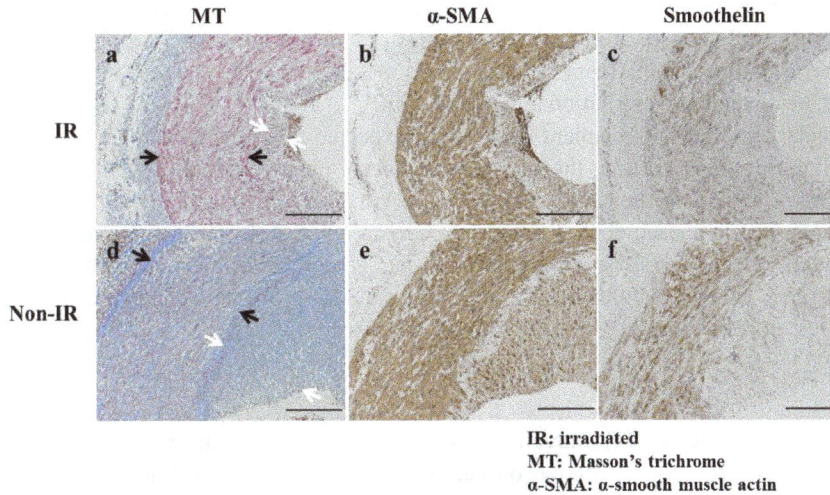

IR: irradiated
MT: Masson's trichrome
α-SMA: α-smooth muscle actin

Figure 2. Evaluation of medial fibrosis using Masson's trichrome and the degree of differentiation of medial smooth muscle cells using immunohistochemistry for α-smooth muscle actin and smoothelin. Representative images of Masson's trichrome, α-smooth muscle actin and smoothelin in the irradiated cases (a)-(c) and non-irradiated cases (d)-(f) are shown. The black arrows indicate the media. The white allows indicate the intima. (a)-(f): Scale bar = 200 μm).

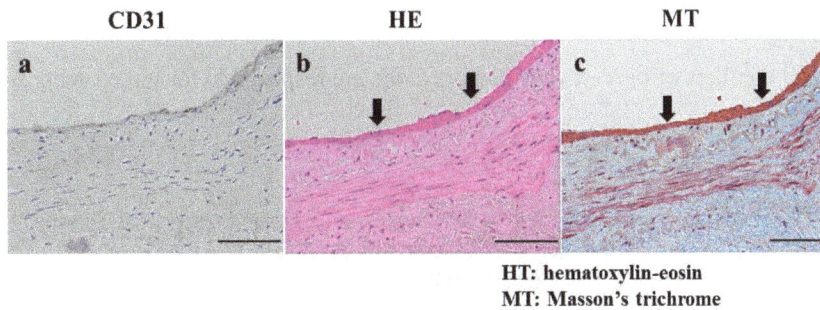

HT: hematoxylin-eosin
MT: Masson's trichrome

Figure 3. Lack of endothelial cell coverage with mural fibrin thrombus formation. CD31 immunohistochemistry revealed a lack of endothelial cells (a). Serial sections of CD31 immunohistochemistry stained with hematoxylin-eosin (b) and Masson's trichrome (c) demonstrated mural fibrin thrombus formation. The arrows indicate mural fibrin thrombus. (a)-(c): Scale bar = 100 μm).

than those with less than five years of follow-up [12]. Although the present study showed no significant differences between the IR and non-IR groups with regard to medial atrophy and fibrosis, the distribution of differentiated SMC in the media showed a tendency to be lower in the IR group, without statistical significance. This result may be derived from the relatively small number of cases in the IR group, and we believe that a larger number of cases in the IR group would have resulted in a significant difference. The phenotypic modulation of SMCs without atrophy and fibrosis of the media in the IR group may be correlated with the short interval between the completion of radiotherapy and vascular resection. There were no significant differences in the intimal thickness or distribution of the dedifferentiated SMC population in the intima between the two groups, yet the EC coverage was significantly decreased in the IR group. Angiopathy is mainly considered to be a delayed type of radiation injury. Small arteries are fairly rigid structures in comparison to capillaries and arterioles, and thus early changes after irradiation tend to be less pronounced [13]. However, it is also known that ECs are sensitive and damaged in the initial process of radiation-induced angiopathy [13]-[15]. Furthermore, Menendez *et al*. [16] reported that endothelial damage occurs almost immediately after irradiation by decreasing the synthesis of endothelial nitric oxide, which protects the vascular wall. Medial atrophy, intimal thickening and fibrosis of the vascular wall are considered to occur thereafter. This study clearly shows that radiation therapy for head and neck cancer is responsible for the initial changes associated with radiation angiopathy, as confirmed based on the lack of CD31-positive ECs with mural thrombus adhesion. Further examinations should be conducted with an increased number of patients and a longer interval. This makes it possible to evaluate the degree of SMC differentiation during the development radiation angiopathy.

Gradual neovascularization of the recipient bed may be expected after microvascular free tissue transfer [17]. Therefore, preventing thrombosis during the postoperative acute phase is of greatest importance in the clinical setting. Various factors, including the surgical skills of the surgeon, vascular diameter and vascular flow, contribute to the success of microvascular free tissue transfer. In addition to these risk factors, the current study shows that irradiation may be a risk factor for thrombosis. Therefore, in patients with a history of radiation therapy, careful surgery and the administration of appropriate medications for preventing vascular occlusion play an important role in achieving successful microvascular anastomosis.

5. Conclusion

In this study, a significant decrease in EC coverage was observed in the irradiated cervical vessels. By providing information about the influence of irradiation on cervical vessels, the current findings may contribute to improving the surgical safety of microvascular anastomosis as well as determining the treatment strategy.

Acknowledgements

We would like to acknowledge all medical laboratory technologists at the Department of Surgical Pathology, Hyogo College of Medicine for their technical assistance. This study was supported by a Grant-in-Aid for Researchers, Hyogo College of Medicine, 2012 for N.U. and 2007 for H.H.

Declaration of Interest

The authors report no conflicts of interest. The authors alone are responsible for the contents and writing of the paper.

References

[1]   Sassler, A.M., Esclamado, R.M. and Wolf, G.T. (1995) Surgery after Organ Preservation Therapy. Analysis of Wound Complications. *Archives of Otolaryngology—Head and Neck Surgery*, **121**, 162-165. http://dx.doi.org/10.1001/archotol.1995.01890020024006

[2]   Kruse, A.L., Luebbers, H.T., Grätz, K.W. and Obwegeser, J.A. (2010) Factors Influencing Survival of Free-Flap in Reconstruction for Cancer of the Head and Neck: A Literature Review. *Microsurgery*, **30**, 242-248.

[3]   Krag, C., De Rose, G., Lyczakowski, T., Freeman, C.R. and Shapiro, S.H. (1982) Free Flaps and Irradiated Recipient Vessels: An Experimental Study in Rabbits. *British Journal of Plastic Surgery*, **35**, 328-336. http://dx.doi.org/10.1016/0007-1226(82)90122-9

[4]   Kiener, J.L., Hoffman, W.Y. and Mathes, S.J. (1991) Influence of Radiotherapy on Microvascular Reconstruction in the Head and Neck Region. *American Journal of Surgery*, **162**, 404-407. http://dx.doi.org/10.1016/0002-9610(91)90159-B

[5]   Klug, C., Berzaczy, D., Reinbacher, H., Voracek, M., Rath, T., Millesi, W. and Ewers, R. (2006) Influence of Previous Radiotherapy on Free Tissue Transfer in the Head and Neck Region: Evaluation of 455 Cases. *Laryngoscope*, **116**, 1162-1167. http://dx.doi.org/10.1097/01.mlg.0000227796.41462.a1

[6]   Hao, H., Gabbiani, G., Camenzind, E., Bacchetta, M., Virmani, R. and Bochaton-Piallat, M.L. (2006) Phenotypic Modulation of Intima and Media Smooth Muscle Cells in Fatal Cases of Coronary Artery Lesion. *Arteriosclerosis, Thrombosis, and Vascular Biology*, **26**, 326-332. http://dx.doi.org/10.1161/01.ATV.0000199393.74656.4c

[7]   Brisset, A.C., Hao, H., Camenzind, E., Bacchetta, M., Geinoz, A., Sanchez, J.C., Chaponnier, C., Gabbiani, G. and Bochaton-Piallat, M.L. (2007) Intimal Smooth Muscle Cells of Porcine and Human Coronary Artery Express S100A4, a Marker of the Rhomboid Phenotype *in Vitro*. *Circulation Research*, **100**, 1055-1062. http://dx.doi.org/10.1161/01.RES.0000262654.84810.6c

[8]   van der Loop, F.T., Schaart, G., Timmer, E.D., Ramaekers, F.C. and van Eys, G.J. (1996) Smoothelin, a Novel Cytoskeletal Protein Specific for Smooth Muscle Cells. *Journal of Cell Biology*, **134**, 401-411. http://dx.doi.org/10.1083/jcb.134.2.401

[9]   Guelinckx, P.J., Boeckx, W.D., Fossion, E. and Gruwez, J.A. (1984) Scanning Electron Microscopy of Irradiated Re-

cipient Blood Vessels in Head and Neck Free Flaps. *Plastic and Reconstructive Surgery*, **74**, 217-226. http://dx.doi.org/10.1097/00006534-198408000-00008

[10] Schultze-Mosgau, S., Erbe, M., Keilholz, L., Radespiel-Tröger, M., Wiltfang, J., Minge, N. and Neukam, F.W. (2000) Histomorphometric Analysis of Irradiated Recipient Vessels and Transplant Vessels of Free Flaps in Patients Undergoing Reconstruction after Ablative Surgery. *International Journal of Oral and Maxillofacial Surgery*, **29**, 112-118. http://dx.doi.org/10.1016/S0901-5027(00)80007-7

[11] Doi, H., Kamikonya, N., Takada, Y., Fujiwara, M., Tsuboi, K., Miura, H., Inoue, H., Tanooka, M., Nakamura, T., Shikata, T., Kimura, T., Tsujimura, T. and Hirota, S. (2012) Long-Term Sequential Changes of Radiation Proctitis and Angiopathy in Rats. *Journal of Radiation Research*, **53**, 217-224. http://dx.doi.org/10.1269/jrr.11075

[12] Cheng, S.W., Wu, L.L., Ting, A.C., Lau, H., Lam, L.K. and Wei, W.I. (1999) Irradiation-Induced Extracranial Carotid Stenosis in Patients with Head and Neck Malignancies. *American Journal of Surgery*, **178**, 323-328. http://dx.doi.org/10.1016/S0002-9610(99)00184-1

[13] Damjanov, I. and Linder, J. (1996) Anderson's Pathology. 10th Edition, Mosby, New York, 496-499.

[14] Murros, K.E. and Toole, J.F. (1989) The Effect of Radiation on Carotid Arteries. A Review Article. *Archives of Neurology*, **46**, 449-455. http://dx.doi.org/10.1001/archneur.1989.00520400109029

[15] Fonkalsrud, E.W., Sanchez, M., Zerubavel, R. and Mahoney, A. (1977) Serial Changes in Arterial Structure Following Radiation Therapy. *Surgery, Gynecology & Obstetrics*, **145**, 395-400.

[16] Menendez, J.C., Casanova, D., Amado, J.A., Salas, E., García-Unzueta, M.T., Fernandez, F., de la Lastra, L.P. and Berrazueta, J.R. (1998) Effects of Radiation on Endothelial Function. *International Journal of Radiation Oncology Biology Physics*, **41**, 905-913. http://dx.doi.org/10.1016/S0360-3016(98)00112-6

[17] Wise, S.R., Harsha, W.J., Kim, N. and Hayden, R.E. (2011) Free Flap Survival Despite Early Loss of the Vascular Pedicle. *Head and Neck*, **33**, 1068-1071.

19

Intratympanic Injections: An Unsolved Mystery

Kartik Parelkar, Vandana Thorawade, Mohan Jagade, Smita Nagle, Rajanala Nataraj, Madhavi Pandare, Reshma Hanwate, Bandu Nagrale, Kiran Kulsange, Devkumar Rangaraja, Arpita Singhal

Department of ENT, Grant Government Medical College & Sir J.J. Group of Hospitals, Mumbai, India
Email: kartikparelkar@ymail.com

Abstract

Aims: The aim of this study was to test the effectiveness of intratympanic dexamethasone injections as a treatment for severe disabling tinnitus and also observe its effect on hearing loss if any. **Materials and Methods:** Thirty patients with severe disabling tinnitus in the age group 20 to 60 years were selected and randomly assigned to receive intratympanic injections of a dexamethasone solution 4 mg/ml (0.5 ml) or isotonic saline (0.5 ml) solution under topical anaesthesia, once per week for 4 weeks using a zero degree endoscope. Improvement in tinnitus was assessed using a visual analog scale, considering 2-point improvement as significant and alteration in hearing if any was noted by pure tone audiometery before and after the therapy. **Results:** The improvement in tinnitus was not significant, with no alteration in audiometery reports. **Conclusions:** Intratympanic therapy is an attractive mode of treatment because of its highly targeted delivery, low concentration of the drugs required and a very good patient tolerance. Although there has been no breakthrough in intratympanic therapy for tinnitus or other otological conditions, accessibility to the inner ear through the semipermeable round window membrane holds many promises in the near future.

Keywords

Intratympanic Injection, Round Window, Tinnitus, Dexamethasone

1. Introduction

One of the principal advantages of intratympanic (IT) therapy is the ability to deliver therapeutic concentrations of the drug in a highly targeted fashion to the inner ear, thus avoiding systemic side effects.

Diffusion occurs across the round window membrane (RWM) into the cochlea, driven by the concentration gradient between the middle ear and the perilymph-filled scala tympani. The diffusion rate is determined by various factors, such as size, configuration, concentration, liposolubility and electrical charge of the active substance, as well as by the thickness of the RWM [1].

A cochleostomy for direct drug delivery entails a substantial risk of permanent damage, whereas RWM provides an attractive gateway to the inner ear. It consists of three layers: an outer epithelium facing the middle ear, a core of connective tissue, and an inner-ear epithelium bordering the inner ear [2].

Compared with IT doses, much higher systemic doses are required when action is intended on the inner ear which is an end organ with blood brain barrier [3].

In 1996, Sakata et al. treated 1214 patients who had tinnitus by infusing dexamethasone solution into their middle ear. The authors reported good overall results in 77% of the ears immediately after the treatment and in 68% after 6 months [4].

In 2000, Shulman and Goldstein treated 10 patients having tinnitus with intratympanic dexamethasone injections [5]. Five patients experienced tinnitus control for at least 1 year and 2 had tinnitus control for only a few hours. Three patients experienced no improvement.

In 2002, Cesarani et al. described 54 patients treated with intratympanic dexamethasone injections [6]. Of these patients, 34% experienced complete resolution of tinnitus, 40% experienced significant improvement, and 26% experienced no change.

However, it should be noted that placebo effect is very high with tinnitus and having a control group is essential. Hence, we conducted this study and would like to report our experience regarding IT therapy for refractory tinnitus.

2. Methodology

Patients having severe disabling tinnitus (SDT) for at least 6 months, refractory to medical line of management in the age group of 20 to 60 years were selected from the ENT out patient department at the Grant Government Medical College and J.J. Group of Hospitals, Mumbai.

Study was conducted from July to December 2014, however it is an ongoing study and we intend to try different molecules for management of refractory tinnitus via the intratympanic route.

Patients with sensorineural, mixed and conductive hearing loss were all included and their pure tone audiogram findings noted prior to the study. Patients with h/o trauma to the ear and carcinomas were excluded from the study.

Detailed history taking, otomicroscopic examination and audiologic testing were also performed to identify the presence of otological diseases associated with the symptom of tinnitus apart from the hearing loss.

The patients were given a specific tinnitus questionnaire regarding: tinnitus duration, ear affected, subjective hearing loss, description of the sound heard and known otologic diseases/previous treatments. The patients were then asked to indicate the intensity of tinnitus on a visual analog scale graded from 1 to 10 (1 was low and 10 was an unbearable level of intensity). Informed consent was obtained from all patients.

The patients were then randomly assigned to receive 0.5-ml IT injection of either a 4-mg/ml dexamethasone solution or isotonic saline. They were placed in a supine position with their heads turned about 45° towards the unaffected ear. Topical anaesthesia of the tympanic membrane was administered using 10 percent lignocaine spray, complete clearance of which was done using suction after 2 to 3 minutes. Using a 2 ml syringe and a 26-gauge one and half inch needle, the assigned solution was injected under direct vision using a zero degree endoscope in the postero-inferior quadrant of the tympanic membrane (**Figure 1** and **Figure 2**). Each patient remained for about 30 minutes in the described position. Four injections were performed, 1 per week for 4 weeks.

In case of Meniere's disease grommet insertion was done and IT therapy was given through the grommet.

After finishing the treatment, the patients indicated, on the visual analog scale, the level of tinnitus intensity following the treatment. We considered that improvement was significant when a lowering of at least 2 points on the visual analog scale was reported.

Also patients pure tone audiometery was repeated after completion of the therapy. Five patients who started treatment were excluded from analysis (3 from the study group and 2 from the control group) because they did not complete treatment or failed to return for follow-up. Of the 25 patients who remained, 5 had both ears treated. Thus, a total of 30 ears were treated and evaluated.

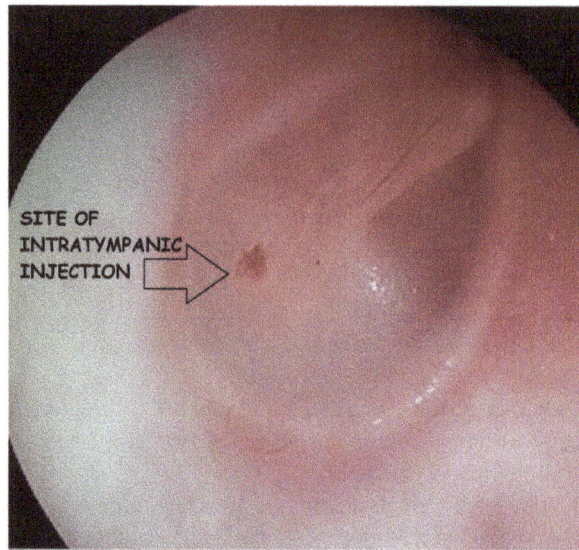

Figure 1. Site of injection showing a blood clot as a result of previous injection.

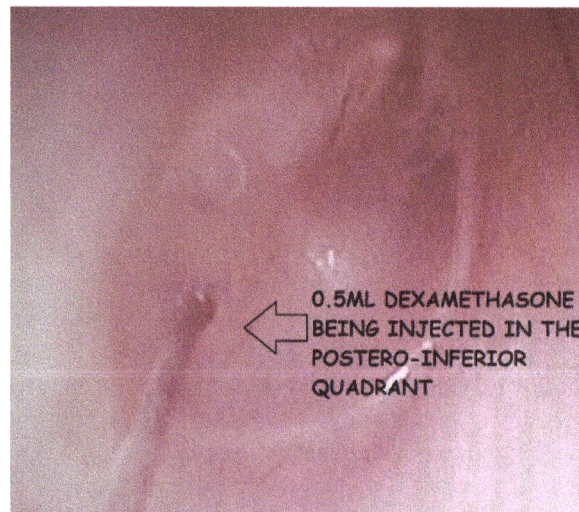

Figure 2. IT injection.

3. Results

From the data provided in **Tables 1-3**; ×2 test (with a significance level of 0.05) showed no significant difference between the groups regarding sex, age and laterality of the tinnitus (**Tables 4-6** respectively). There was no significant difference between the results of treatment with a dexamethasone solution and treatment with a saline solution (**Table 7**). There was no change in the hearing levels before and after treatment as per the pure tone audiogram reports in both the groups.

4. Discussion

The fact that intratympanic therapy was first used for tinnitus and not Meniere's has probably been forgotten.

Harold Schuknecht proposed the use of streptomycin in Meniere's disease as an alternative to surgical labyrinthine ablation in 1956 [7]. 5% ethylmorphine hydrochloride, was used for intratympanic injections in cases of tinnitus by Trowbridge. He treated 20 patients and claimed complete tinnitus relief in 11 of them, partial improvement in seven and no change in the remaining two [8] [9].

Table 1. Gives the otologic diagnosis for the 30 ears, with the number and percentage of ears with each diagnosis.

Diagnosis	Ears No.	Percentage %
Presbyacusis	10	33%
Idiopathic	8	27%
CSOM	4	13%
Menieres disease	2	7%
Otosclerosis	2	7%
NIHL	2	7%
Ototoxicity	1	3%
Sudden deafness	1	3%

CSOM: chronic suppurative otitis media. NIHL: noise induced hearing loss.

Table 2. Gives the otologic diagnoses in the 16 ears of the study group (who received 0.5 ml dexamethasone).

Patients No.	Sex/age	Side of symptom	Visual analog scale score		Complications	Diagnosis
			Pre-treatment	Post-treatment		
1	M/53	R	8	7	-	Presbyacusis
2	M/47	L	6	6	-	Presbyacusis
3	M/60	L	7	5*	Vertigo	Presbyacusis
4	M/60	R	7	5*	Vertigo	Presbyacusis
5	F/55	L	7	7	-	Presbyacusis
6	F/55	R	7	7	-	Presbyacusis
7	F/32	R	6	6	-	Idiopathic
8	M/22	L	8	8	-	Idiopathic
9	M/27	L	6	5	Vertigo	Idiopathic
10	M/27	R	6	5	Vertigo	Idiopathic
11	M/45	L	7	6	-	CSOM
12	M/35	R	7	7	-	CSOM
13	M/42	L	7	7	-	Menieres d.
14	M/30	R	6	5	-	NIHL
15	F/43	R	6	6	-	SSNHL
16	F/36	L	8	6*	-	Otosclerosis

M: male; F: female; R: right ear; L: left ear. CSOM: chronic supppurative otitis media; NIHL: noise induced hearing loss; SSNHL: sudden sensory neural hearing loss. *Significant improvement in tinnitus. Mean score improvement is 0.62. Mean of pre-treatment score is 6.81. Mean of post-treatment score is 6.12.

Lidocaine was tested in the treatment of Meniere's disease by way of systemic administration [10] [11]. Following which, in the 1970s, Eiji Sakata administered lidocaine and dexamethasone intratympanically [10] [12]. However lignocaine had an unacceptable vertigo as its side-effect.

Table 3. Gives the otologic diagnoses in the 14 ears of the control group (who received 0.5 ml saline).

Patients No.	Sex/age	Side of symptom	Visual analog scale score		Complications	Diagnosis
			Pre-treatment	Post-treatment		
1	M/55	L	7	5*	-	Presbyacusis
2	M/55	R	7	5*	-	Presbyacusis
3	F/52	R	6	6	-	Presbyacusis
4	M/60	R	7	7	-	Presbyacusis
5	F/32	L	5	5	Vertigo	Idiopathic
6	F/32	R	5	5	Vertigo	Idiopathic
7	M/27	R	8	5*	-	Idiopathic
8	F/22	L	7	6	-	Idiopathic
9	M/33	R	7	7	-	Idiopathic
10	M/47	L	6	6	-	CSOM
11	M/35	R	8	6*	-	CSOM
12	M/40	L	7	6	-	Menieres d.
13	M/40	R	5	5	Vertigo	Ototoxicity
14	M/34	L	6	5	-	NIHL

M: male; F: female; R: right ear; L: left ear. CSOM: chronic supppurative otitis media; NIHL: noise induced hearing loss; *Significant improvement in tinnitus. Mean score improvement is 0.83. Mean of pre-treatment score is 6.58. Mean of post-treatment score is 5.75.

Table 4. Sex.

Test	Value	df	p-value	Association is
Pearson chi-square	11.04	1	0.13	Not significant
Fisher's exact test	9.76		0.16	

Table 5. Age.

Test	Value	df	p-value	Association is
Pearson chi-square	17.50	9	0.393	Not significant
Fisher's exact test	16.67		0.479	

Table 6. Laterality.

Test	Value	df	p-value	Association is
Pearson chi-square	8.09	1	0.573	Not significant
Fisher's exact test	7.16		0.705	

Table 7. Treatment.

Test	Value	df	p-value	Association is
Pearson chi-square	32.86	6	0.77	Not significant
Fisher's exact test	40.18		0.44	

There are different methods of IT injections. Tympanopunction *i.e.* Direct injection of the drug into the middle ear or myringotomy first followed by endoscopic examination of round window region followed by injection [13] [14]. In our study tympanopunction was done and a slow and steady injection was found to be a feasible mode of delivering the drug.

Actually, about 5 µl is usually sufficient to fill the entire round window niche [15]. In IT therapy concentration of the drug and the duration for which it stays over the RWM is more important than the volume [16]. Injected volumes in published studies range from <0.3 ml [17] to 1 ml [18] [19] at the higher end.

Even in sudden deafness a high-rate of spontaneous recovery of hearing loss and accompanying tinnitus is a hallmark, which necessitates appropriate controls and there is still a lack of clear evidence of a therapeutic benefit of steroids with regard to tinnitus [20] [21].

In a placebo-controlled, double-blind crossover study in 20 patients with unilateral Meniere's disease, three consecutive daily i.t. injections of dexamethasone in a hyaluronate formulation showed no better effect on tinnitus than a placebo [22].

Simple placement of ventilation tube with no additional therapy has been reported in control of vertigo in many patients with menieres disease to a degree similar to endolymphatic sac surgery [23] [24]. Hence in our study, for patients with Meniere's disease grommet insertion was done and IT injections were given through the ventilation tube. These patients however didn't show significant improvement in tinnitus or other symptoms of the disease per se.

Other than steroids, i.v. administration of caroverine, has been tried [22] [25] but has failed. The compound has also been tried in form of local ear drops with claimed improvement of tinnitus [26].

AM-101, an NDMA receptor antagonist formulated in a hyaluronic acid gel, showed good tolerance and improvement in tinnitus status [17]. An open trial with IT administration of pilocarpine and carbachol showed a transient effect on the tinnitus [27].

RWM thickness (on average 70 µm) and, especially, its size varies widely in humans [2] and in some cases, its covered by an "false" membrane or by fibrous or fatty plugs within the niche itself [28]. False membranes are sometimes perforated or reticular [29]. Magnetic resonance imaging studies have shown no round window permeability in 5% of ears, and poor permeability in 13% [30].

Also animal data has shown basal-apical concentration differences of over 1000-fold [16]. While direct determination of the gradient in a human cochlea is not feasible, it has been estimated in a computer-based simulation for IT gentamicin at around 100:1 (basal to apical levels) [31].

Since the sampling of inner ear fluids places hearing at risk [32]. Three studies with patients undergoing cochlear implantation, labyrinthectomy or translabyrinthine surgery found that perilymph concentrations varied significantly following IT injections of methylprednisolone [18], dexamethasone [33] or gentamicin [34].

Formulations or devices that ensure retention at RWM are preferable. This may be achieved by injecting viscous gel formulations, or by placing wicks, microcatheters [35] into, or close to, the round window niche. Gel-based formulations include hyaluronates [36], collagens [37], chitosans [38], fibrins [39], starch, celluloses, 6 elatin [40], poloxamers [41], and many others. Viscosity that is too high may also result in the formation of an air bubble on the RWM, thus preventing effective diffusion, or may temporarily impair the ossicular mobility.

It seems tempting, to enhance RWM diffusion of a drug by incorporating formulations that are known to enhance permeability, such as histamine or dimethylsulfoxide (DMSO) [42], prostaglandins or leukotrienes, or to use microsphere or nanoparticle formulations. However DMSO has been shown to be cytotoxic in cochlear organotypic cultures at concentrations between 0.5% and 6% [43] and may lead to reduced permeability [44].

Unlike dexamethasone, hydrocortisone has led to RWM inflammation after topical instillation [45]. In our study too, 4 cycles of IT dexamethasone injections didn't cause inflammation of the middle ear mucosa (**Figure 3**).

Local side effects, may include injection-site pain, dizziness, caloric vertigo, infection, persistent tympanic membrane perforation, or possible vasovagal or syncopal episodes during injection [14] [19] [46]. In our study no side-effects except for transient vertigo in few patients were noted. Sufficient warming of the drug, the use of fine needles [45] and appropriate local anaesthesia, a gentle rate of injection, and avoidance of excessive injection volumes seem to be key factors for good local tolerance.

5. Conclusions

Though IT therapy is a highly efficacious and tempting mode of drug delivery, IT dexamethasone injections are

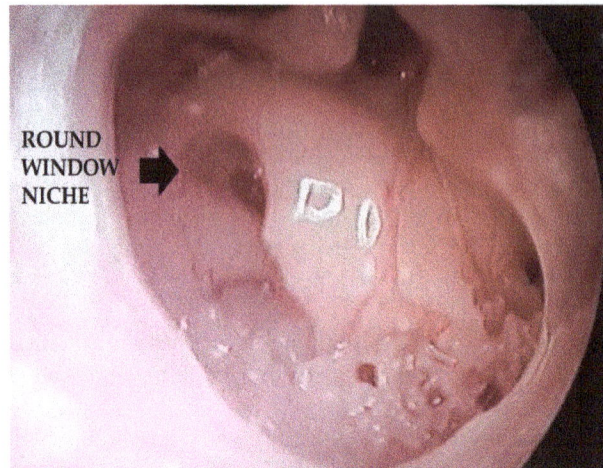

Figure 3. Normal mucosa after it dexamethasone injections.

not effective for refractory tinnitus and don't alter the hearing loss as per our study.

The lack of specific effective drugs must be considered the first and foremost obstacle for a more widespread use of the IT therapy.

The quest for the discovery of effective and safe therapeutic molecules should continue and hopefully there should be breakthrough in tinnitus therapy by intratympanic route in the near future.

References

[1] Goycoolea, M.V. and Lundman, L. (1997) Round Window Membrane. Structure Function and Permeability: A Review. *Microscopy Research and Technique*, **36**, 201-211. http://dx.doi.org/10.1002/(SICI)1097-0029(19970201)36:3<201::AID-JEMT8>3.0.CO;2-R

[2] Goycoolea, M.V. (2001) Clinical Aspects of Round Window Membrane Permeability under Normal and Pathological Conditions. *Acta Oto-Laryngologica*, **121**, 437-447. http://dx.doi.org/10.1080/000164801300366552

[3] Jahnke, K. (1980) The Blood-Perilymph Barrier. *Archives of Otorhinolaryngology*, **228**, 29-34. http://dx.doi.org/10.1007/BF00455891

[4] Sakata, E., Itoh, A. and Itoh, Y. (1996) Treatment of Cochlear-Tinnitus with Dexamethasone Infusion into the Tympanic Cavity. *International Tinnitus Journal*, **2**, 129-135.

[5] Shulman, A. and Goldstein, B. (2000) Intratympanic Drug Therapy with Steroids for Tinnitus Control: A Preliminary Report. *International Tinnitus Journal*, **6**, 10-20.

[6] Cesarani, A., Capobianco, S., Soi, D., Giuliano, D.A. and Alpini, D. (2002) Intratympanic Dexamethasone Treatment for Control of Subjective Idiophatic Tinnitus: Our Clinical Experience. *International Tinnitus Journal*, **8**, 11-113.

[7] Lustig, L.R. (2004) The History of Intratympanic Drug Therapy in Otology. *Otolaryngologic Clinics of North America*, **37**, 1001-1017. http://dx.doi.org/10.1016/j.otc.2004.04.001

[8] Trowbridge, B.C. (1944) Injection of the Tympanum for Chronic Conductive Deafness and Associated Tinnitus Aurium: A Preliminary Report on the Use of Ethylmorphine Hydrochloride. *Archives of Otolaryngology*, **39**, 523. http://dx.doi.org/10.1001/archotol.1944.00680010542012

[9] Trowbridge, B.C. (1949) Tympanosympathetic Anesthesia for Tinnitus Aurium and Secondary Otalgia. *Archives of Otolaryngology*, **50**, 200-215. http://dx.doi.org/10.1001/archotol.1949.00700010209005

[10] Coles, R.R., Thompson, A.C. and O'Donoghue, G.M. (1992) Intra-Tympanic Injections in the Treatment of Tinnitus. *Clinical Otolaryngology and Allied Sciences*, **17**, 240-242. http://dx.doi.org/10.1111/j.1365-2273.1992.tb01835.x

[11] Dodson, K.M. and Sismanis, A. (2004) Intratympanic Perfusion for the Treatment of Tinnitus. *Otolaryngologic Clinics of North America*, **37**, 991-1000. http://dx.doi.org/10.1016/j.otc.2004.03.003

[12] Sakata, E. and Umeda, Y. (1976) Treatment of Tinnitus by Transtympanic Infusion of Lidocaine. *Auris Nasus Larynx*, **3**, 133-138. http://dx.doi.org/10.1016/S0385-8146(76)80014-4

[13] Gouveris, H., Schuler-Schmidt, W., Mewes, T. and Mann, W. (2011) Intratympanic Dexamethasone/Hyaluronic Acid Mix as an Adjunct to Intravenous Steroid and Vasoactive Treatment in Patients with Severe Idiopathic Sudden Sensorineural Hearing Loss. *Otology & Neurotology*, **32**, 756-760. http://dx.doi.org/10.1097/MAO.0b013e31821a3fc3

[14] Topak, M., Sahin-Yilmaz, A., Ozdoganoglu, T., Yilmaz, H.B., Ozbay, M. and Kulekci, M. (2009) Intratympanic Methylprednisolone Injections for Subjective Tinnitus. *Journal of Laryngology & Otology*, **123**, 1221-1225. http://dx.doi.org/10.1017/S0022215109990685

[15] Takahashi, H., Sando, I. and Takagi, A. (1989) Computer-Aided Three-Dimensional Reconstruction and Measurement of the Round Window Niche. *Laryngoscope*, **99**, 505-509. http://dx.doi.org/10.1288/00005537-198905000-00008

[16] Salt, A.N. and Plontke, S.K. (2009) Principles of Local Drug Delivery to the Inner Ear. *Audiology Neurotology*, **14**, 350-360. http://dx.doi.org/10.1159/000241892

[17] Muehlmeier, G., Biesinger, E. and Maier, H. (2011) Safety of Intratympanic Injection of AM-101 in Patients with Acute Inner Ear Tinnitus. *Audiology Neurotology*, **16**, 388-397. http://dx.doi.org/10.1159/000322641

[18] Bird, P.A., Begg, E.J., Zhang, M., Keast, A.T., Murray, D.P. and Balkany, T.J. (2007) Intratympanic versus Intravenous Delivery of Methylprednisolone to Cochlear Perilymph. *Otology & Neurotology*, **28**, 1124-1130. http://dx.doi.org/10.1097/MAO.0b013e31815aee21

[19] Rauch, S.D., Halpin, C.F., Antonelli, P.J., Babu, S., Carey, J.P., Gantz, B.J., *et al.* (2011) Oral vs Intratympanic Corticosteroid Therapy for Idiopathic Sudden Sensorineural Hearing Loss: A Randomized Trial. *Journal of the American Medical Association*, **305**, 2071-2079. http://dx.doi.org/10.1001/jama.2011.679

[20] Conlin, A.E. and Parnes, L.S. (2007) Treatment of Sudden Sensorineural Hearing Loss: I. A Systematic Review. *Archives of Otolaryngology—Head & Neck Surgery*, **133**, 573-581. http://dx.doi.org/10.1001/archotol.133.6.573

[21] Conlin, A.E. and Parnes, L.S. (2007) Treatment of Sudden Sensorineural Hearing Loss: II. A Meta-Analysis. *Archives of Otolaryngology—Head & Neck Surgery*, **133**, 582-586. http://dx.doi.org/10.1001/archotol.133.6.582

[22] Denk, D.M., Heinzl, H., Franz, P. and Ehrenberger, K. (1997) Caroverine in Tinnitus Treatment. A Placebo-Controlled Blind Study. *Acta Oto-Laryngologica*, **117**, 825-830. http://dx.doi.org/10.3109/00016489709114208

[23] Montandon, P., Guillemin, P. and Hausler, R. (1988) Prevention of Vertigo in Ménière's Syndrome by Means of Transtympanic Ventilation Tubes. *ORL Journal of Oto-Rhino-Laryngology and Its Related Specialties*, **50**, 377-381. http://dx.doi.org/10.1159/000276016

[24] Sugawara, K., Kitamura, K., Ishida, T. and Sejima, T. (2003) Insertion of Tympanic Ventilation Tubes as a Treating Modality for Patients with Meniere's Disease: A Short- and Long-Term Follow up Study in Seven Cases. *Auris Nasus Larynx*, **30**, 25-28. http://dx.doi.org/10.1016/S0385-8146(02)00105-0

[25] Domeisen, H., Hotz, M.A. and Häusler, R. (1998) Caroverine in Tinnitus Treatment. *Acta Oto-Laryngologica*, **118**, 606-608. http://dx.doi.org/10.1080/00016489850154801

[26] Ehrenberger, K. (2005) Topical Administration of Caroverine in Somatic Tinnitus Treatment: Proof-of-Concept Study. *International Tinnitus Journal*, **11**, 34-37.

[27] DeLucchi, E. (2000) Transtympanic Pilocarpine in Tinnitus. *International Tinnitus Journal*, **6**, 37-40.

[28] Alzamil, K.S. and Linthicum, Jr., F.H. (2000) Extraneous Round Window Membranes and Plugs: Possible Effect on Intratympanic Therapy. *Annals of Otology, Rhinology & Laryngology*, **109**, 30-32. http://dx.doi.org/10.1177/000348940010900105

[29] Nomura, Y. (1984) Round Window Niche and Round Window Membrane. In: Pfaltz, C.R., Ed., *Otological Significance of the Round Window. Advances in Oto-Rhino-Laryngology*, Vol. 33, S. Karger AG, Basel, 27-37.

[30] Yoshioka, M., Naganawa, S., Sone, M., Nakata, S., Teranishi, M. and Nakashima, T. (2009) Individual Differences in the Permeability of the Round Window: Evaluating the Movement of Intratympanic Gadolinium into the Inner Ear. *Otology & Neurotology*, **30**, 645-648. http://dx.doi.org/10.1097/MAO.0b013e31819bda66

[31] Plontke, S.K., Wood, A.W. and Salt, A.N. (2002) Analysis of Gentamicin Kinetics in Fluids of the Inner Ear with Round Window Administration. *Otology & Neurotology*, **23**, 967-974. http://dx.doi.org/10.1097/00129492-200211000-00026

[32] Banerjee, A. and Parnes, L.S. (2004) The Biology of Intratympanic Drug Administration and Pharmacodynamics of Round Window Drug Absorption. *Otolaryngologic Clinics of North America*, **37**, 1035-1051. http://dx.doi.org/10.1016/j.otc.2004.04.003

[33] Bird, P.A., Murray, D.P., Zhang, M. and Begg, E.J. (2011) Intratympanic versus Intravenous Delivery of Dexamethasone and Dexamethasone Sodium Phosphate to Cochlear Perilymph. *Otology & Neurotology*, **32**, 933-936. http://dx.doi.org/10.1097/MAO.0b013e3182255933

[34] Becvarovski, Z., Bojrab, D.I., Michaelides, E.M., Kartush, J.M., Zappia, J.J. and LaRouere, M.J. (2002) Round Window Gentamicin Absorption: An *in Vivo* Human Model. *Laryngoscope*, **112**, 1610-1613. http://dx.doi.org/10.1097/00005537-200209000-00015

[35] Borkholder, D.A. (2008) State-of-the-Art Mechanisms of Intracochlear Drug Delivery. *Current Opinion in Otolaryngology & Head & Neck Surgery*, **16**, 472-477. http://dx.doi.org/10.1097/MOO.0b013e32830e20db

[36] Borden, R.C., Saunders, J.E., Berryhill, W.E., Krempl, G.A., Thompson, D.M. and Queimado, L. (2011) Hyaluronic Acid Hydrogel Sustains the Delivery of Dexamethasone across the Round Window Membrane. *Audiology Neurotology*, **16**, 1-11. http://dx.doi.org/10.1159/000313506

[37] Iwai, K., Nakagawa, T., Endo, T., Matsuoka, Y., Kita, T., Kim, T.S., *et al.* (2006) Cochlear Protection by Local Insulin-Like Growth Factor-1 Application Using Biodegradable Hydrogel. *Laryngoscope*, **116**, 529-533. http://dx.doi.org/10.1097/01.mlg.0000200791.77819.eb

[38] Paulson, D.P., Abuzeid, W., Jiang, H., Oe, T., O'Malley, B.W. and Li, D. (2008) A Novel Controlled Local Drug Delivery System for Inner Ear Disease. *Laryngoscope*, **118**, 706-711. http://dx.doi.org/10.1097/MLG.0b013e31815f8e41

[39] Sheppard, W.M., Wanamaker, H.H., Pack, A., Yamamoto, S. and Slepecky, N. (2004) Direct Round Window Application of Gentamicin with Varying Delivery Vehicles: A Comparison of Ototoxicity. *Otolaryngology—Head and Neck Surgery*, **131**, 890-896. http://dx.doi.org/10.1016/j.otohns.2004.05.021

[40] Sakamoto, T., Nakagawa, T., Horie, R.T., Hiraumi, H., Yamamoto, N., Kikkawa, Y.S., *et al.* (2010) Inner Ear Drug Delivery System from the Clinical Point of View. *Acta Oto-Laryngologica*, **563**, 101-104. http://dx.doi.org/10.3109/00016489.2010.486801

[41] Salt, A.N., Hartsock, J., Plontke, S., LeBel, C. and Piu, F. (2011) Distribution of Dexamethasone and Preservation of Inner Ear Function Following Intratympanic Delivery of a Gel-Based Formulation. *Audiology Neurotology*, **16**, 323-335. http://dx.doi.org/10.1159/000322504

[42] Chandrasekhar, S.S., Rubinstein, R.Y., Kwartler, J.A., Gatz, M., Connelly, P.E., Huang, E., *et al.* (2000) Dexamethasone Pharmacokinetics in the Inner Ear: Comparison of Route of Administration and Use of Facilitating Agents. *Otolaryngology—Head and Neck Surgery*, **122**, 521-528.

[43] Mikulec, A.A., Hartsock, J.J. and Salt, A.N. (2008) Permeability of the Round Window Membrane Is Influenced by the Composition of Applied Drug Solutions and by Common Surgical Procedures. *Otology & Neurotology*, **29**, 1020-1026. http://dx.doi.org/10.1097/MAO.0b013e31818658ea

[44] Qi, W., Ding, D. and Salvi, R.J. (2008) Cytotoxic Effects of Dimethyl Sulphoxide (DMSO) on Cochlear Organotypic Cultures. *Hearing Research*, **236**, 52-60. http://dx.doi.org/10.1016/j.heares.2007.12.002

[45] Belhassen, S. and Saliba, I. (2012) Pain Assessment of the Intratympanic Injections: A Prospective Comparative Study. *European Archives of Oto-Rhino-Laryngology*, **269**, 2467-2473. http://dx.doi.org/10.1007/s00405-011-1897-z

[46] Stachler, R.J., Chandrasekhar, S.S., Archer, S.M., Rosenfeld, R.M., Schwartz, S.R., Barrs, D.M., *et al.* (2012) Clinical Practice Guideline: Sudden Hearing Loss. *Otolaryngology—Head and Neck Surgery*, **146**, S1-S35. http://dx.doi.org/10.1177/0194599812436449

20

Schwannoma of the Brachial Plexus Presented as a Neck Mass: A Case Report and Review of the Literature

Aslan Ahmadi, Hengameh Hirbod, Mostafa Cheraghipoor, Farzad Izadi

Department of Ear Nose & Throat, Hazrate Rasool Hospital, Tehran, Iran
Email: dr.aslan_ahmadi@yahoo.com, hehirbod@yahoo.com, mostafa.cheraghipoor@yahoo.com, izadimd@yahoo.com

Abstract

Schwannomas of the head and neck as well as brachial plexus primary tumors are both uncommon entities, and combination of these conditions is quite rare. Schwannomas of the brachial plexus are usually asymptomatic and they present as slowly enlarging masses in the supra- or infraclavicular regions. Although imaging plays a routine role in the detection of these neoplasms, identification of the nerve origin is not often feasible until the time of surgery. Definitive diagnosis is based on histopathological features with presence of spindle-shaped Schwann cells. We report a case of a middle aged woman with left lateral mid-neck mass, which based on the clinical findings, was provisionally diagnosed as a painless lymphadenopathy. Ensuing excisional biopsy revealed the brachial plexus as the origin of a tumor, which subsequently was confirmed to be a schwannoma with microscopic evaluation. The course of disease was complicated with upper brachial plexus injury which was recovered by sural nerve graft.

Keywords

Schwannoma, Cervical Schwannoma, Brachial Plexus Tumors, Extracranial Schwannoma

1. Introduction

Schwannomas, also termed as neurilemmomas, are benign nerve sheath neoplasms that originate from peripheral, cranial or autonomic nerves. These are well encapsulated tumors and malignant transformation is extremely rare. Tumors involving head and neck region consist of around 25% of all cases, usually originated from cranial (V, VII, IV, X, XI and XII) nerves, sympathetic or peripheral nerves [1]-[4]. These lesions are generally presented as a cosmetic deformity, an asymptomatic mass or symptoms related to nerve compression [5]. Advanced imaging investigations, such as magnetic resonance imaging (MRI) and/or computed tomography (CT) scan, are particularly useful in diagnosing these neoplasms and have become the routine studies for these patients [6]. Microscopically, pathological features of these tumors are unique, composed of spindle Schwann cells forming hyper- or hypocellular areas (Antoni A and Antoni B, respectively) [1].

Schwannomas of the brachial plexus are rare and due to their rarity, as well as the complex anatomical situation, they may pose diagnostic or surgical challenges [5] [7]. Proper diagnosis of the tumor must be established prior to surgery as it can be mistaken with a lymphadenopathy [8]. Previous reports showed that a majority of cases with schwannoma involving cranial nerves or sympathetic nerve were associated with a neck mass [2] [6] [9]-[11], while cases with brachial plexus tumors commonly presented as supraclavicular, infraclavicular or neck root swelling, with or without neurological manifestation [3]-[5] [7] [8] [12]-[14].

In this study, we report a middle aged woman with brachial plexus schwannoma who was presented as mid-cervical mass.

2. Case Report

A 42-year-old lady presented with a left neck progressively enlarging swelling for three months duration. There was no history of trauma, pain, hoarseness, dysphagia, syncopal attacks or any constitutional symptoms. Systemic physical examination was normal, however locally; there were a 2 × 2 cm firm, nonpulsatile and fairly mobile mass located at the left mid-cervical region. It was not tender, warm or fluctuant and clinically resembled an anterior cervical lymphadenopathy. Otoscopic and oropharynx examination as well as indirect laryngoscopy revealed no abnormality or any source of infection. She was neurologically intact with no evidence of sensory loss and myotomal weakness or abnormal reflexes. Blood investigations showed normal values. A computed tomography (CT) of the neck was performed and discovered a well-defined mass in left lateral cervical region measuring 2 × 2 cm at the level of fourth to fifth cervical vertebra (**Figure 1**). A fine-needle aspiration was performed, which was inconclusive.

Patient was planned for an excisional biopsy and using a left transcervical approach, the entire mass was resected. Intraoperatively, a well-circumscribed mass, measuring 1.5 × 2 × 2 cm was identified, with its bundles passing through the fascicles of the brachial plexus.

Postoperatively she sustained weakness of shoulder abduction, elbow flexion and supination and an upper brachial plexus injury was suspected. She underwent the second operation aiming to explore the existing neural defect and a partially injured C5 nerve root and upper trunk of the brachial plexus was detected. The injured nerves were resected and sural nerve graft was carried out using a microsurgical technique.

Pathological assessment revealed encapsulated lesion composed of neoplastic spindle cells with basophilic nuclei (Schwann cells), organized in patternless alternative hyper and hypo-cellular areas, representing Antoni A and Antoni B patterns, respectively (**Figure 2**). There were no mitotic figures or necrosis. The final diagnosis

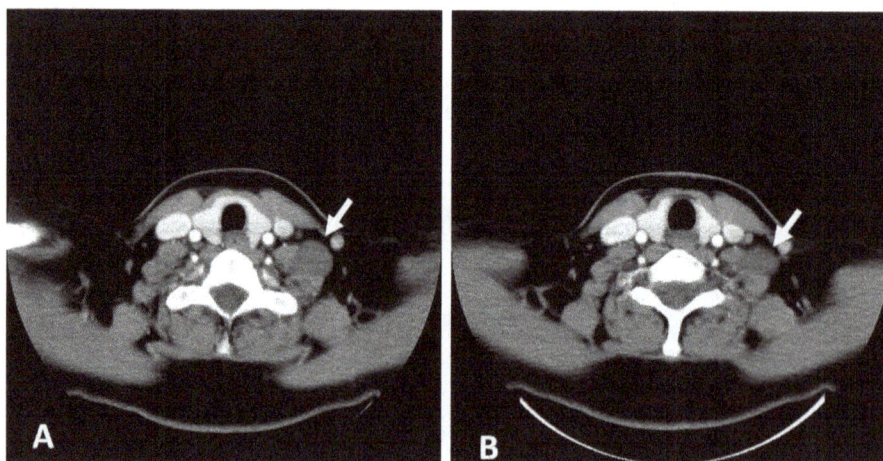

Figure 1. Contrast enhanced computed tomography (CT) scan (axial view) showing the isodense lesion in left cervical region with minimal enhancement (white arrows).

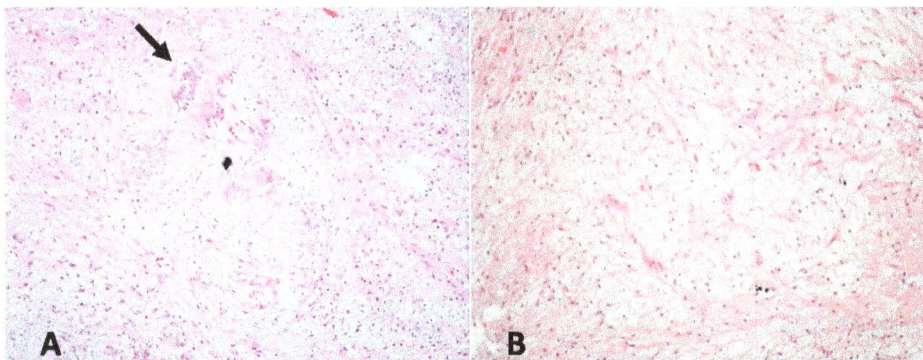

Figure 2. Microscopic examination showed a spindle cell neoplasm with the composition of a hypercellular area, Antoni A (A) and a hypocellular area, Antoni B (B) (H & E stain, ×400). Note the palisading nuclei of the spindle cells surrounding pink areas, known as verocay bodies, representing Antoni A pattern (black arrow).

was schwannoma.

At 4 months follow up after discharge, she was symptom free, without any residual neurological deficit.

3. Discussion

Primary tumors arising in the brachial plexus are rare [15]. These neoplasms may manifest as pain in the shoulder or upper limb, sensory/motor disturbances or an asymptomatic swelling. Among these primary tumors, schwannoma and neurofibromatosis are the two most common neoplasms and both of which are benign and eccentrically arise from neural sheath [5] [15] [16]. Although schwannomas typically present as a solitary tumor, neurofibromas usually occur in the context of neurofibromatosis type I [5].

Schwannomas are usually indolent neoplasms that originate from cranial, peripheral or autonomic nerve sheaths. The eccentric position of the tumor in the nerve is probably contributing to the reason why the majority of cases with schwannoma, as in our case, are neurologically spared. However, these tumors may have been investigated for space occupying lesion or nerve compression, months or even years prior to final diagnosis [3] [4]. Even more complicated presentations, such as a cystic pectoral lesion [12] or axillary [7] masses have also been reported. Considering the complexity of the regional anatomy, surgical resection of this tumor is a technically challenging procedure that has the potential for devastating neurological complications. In order to achieve the best result, an accurate preoperative planning, using imaging techniques such as MRI or CT scan is highly recommended.

We could not find any published evidence regarding the precise incidence of postoperative neurological complications; however, the review of the reported cases shows that temporary sensory or motor deficit frequently occurs after surgical resection of the schwannoma [3] [5]-[7]. There are scattered reports of long term or permanent motor impairment after this operation as well [5]. Our patient developed a neurological deficit postoperatively that required us to perform the surgical exploration to find out underlying reason, which was discontinuation of the C5 nerve root and upper trunk of the plexus. Neurological and functional outcome of this patient was evaluated as excellent, four months after operation, with full muscle power and no sensory impairment.

4. Conclusion

Brachial plexus primary tumors as well as schwannomas of the head and neck are both uncommon entities, and combination of these conditions is quite rare. A majority of cases are presented as supraclavicular masses. However, if it arises from upper nerve roots of the brachial plexus, as our case, it may manifest as a mid-neck swelling that can be clinically indistinguishable from a lymph node. Close anatomical relations of the brachial plexus schwannoma with the critical structures in the cervical region, require an accurate preoperative planning to avoid catastrophic neurovascular complications. Despite the best precautions, a postoperative sensory or motor deficit commonly may occur. Although, fortunately, the vast majority of sensory injuries resolve spontaneously, motor injuries may require repair and nerve grafting, as in our case happened.

Consent

Written informed consent was obtained from the patient for publication of this case report and any accompanying images. A copy of the written consent is available for review by the Editor-in-Chief of this journal.

Competing Interest

We declare that we have no financial or non-financial competing interests.

Authors' Contributions

AA was the primary surgeon, conceived of the report and obtained the patient's history and physical exam. HH assisted the surgery, reviewed the literature and drafted the manuscript. MC was surgeon's assistant and provided the images and their interpretations. FI reviewed the manuscript and contributed to its final form. All authors have been involved in writing this manuscript and have approved the final manuscript and its submission.

References

[1]   Bradley, W. and Midah, R. (2008) Chap 49: Schwannoma. In: Midah, R., Ed., *Surgery of Peripheral Nerve: A Case Based Approach*, Thieme, New York, 231.

[2]   Bocciolini, C., *et al.* (2005) Schwannoma of Cervical Sympathetic Chain: Assessment and Management. *Acta Otorhinolaryngologica Italica*, **25**, 191-194.

[3]   Jaafar, R., *et al.* (2012) Cervical Schwannoma: Report of Four Cases. *Medical Journal of Malaysia*, **67**, 345-348.

[4]   Patel, M.L., Sachan, R., Seth, G., *et al.* (2014) Schwannoma of the Brachial Plexus: A Rare Cause of Monoparesis. *BMJ Case Reports*.

[5]   Soltani, A.M., *et al.* (2013) Neural Sheath Tumors of the Brachial Plexus: A Multidisciplinary Team-Based Approach. *Annals of Plastic Surgery*, **71**, 80-83. http://dx.doi.org/10.1097/SAP.0b013e31827100d8

[6]   Chiofalo, M.G., Longo, F., Marone, U., Franco, R., Petrillo, A. and Pezzullo, L. (2009) Cervical Vagal Schwannoma: A Case Report. *Acta Otorhinolaryngologica Italica*, **29**, 33-35.

[7]   Kumar, A. and Akhtar, S. (2011) Schwannoma of Brachial Plexus. *Indian Journal of Surgery*, **73**, 80-81. http://dx.doi.org/10.1007/s12262-010-0141-1

[8]   Rashid, M., *et al.* (2013) Schwannoma of the Brachial Plexus; Report of Two Cases Involving the C7 Root. *Journal of Brachial Plexus and Peripheral Nerve Injury*, **8**, 12. http://dx.doi.org/10.1186/1749-7221-8-12

[9]   Iaacconi, P., *et al.* (2012) Cervical Sympathetic Chain Schwannoma: A Case Report. *Acta Otorhinolaryngologica Italica*, **32**, 133-136.

[10]   Sérémé, M., Ouédraogo, A., Gyébré, Y. and Ouoba, K. (2014) Cervical Vagal Schwannoma: Difficulty of Diagnosis and Particularity of Treatment. *The Internet Journal of Otorhinolaryngology*, **16**.

[11]   Ahmadi-Yazdi, C. and Habashi, S. (2005) Schwannoma of Accessory Nerve: A Case Report. *The Internet Journal of Otorhinolaryngology*, **4**.

[12]   Chen, F., Miyahara, R., Matsunaga, Y. and Koyama, T. (2008) Schwannoma of the Brachial Plexus Presenting as an Enlarging Cystic Mass: Report of a Case. *Annals of Thoracic and Cardiovascular Surgery*, **14**, 311-313.

[13]   Somayaji, K.S.G., Rajeshwari, A. and Gangadhara, K.S. (2004) Schwannoma of the Brachial Plexus Presenting as a Cystic Swelling. *Indian Journal of Otorhinolaryngology and Head & Neck Surgery*, **56**, 228-230.

[14]   Haghari, S., İmerci, A., Koçak, M., Sürer, L. and Güney, E. (2013) A Case of Schwannoma Arising from Brachial Plexus in an Operated Patient with the Diagnosis of Cubital Tunnel Syndrome. *Türkiye Fiziksel Tıp ve Rehabilitasyon Dergisi*, **59**, 165-166. http://dx.doi.org/10.4274/tftr.10693

[15]   Binder, D.K., Smith, J.S. and Barbaro, N.M. (2004) Primary Brachial Plexus Tumors: Imaging, Surgical, and Pathological Findings in 25 Patients. *Neurosurgical Focus*, **16**, E11.

[16]   Lusk, M.D., Kline, D.G. and Garcia, C.A. (1987) Tumors of the Brachial Plexus. *Neurosurgery*, **21**, 439-453. http://dx.doi.org/10.1227/00006123-198710000-00001

21

Charge Syndrome—A Case Report

A. Ravindran, A. Amirthagani, Prince Peter Dhas, S. Nagarajan, Senthil Kumar, Satheesh Kumar, Venkatesh

Department of Otorhonolaryngology, Thanjavur Madical College, Thanjavur, India
Email: ravindranent2@gmail.com

Abstract

CHARGE syndrome is a rare, recently well recognized entity with non-random pattern of congenital anomalies. The syndrome associations consist of C-coloboma of the eyes, H-heart disease, A-atresia of the choanae, R-retarded growth and development, G-genital hypoplasia/genitourinary anomalies and E-ear anomalies and/or hearing loss. All anomalies are not seen in every case and a varied spectrum of associations is seen in most of the cases. The exact incidence is not known. However, the reported prevalence is approximately 1:10,000 births. We report one such case.

Keywords

Charge Syndrome, Choanal Atresia, Coloboma

1. Introduction

CHARGE syndrome was initially defined as a non-random association of anomalies (coloboma, heart defect, atresia choanae, retarded growth and development, genital hypoplasia, ear anomalies/deafness). In 1998, an expert group defined the major (the classical 4C's: Choanal atresia, Coloboma, Characteristic ears and Cranial nerve anomalies) and minor criteria of CHARGE syndrome. Individuals with all four major characteristics or three major and three minor characteristics are highly likely to have CHARGE syndrome. However, there have been individuals genetically identified with CHARGE syndrome without the classical choanal atresia and coloboma. The reported incidence of CHARGE syndrome ranges from 0.1 - 1.2/10,000 and depends on professional recognition. Coloboma mainly affects the retina. Major and minor congenital heart defects (the commonest cyanotic heart defect is tetralogy of Fallot) occur in 75% - 80% of patients. Choanal atresia may be membranous or bony, bilateral or unilateral. Mental retardation is variable with intelligence quotients (IQ) ranging from normal to profound retardation. Under-development of the external genitalia is a common finding in males but it is less apparent in females. Ear abnormalities include a classical finding of unusually shaped ears and hearing loss (conductive and/or nerve deafness that ranges from mild to severe deafness). Multiple cranial nerve dysfunctions are common. A behavioral phenotype for CHARGE syndrome is emerging. Mutations in the *CHD*7 gene (member of the chromodomain helicase DNA protein family) are detected in over 75% of patients with CHARGE syndrome. Children with CHARGE syndrome require intensive medical management as well as numerous surgical interventions. They also need multidisciplinary follow-up.

Some of the hidden issues of CHARGE syndrome are often forgotten, one being the feeding adaptation of these children, which needs an early aggressive approach from a feeding team. As the child develops, challenging behaviors become more common and require adaptation of educational and therapeutic services, including behavioral and pharmacological interventions.

2. Case Report

A female child aged 14, was brought to the OPD by the grand mother, with the complaints of discharge from left side of nose since birth. There was history of hard of hearing both ears, difficulty in speech, defective vision on left eye. Otherwise, the perinatal and developmental history was normal.

On examination, pt had unilateral choanal atresia, sensorineural hearing loss on both side. Eye examination revealed left eye micro cornea with typical coloboma (**Figure 1**) choroid involving optic disc and iris, squint, spontaneous nystagmus, loss of left eye vision. General examination of the patient showed facial asymmetry (**Figure 2**), polydactyly (**Figure 3**), poor breast development on left side, systemic examination revealed, wide fixed split on auscultation, abdominal and respiratory systems are normal.

Child was investigated. Diagnostic nasal endoscopy showed complete choanal atresia on left side. Severe sensorineural hearing loss on both sides on Pure Tone Audiogram. CT PNS and temporal bone showed posterior coloboma left eye, left osseous choanal atresia (**Figure 4**).

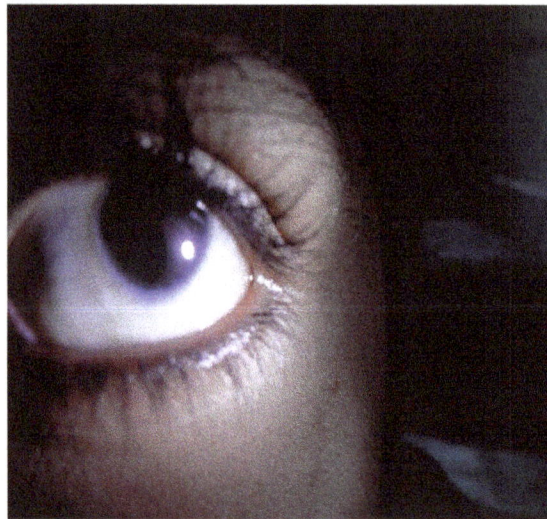

Figure 1. Coloboma left eye.

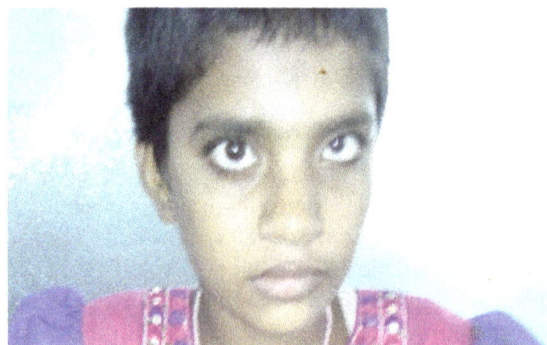

Figure 2. Showing facial asymmetry.

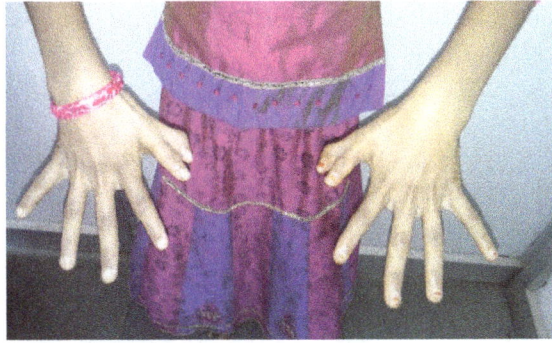

Figure 3. Showing polydactyly.

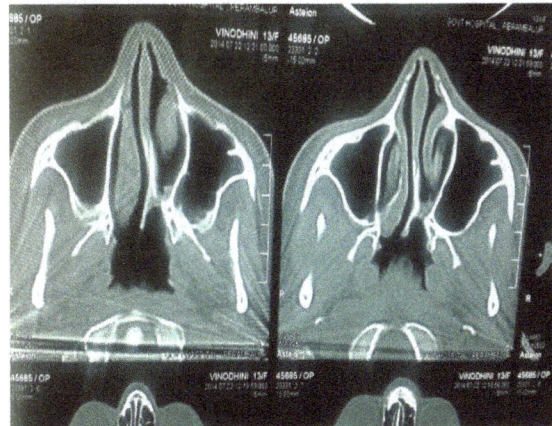

Figure 4. CT PNS showing choanal atresia (L).

Ultra sonogram of abdomen showed Left side extra renal pelvis. On echocardiogram moderate size 5 mm ostium secondum type of atrial septal defect with less than 2:1 left to right shunt.

Child has choanal atresia, coloboma of eyes, hearing loss, heart defect thus satisfying the criteria for CHARGE SYNDROME, which is undiagnosed till the age of 14.

3. Discussion

The CHARGE association was first described in 1979 by Hall *et al.*, in 17 children with multiple congenital anomalies who were ascertained by choanal atresia [1] [2]. In the same year, Hittner reported this syndrome in 10 children with ocular colobomas and multiple congenital anomalies [3], hence the syndrome is also called Hall-Hittner syndrome [4]. Pagon *et al.*, in 1981 first coined the acronym CHARGE association [5], (coloboma, heart defect, atresia choanae, retarded growth and development, genital hypoplasia, Ear anomalies/deafness) as a non-random association of anomalies occurring together more frequently than one would expect on the basis of chance. The original diagnostic criteria required the presence of four out of six of the CHARGE characteristics. Over the past 15 years the specificity of this pattern of malformations has reached the level that many clinicians now consider it to be a recognizable CHARGE syndrome [2].

4. Clinical Description

4.1. Coloboma

This feature may be unilateral or bilateral and may affect only the iris or extend to involve the retina, or only the retina. Vision may be normal or impaired. The eye abnormalities range from iris coloboma without visual impairment to microphthalmos and anophthalmos. Retinal coloboma is more prevalent than iris coloboma and can affect the optic nerve. Eye malformations have been reported in as many as 80% of patients with CHARGE syndrome, with retinal involvement being the most common [6]. External inspection is not sufficient and testing for functional vision is important but challenging especially in CHARGE individuals with extensive bilateral chorioretinal coloboma involving the optic nerve [7].

4.2. Heart Defect

Congenital heart defects occur in 75% - 80% of patients with CHARGE syndrome. The most common major heart defect is tetralogy of Fallot (33%). Other frequent anomalies are patent ductus arteriosus, double outlet right ventricle with atrioventricular canal, ventricular septal defect and atrial septal defect with or without cleft mitral valve. Vascular rings and more complex heart defects need to be anticipated [8]-[11].

4.3. Choanal Atresia

Choanal atresia is a narrowing or a blockage of the passages between the nasal cavity and the naso-pharynx. It represents a primary feature with a high index of suspicion for CHARGE syndrome and it should focus attention on other organ systems such as the eye and heart. Choanal atresia may be membranous or bony; bilateral or unilateral. Bilateral posterior choanal atresia (BPCA) was shown to be associated with increased neonatal mortality, especially if associated with major cardiac malformations +\− tracheoesophageal atresia [8]. However, the Canadian epidemiological study data suggests that an individual from this population with a more severe clinical presentation of CHARGE features generally survive [9]. Polyhydramnios in pregnancy is seen commonly in individuals with bilateral posterior choanal atresia, and may also be present without BPCA, probably due to an insufficient swallowing mechanism. Chronic middle ear infections and deafness can be associated complications of choanal atresia [12].

4.4. Retardation of Growth and Development

Growth and developmental retardation become more obvious as the child matures. At birth, children with CHARGE syndrome usually have normal weights and lengths [13]. When growth deceleration is due to cardiac and respiratory problems, there may be catch up growth, and normal height can be obtained [14]. However, the influence of feeding problems on growth in infancy should not be underestimated. Early and continued intervention for feeding difficulties is vitally important [15]; occasionally there is growth hormone deficiency. The majority of school-aged children with CHARGE syndrome are below the third percentile for physical growth norms [13]; feeding with solids and lumpy foods, and risk of aspiration may still exist. Mental retardation is variable with intelligence quotients (IQ) ranging from near-normal to profound retardation. Behavioral issues and an autism-like spectrum disorder are now being recognized as features of the syndrome [16] [17].

4.5. Genitourinary Problems

Under-development of the external genitalia is a common finding in males but it is more difficult to recognize in females. Microphallus, penile agenesis, hypospadias, chordee, cryptorchidism, bifid scrotum, atresia of uterus, cervix and vagina, hypoplastic labia and clitoris are reported genital anomalies in this syndrome. Reported renal anomalies include solitary kidney, hydronephrosis, renal hypoplasia, duplex kidneys and vesicoureteral reflux. Hypogonadotrophic hypogonadism has been reported and is associated with delays in puberty or pubertal arrest [18] [19].

4.6. Ear, Olfactory and Other Cranial Nerve Anomalies

Ear abnormalities include a classical finding of unusually shaped ears [6]. Lack of cartilage to the outer ear with deficient 7th nerve innervation to intrinsic ear muscles produces a prominent lop- or cup-shaped ear with a hypoplastic lobule (**Figure 2**). Hearing loss, conductive and/or nerve deafness, ranges from mild to severe. Ear anomalies were reported in 80% - 100% of cases in different series [10] [20]. Facial nerve palsies were noted to be a reliable predictor of sensorineural hearing loss. The characteristic abnormalities demonstrated by temporal bone computerized tomography (CT) or magnetic resonance imaging (MRI) scan include hypoplastic incus, decreased numbers of turns to the cochlea (mondini defect), and, in particular, absent semicircular canals. These distinctive radiological findings are classical for CHARGE syndrome and can aid diagnosis in a suspected case [21]. For this reason, a neonatal CT scan to look at the choanae and temporal bones can be extremely useful.

Blake *et al.* suggested that a typical clinical diagnosis of CHARGE syndrome requires the presence of at least 4 major features or 3 major features plus at least 3 minor features. Major features include ocular coloboma or microphthalmia, choanal atresia or stenosis, cranial nerve abnormalities, and characteristic auditory and/or auricular anomalies. Minor features include distinctive facial dysmorphology, facial clefting, tracheoesophageal fistula, congenital heart defects, genitourinary anomalies, developmental delay, and short stature. Other frequently associated abnormal findings include characteristic hand dysmorphology, hypotonia, deafness, and dysphagia [1] [22].

In our case, patient has unilateral coloboma, choanal atresia, sensorineural deafness, Left side extra renal pelvis, ostium secondum type of atrial septal defect. Thus fulfilling the criteria for charge syndrome [22]. The peculiar feature of the case is the late diagnosis. Usually patient will present with early symptoms. Here our patient came with the unilateral watery discharge from nose leading to our diagnosis of charge syndrome.

5. Management

Children with CHARGE syndrome require intensive medical Management as well as numerous surgical interventions. The most common neonatal emergencies in CHARGE syndrome involve cyanosis due to bilateral posterior choanal atresia and/or congenital heart defects, or the less common presentation of tracheoesophageal fistula. The primary foci of management should be airway Stabilization and circulatory support [1]. All patients suspected of having CHARGE syndrome should have a cardiology consultation. If the infant has Restrictive pulmonary blood flow and is dependant on a patent ductus arteriosus, the administration of prostaglandin to maintain ductal patency may be life saving. Some children require tracheostomy to manage chronic Airway problems and/or gastroesophageal reflux and aspiration.

Children with CHARGE syndrome require aggressive Medical management of their feeding difficulties, often needing gastrostomy and jejunostomy feeding tubes. Gastrooesophageal fundoplication may be required for GER that does not respond to medical management. As intubation can be difficult in children with CHARGE syndrome, a pediatric anesthesiologist or pediatric Otolaryngologist should be present for planned surgical Procedures.

Any infant suspected of having CHARGE syndrome should have a complete eye examination by an ophthalmologist, with follow-up every three to six months thereafter, depending on the eye involvement. Photophobia is often a significant problem that can be ameliorated with tinted spectacles or by wearing a cap or visor with a dark brim. In the presence of facial palsy, patients should avoid corneal scarring by using artificial tears.

Hearing aids should be used as soon as hearing loss is documented. Frequent re-molding of the earpieces is necessary as the ear canals can be initially very small and ear cartilage may be insufficient to support a hearing aid. Cochlear implantations have been successfully performed in CHARGE syndrome patients. Children with CHARGE syndrome who undergo cochlear implantation should be allowed to continue with their sign language in parallel with their expressive speech training [23]. Adapted educational and therapeutic services to deal with dual auditory and visual sensory impairment should be proposed early in the child's life [23]-[25]. However, this population is unique with respect to their aberrant cranial nerve pathways and problems with expressive language.

In terms of endocrine issues, sex steroid therapy has been used for penile growth and descent of testes in males with CHARGE syndrome. The main use for testosterone is for delayed and incomplete male puberty during adolescence. Females often require hormone replacement at puberty [18]. Sex hormone replacement is also indicated for prevention of osteoporosis [19].

6. Conclusion

The acronym "CHARGE" denotes the nonrandom association of coloboma, heart anomalies, choanal atresia, retardation of growth and development, and genital and ear anomalies, which are frequently present in various combinations and varying degrees in individuals with CHARGE syndrome [3] [4]. No single feature is universally present or sufficient for the clinical diagnosis of CHARGE syndrome, and numerous guidelines have been published to aid in establishing a likely clinical diagnosis. The peculiar feature of the case is the late diagnosis. Usually patient will present with early symptoms. Here our patient came with the unilateral watery discharge from nose leading to our diagnosis of charge syndrome. With the permission of the patient and her parent, we are publishing this article due to the peculiarity of the case.

References

[1]   Blake, K.D., Davenport, S.L.H., Hall, B.D., Hefner, M.A., Pagon, R.A., Williams, M.S., Lin, A.E. and Graham Jr., J.M. (1998) CHARGE Association: An Update and Review for the Primary Pediatrician. *Clinical Pediatrics*, **37**, 159-173. http://dx.doi.org/10.1177/000992289803700302

[2]   Hall, B.D. (1979) Choanal Atresia and Associated Multiple Anomalies. *Journal of Pediatrics*, **95**, 395-398. http://dx.doi.org/10.1016/S0022-3476(79)80513-2

[3]   Hittner, H., Hirsch, N., Kreh, G. and Rudolph, A. (1979) Colobomatous Microphthalmia, Heart Disease, Hearing Loss, and Mental Retardation: A Syndrome. *Journal of Pediatric Ophthalmology and Strabismus*, **16**, 122-128.

[4]   Graham Jr., J.M. (2001) A Recognizable Syndrome within CHARGE Association: Hall-Hittner Syndrome. *American Journal of Medical Genetics*, **99**, 120-123. http://dx.doi.org/10.1002/1096-8628(2000)9999:9999<00::AID-AJMG1132>3.0.CO;2-J

[5]   Pagon, R.A., Graham Jr., J.M., Zonana, J. and Young, S.L. (1981) Coloboma, Congenital Heart Disease, and Choanal Atresia with Multiple Anomalies: CHARGE Association. *Journal of Pediatrics*, **99**, 223-227. http://dx.doi.org/10.1016/S0022-3476(81)80454-4

[6]   Russell-Eggitt, I.M., Blake, K.D., Taylor, D. and Wyse, R.K. (1990) The Eye in CHARGE Association. *British Journal of Ophthalmology*, **74**, 421-426. http://dx.doi.org/10.1136/bjo.74.7.421

[7]   McMain, K., Robitalle, J., Blake, K., Wood, E., Smith, I., Temblay, F., Johnston, J. and Beis, J. (2005) Eye in Charge. http://www.chargesyndrome.ca/TheEyeInCHARGE.htm

[8]   Blake, K.D., Russell-Eggitt, I.M., Morgan, D.W., Ratcliffe, J.M. and Wyse, R.K.H. (1990) Who's in CHARGE? Multidisciplinary Management of Patients with CHARGE Association. *Archives of Disease in Childhood*, **65**, 217-223. http://dx.doi.org/10.1136/adc.65.2.217

[9]   Lin, A.E., Siebert, J.R. and Graham Jr., J.M. (1990) Central Nervous System Malformations in the CHARGE Association. *American Journal of Medical Genetics*, **37**, 304-310. http://dx.doi.org/10.1002/ajmg.1320370303

[10]   Tellier, A.L., Cormier-Daire, V., Abadie, V., Amiel, J., Sigaudy, S., Bonnet, D., de Lonlay-Debeney, P., Morrisseau-Durand, M.P., Hubert, P., Michel, J.L., Jan, D., Dollfus, H., Baumann, C., Labrune, P., Lacombe, D., Philip, N., Le-Merrer, M., Briard, M.L., Munnich, A. and Lyonnet, S. (1998) CHARGE Syndrome: Report of 47 Cases and Review. *American Journal of Medical Genetics*, **76**, 402-409. http://dx.doi.org/10.1002/(SICI)1096-8628(19980413)76:5<402::AID-AJMG7>3.0.CO;2-O

[11]   Cyran, S.E., Martinez, R., Daniels, S., Dignan, P.S.J. and Kaplan, S. (1987) Spectrum of Congenital Heart Disease in CHARGE Association. *Journal of Pediatrics*, **110**, 576-580. http://dx.doi.org/10.1016/S0022-3476(87)80555-3

[12]   Keller, J.L. and Kacker, A. (2000) Choanal Atresia, CHARGE Association, and Congenital Nasal Stenosis. *Otolaryngologic Clinics of North America*, **33**, 1343-1351. http://dx.doi.org/10.1016/S0030-6665(05)70285-1

[13]   Blake, K.D., Kirk, J.M. and Ur, E. (1993) Growth in CHARGE Association. *Archives of Disease in Childhood*, **68**, 508-509. http://dx.doi.org/10.1136/adc.68.4.508

[14]   Searle, L. and Blake, K.D. (2005) CHARGE Syndrome from Birth to Adulthood: An Individual Reported on from 0 to 33 Years. *American Journal of Medical Genetics Part A*, **133**, 344-349. http://dx.doi.org/10.1002/ajmg.a.30565

[15]   Dobbelsteyn, C., Marche, D.M., Blake, K.D. and Rashid, M. (2005) Early Oral Sensory Experiences and Feeding Development in Children with CHARGE Syndrome: A Report of Five Cases. *Dysphagia*, **20**, 89-100. http://dx.doi.org/10.1007/s00455-004-0026-1

[16]   Smith, I.M., Nichols, S.L., Issekutz, K. and Blake, K. (2005) Behavioral Profiles and Symptoms of Autism in CHARGE Syndrome: Preliminary Canadian Epidemiological Data. *American Journal of Medical Genetics Part A*, **133**, 248-256. http://dx.doi.org/10.1002/ajmg.a.30544

[17]   Hartshorne, T.S., Grialou, T.L. and Parker, K.R. (2005) Autistic-like behavior in CHARGE syndrome. *American Journal of Medical Genetics Part A*, **133**, 257-261. http://dx.doi.org/10.1002/ajmg.a.30545

[18]   Blake, K.D., Salem-Hartshorne, N., Abi Daoud, M. and Gradstein, J. (2005) Adolescent and Adult Issues in CHARGE Syndrome. *Clinical Pediatrics*, **44**, 151-159. http://dx.doi.org/10.1177/000992280504400207

[19]   Forward, K., Cummings, E. and Blake, K. (2005) Bone Health in Adolescents and Adults with CHARGE Syndrome. In Press.

[20]   Lalani, S.R., Safiullah, A.M., Fernbach, S.D., Harutyunyan, K.G., Thaller, C., Peterson, L.E., McPherson, J.D., Gibbs, R.A., White, L.D., Hefner, M., Davenport, S.L., Graham, J.M., Bacino, C.A., Glass, N.L., Towbin, J.A., Craigen, W.J., Neish, S.R., Lin, A.E. and Belmont, J.W. (2006) Spectrum of *CHD7* Mutations in 110 Individuals with CHARGE Syndrome and Genotype-Phenotype Correlation. *The American Journal of Human Genetics*, **78**, 303-314. http://dx.doi.org/10.1086/500273

[21]   Amiel, J., Attiee-Bitach, T., Marianowski, R., Cormier-Daire, V., Abadie, V., Bonnet, D., Gonzales, M., Chemouny, S.,

Brunelle, F., Munnich, A., Manach, Y. and Lyonnet, S. (2001) Temporal Bone Anomaly Proposed as a Major Criterion for Diagnosis of CHARGE Syndrome. *American Journal of Medical Genetics*, **99**, 124-127. http://dx.doi.org/10.1002/1096-8628(20010301)99:2<124::AID-AJMG1114>3.0.CO;2-9

[22] Verloes, A. (2005) Updated Diagnostic Criteria for CHARGE Syndrome: A Proposal. *American Journal of Medical Genetics Part A*, **133A**, 306-308. http://dx.doi.org/10.1002/ajmg.a.30559

[23] Blake, K.D. and Brown, D. (1993) CHARGE Association Looking at the Future—The Voice of a Family Support Group. *Child: Care, Health and Development*, **19**, 395-409. http://dx.doi.org/10.1111/j.1365-2214.1993.tb00744.x

[24] Tellier, A.L., Lyonnet, S., Cormier-Daire, V., de Lonlay, P., Abadie, V., Baumann, C., Bonneau, D., Labrune, P., Lacombe, D., Le Merrer, M., Nivelon, A., Philip, N., Briard, M.L. and Munnich, A. (1996) Increased Paternal Age in CHARGE Association. *Clinical Genetics*, **50**, 548-550. http://dx.doi.org/10.1111/j.1399-0004.1996.tb02736.x

[25] Thelin, J.W. and Fussner, J.C. (2005) Factors Related to the Development of Communications in CHARGE Syndrome. *American Journal of Medical Genetics Part A*, **133**, 282-290. http://dx.doi.org/10.1002/ajmg.a.30550

22

A Unified Management for Spontaneous CSF Leak

Lobna El Fiky[1], Ali Kotb[2], Badr Eldin Mostafa[1]

[1]Otolaryngology Department, Ain Shams University, Cairo, Egypt
[2]Neurosurgery Department, Ain Shams University, Cairo, Egypt
Email: elfikylobna@hotmail.com, elfikylobna@gmail.com

Abstract

Background: Spontaneous CSF leak represents less frequent cause of CSF leak, but cases are more difficult to control, with the highest failure rate and recurrence despite adequate repair. The problems in these cases might be related to an underlying undiagnosed associated intracranial hypertension. Recognition and long-term treatment of elevated ICP is therefore critical to the successful management of these patients. Objective: To evaluate the CSF pressure in cases of spontaneous CSF rhinorrhea and to describe our same setting combined protocol to the repair of the leak, measurement and management of CSF pressure. Patients and Methods: All patients presenting to Ain Shams University Hospitals, Cairo, Egypt, with spontaneous CSF leak were included prospectively in the study. Clinical and radiologic data were collected to suspect elevated intracranial pressure. After CSF repair, CSF pressure was measured and if found to be more than 20 cmH$_2$O, a lumboperitoneal shunt was used. Results: Twenty-seven cases, 23 women and 4 men, presented with spontaneous CSF leak. 23 patients had BMI above 30. All patients had empty sella syndrome (100%), and a meningoencephalocele was found in 13 cases (48%). CSF pressure ranged from 5 to 39 cmH$_2$O (mean = 28.7). A pressure above 21 cmH$_2$O was found in19 patients (70%) and subsequently had lumboperitoneal shunt in the same setting. No recurrence occurred in this subset of patients with 6 - 60 months follow-up period. Conclusion: A selective and specific same setting protocol can result in a better diagnosis and control of the accompanying elevated ICP in cases of spontaneous CSF leak. It avoids a second operative intervention, and shortens the hospital stay, with an increase in the success rate. In the same time, the smaller number of patients with normal ICP can avoid further drainage.

Keywords

CSF Rhinorrhea, Elevated ICP, Spontaneous CSF Leak, Lumbar Drain, Acetazolamide, Empty Sella Syndrome, Intracranial Hypertension, Endoscopic CSF Repair, CSF Diversion, Lumboperitoneal Shunts

1. Introduction

Spontaneous CSF leak represents a distinct clinical entity that warrants a separate designation [1]. Although less frequent than other causes of CSF leak, cases are more difficult to control, with the highest failure rate and recurrence despite adequate repair [2].

Although the precise cause and mechanism of spontaneous CSF leaks are not fully understood, the knowledge and experience with spontaneous CSF leaks have increased dramatically over the last decade [3]. The problems in these cases might be related to an underlying undiagnosed associated intracranial hypertension and its correction may be warranted [4]-[8].

The majority of these patients exhibit demographics, clinical symptoms and radiographic signs of elevated intracranial pressure (ICP) and should be considered as a high-pressure condition [1] [3] [5] [9]-[12]. Similarities include middle age obese females and empty sella [13]. Direct evidence of elevated ICP in most patients with spontaneous CSF leaks was also found [3] [7] [13] [14].

The pressure usually exceeds 20 cmH$_2$O fitting with modified Dandy's criteria for intracranial hypertension [1]. The high ICP has been identified as a negative risk factor for successful repair [2] [15]. However, the raised ICP does not become evident until the pressure is rechecked after the leak is closed [16].

Worsening of pressure-type headaches and pulsatile tinnitus can occur after successful repair of CSF leak probably due to elimination of nasal CSF diversion via the leak and the resultant rise in the ICP post-operatively [5].

Several reports initiated a protocol to prospectively identify and treat patients with CSF leaks and elevated ICP and therefore at risk for recurrence of the leak [17]. Recognition and long-term treatment of elevated ICP is therefore critical to the successful management of these patients.

The purpose of our study was to evaluate the CSF pressure in cases of spontaneous CSF rhinorrhea and to report the outcome of repair of these cases when the elevated ICP was addressed. We also describe our same setting combined protocol to the repair of the leak, measurement and management of CSF pressure in this subset of patients.

2. Materials and Methods

In this prospective descriptive study, all patients presenting with primary or recurrent spontaneous CSF leak, to Ain Shams University Hospitals, Otolaryngology and Neurosurgical Departments between September 2008 and September 2013 were included. Patients with traumatic or iatrogenic causes were excluded. This study was approved by the Ethical committee for Ain Shams University, Cairo, Egypt and all patients signed a written consent for inclusion.

All demographic data, clinical presentation, body mass index (BMI), comorbidities and duration of leak were collected as well as chemical confirmation of the leaked fluid. All patients had visual acuity and fundus examination evaluation. Radiological workup included a CT scan paranasal sinuses without contrast, thin cuts, bony window, axial and coronal views in addition to an MRI, T1W, T1Gd and heavily weighted T2W sequences to localize the leak in the nasal cavity. A CT scan with metrizamide was also done for all patients.

The protocol for treatment included: decision on route of access, whether endoscopic, external or cranial approach; measurement of CSF pressure after completion of the repair; insertion of a lumboperitoneal shunt if the pressure exceeded 20 cmH$_2$O at the end of the operation.

All patients were discharged within 48 - 72 hours postoperatively with a Merocel pack in place and instructions to avoid increase intracranial pressure. The pack was removed on the 5th day in the outpatient clinic.

A routine paranasal sinus CT scan and abdominal plain X-ray were performed the next day of the operation. Patients with an intraoperative CSF pressure of 11 - 19 cmH$_2$O, had a re-measuring of the pressure 3 days after operation and if the pressure was still high a shunt was immediately performed (**Figure 1**). All patients were followed up and all postoperative complications were documented.

3. Results

Twenty-seven cases presented with spontaneous CSF leak during the study period. They were 23 women and 4 men. Their age ranged from 29 to 68 years old (mean = 45.3 years). Their BMI ranged from 26.6 to 43 (mean = 38.5). Four patients had a BMI of 25 - 30, 9 patients had a BMI between 31 and 35 and 14 patients had a BMI above 36. Five patients had hypertension, while 2 patients were diabetic. Four patients had recurrent leak after previous endoscopic repair. Most of the patients either received or were intolerant to acetazolamide treatment

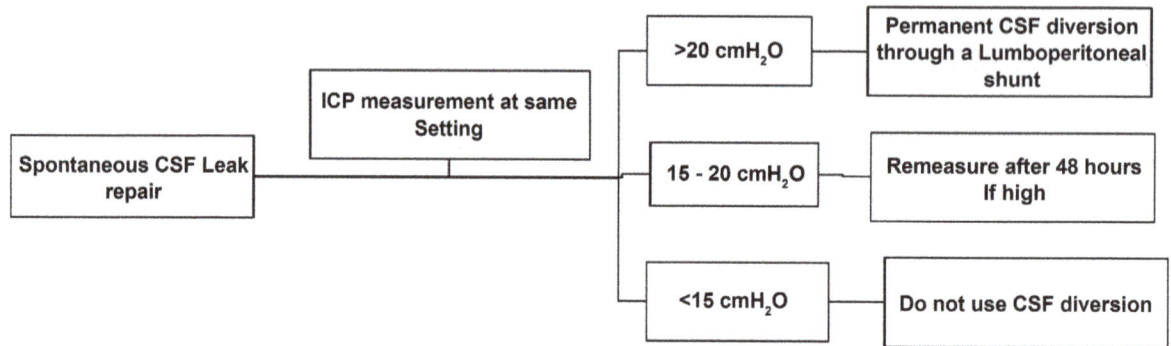

Figure 1. Protocol for management of spontaneous CSF leak and ICP.

before presenting to us without response.

The site of the leak was localized preoperatively in the radiological examination in all cases (**Table 1**). No cases had multiple sites of leak in our series. A meningoencephalocele was found in 13 cases (48%) (**Figure 2**).

The radiological data suspicious of increased intracranial pressure were looked for in CT scan and MRI. All patients had empty sella syndrome (100%) whether partial or complete (**Figure 3**). Ten patients had slit-like ventricles and tight subarachnoid spaces, while only 5 patients had tortuous optic nerve (**Figure 4**).

Surgery: All the repairs were performed extracranially: Endoscopic repair in 24 cases and external frontoeth-moidectomy approach in 3 cases for a defect in the posterior table of the frontal sinus. The same technique was used in all cases for repair: underlay and overlay fascia lata graft with tissue glue use. Gel foam packing and Merocel® nasal pack were further used. In large size defects more than 1.5 cm, a septal cartilage graft was also added.

At the end of the procedure, after graft placement and nasal packing, the patient was repositioned in the lateral decubitus and CSF pressure measurement was done using a wide bore lumbar drain needle. A collecting chamber with a pressure transducer was connected to the drain and zeroed at the spinal cord and the pressure was read when the flow stabilized. CSF pressure ranged from 5 to 39 cmH_2O (mean = 28.7). Only 2 patients had a pressure below 10 cmH_2O (7%), 6 had pressure between 11 - 20 cmH_2O (22%) and 19 patients (70%) had a pressure above 21 cmH_2O.

A lumboperitoneal shunt (Johnson® 84cm) was inserted in all patients with a pressure > 21 cmH_2O (n = 19). These patients stayed 48 - 72 hours in the hospital and were then discharged with the nasal pack in situ. Patients with a pressure between 11 and 20 cmH_2O (n = 6) had a repeat measurement 3 days post-operatively. Only 2 patients had a pressure above 20 cmH_2O and had the shunt inserted 4 days after the operation. The remaining 4 patients had a lower CSF pressure and had no further interventions and were discharged accordingly.

Complications: Minimal pneumocephalus occurred in 2 cases and resolved spontaneously without neurological affection. Postoperative headache for up to one month occurred in 6 cases. Those patients received Acetazolamide 500 mg twice daily for at least one month for postoperative headache development.

There were 5 cases of intranasal adhesions, 2 cases of abdominal wound gaping, one case of incisional hernia, and one case of shunt infection necessitating removal after 2 months.

A delayed frontal mucocele occurred in a patient treated externally after 8 months necessitating reoperation. All patients had successful repair with no recurrences with follow up period of 6 - 60 months (mean = 30 months) (**Figures 2-5**).

4. Discussion

Spontaneous CSF leak is a challenging clinical condition, with frequent recurrences following attempted surgical closure [12]. These recurrences should be considered as failure of management of elevated ICP rather than failure of operative repair 3. Decreasing ICP may have a beneficial adjuvant role to endoscopic repair of CSF rhinorrhea. Better management of the elevated ICP in this specific group of patients may lead to higher success rates [2]. The art of repairing these defects lies in knowing which patients will require CSF diversion and which who would not need it.

Patients with elevated ICP should preferably be identified upfront avoiding a second operation [17]. Although

Table 1. Preoperative localization of the site of leak.

Site of leak	Number
Cribriform plate	8
Fovea ethmoidalis	5
Cribriform + fovea	5
Frontal sinus	4
Sphenoid sinus	4
Sellaturcica	1

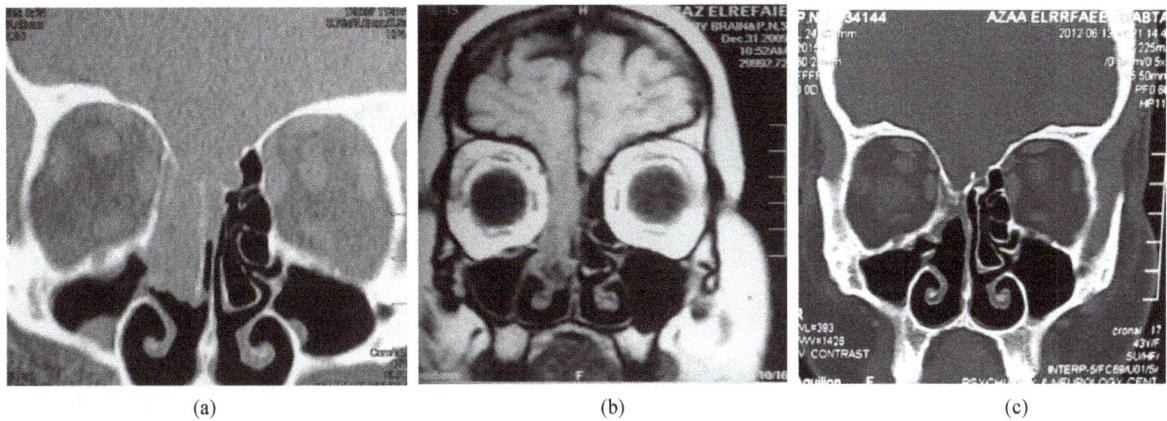

(a)　　　　　　　　　　(b)　　　　　　　　　　(c)

Figure 2. (a) Coronal CT scan PNS; (b) Coronal T1 weighted MRI showing a right sided huge meningoencephalocele, involving right fovea ethmoidalis and cribrifom plate; (c) Follow up CT scan 12 months after the repair showing success of the repair.

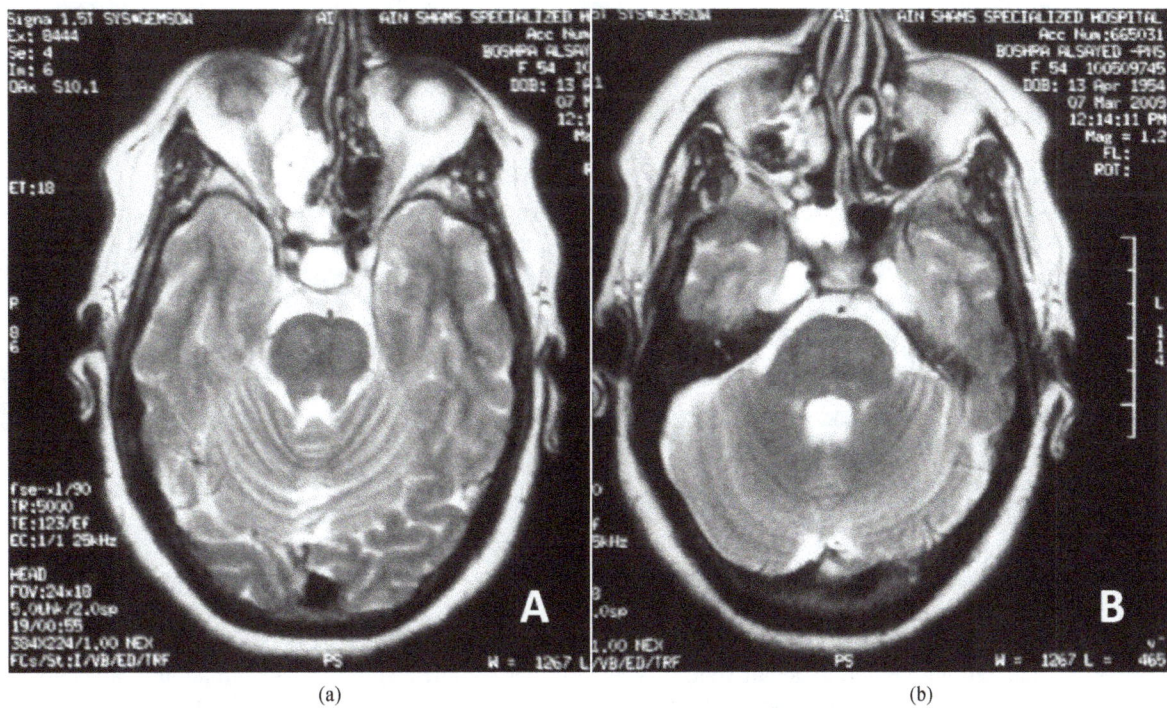

(a)　　　　　　　　　　(b)

Figure 3. Axial T2 weighted MRI of paranasal sinuses showing (a) empty sella syndrome; bilaterally distended Meckel's cave (b). CSF leak is seen in the right ethmoid air cells and nasal cavity (a) & (b).

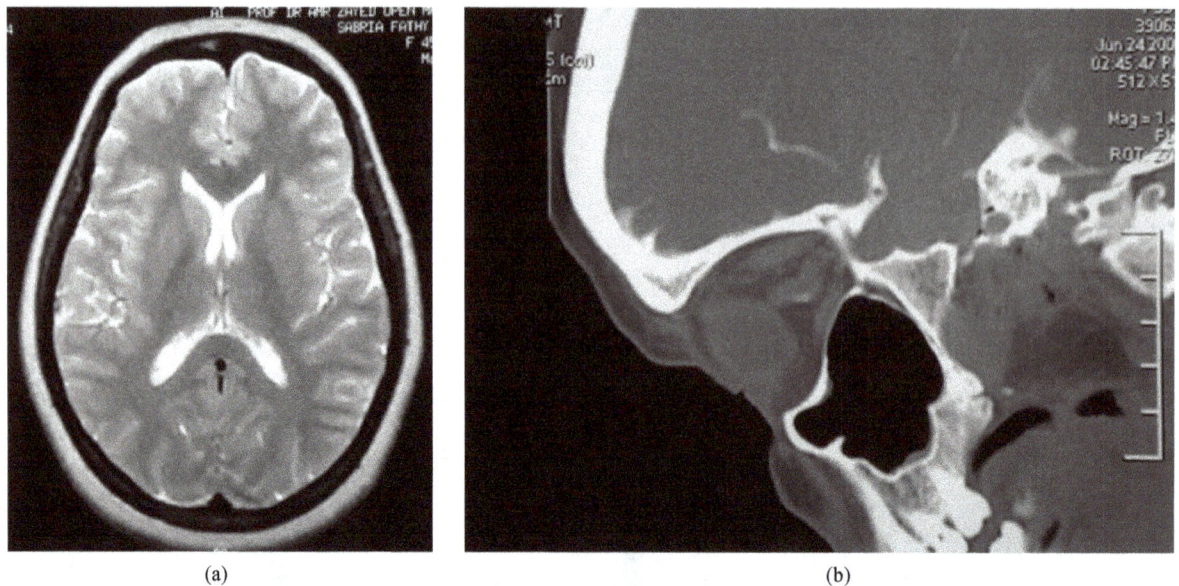

(a)   (b)

Figure 4. Radiologic criteria of elevated ICP (a) T2 weighted MRI showing slit-like ventricles and tight subarachnoid spaces (b) Sagittal CT scan showing tortuous optic nerve.

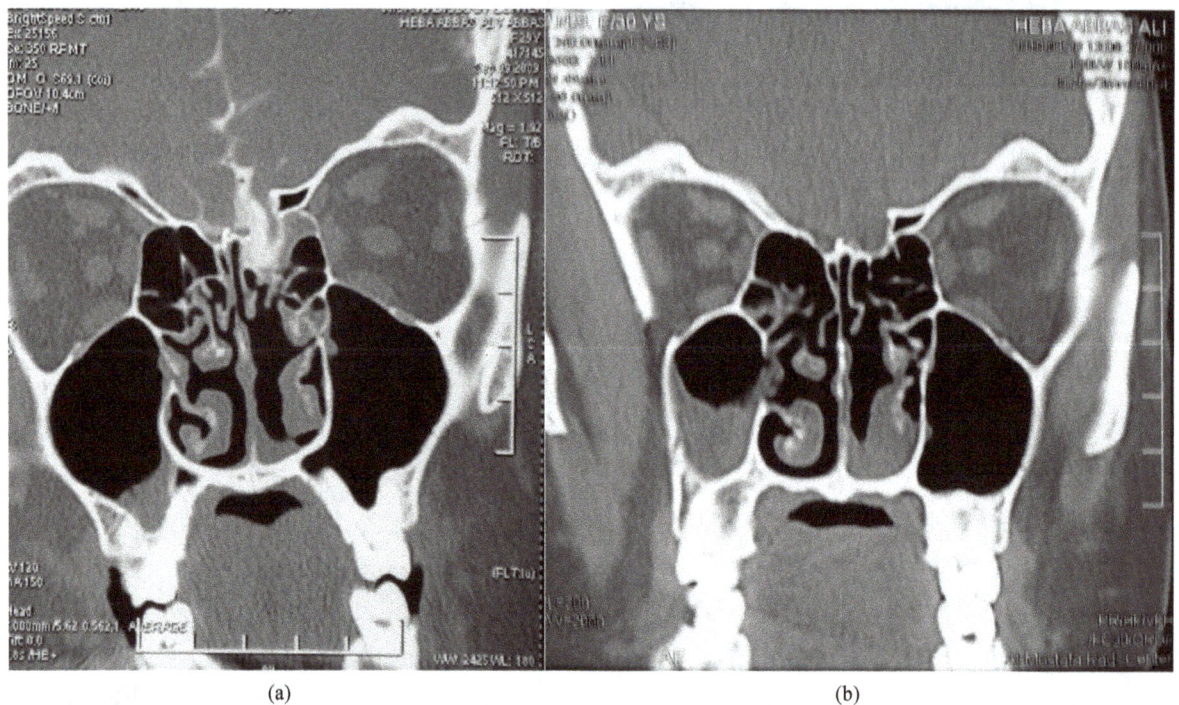

(a)   (b)

Figure 5. (a) CT cisternography with metrizamide showing a left sided large skull base defect in the fovea ethmoidalis; (b) Follow up CT scan after 12 months showing successful repair.

there are several clinical and radiologic clues, there are no rules [18]. Regarding the clinical clues, most of patients were females and BMI was above 30.

Radiologic findings may serve as a non-invasive indicator of elevated ICP. Radiographic evidence of elevated ICP include, but not limited to, small ventricles, a partial or complete empty sella, formation of arachnoid pits, abnormalities of the optic nerve sheath complex and meningoencephaloceles [1] [2] [4] [13] [15] [19]-[22]. Regarding radiologic clues in our patients, several were found especially the empty sella syndrome.

The pressure can be directly measured at the time of operation or post-operatively. Whenever the ICP is high, several authors resort to temporary or permanent CSF lowering. This can be achieved temporarily via medical treatment with acetazolamide, or through a lumbar drain [12] [23] [24]. However, inadequate response or intolerance to acetazolamide has been increasingly documented. A large number of our cases received prolonged treatment before presenting to us with no control. Lumbar drains have been advocated to transiently reduce CSF pressure in the immediate postoperative period and may also serve to determine which patients require long-term management of increased ICP2. Little is known about the indications or efficacy of post-operative lumbar drains to control CSF pressure after endoscopic repair of CSF rhinorrhea and its use remains controversial [24] [25]. Most authors use a lumbar drain during surgery and maintain it in the postoperative period for CSF diversion and measurement [5] [13] [17] [18]. If CSF pressure is high they recommend medical treatment but if the pressure is higher than 35 they consider permanent shunting [5].

However, not only is there a potential for associated complications, but there is also the need for hospitalization when these drains are used [26]. These are the same complications occurring when using a permanent lumboperitoneal shunt, and we find the benefits far outweigh the risks of such a minor procedure in well trained hands. In the same time, cases with refractory elevated ICP to a combination of medical management by acetazolamide and lumbar drain in spontaneous CSF leak has been shown to occur [14]. These patients usually have delayed recurrent leakage that may require permanent diversion procedures in a revision setting [5] [16]. This failure usually occurs later than 14 months, which implies the need of a long-term solution rather than a temporary one.

In our protocol, we prefer to measure the CSF pressure at the end of the repair, after depletion of the CSF during the repair. If the pressure is still high, we resort to permanent CSF diversion through a lumboperitoneal shunt in the same setting, sparing a second operation, allowing early ambulance, shortening hospital stay, increasing the success rate of the graft and decreasing recurrence rate. However, shunts are not without associated morbidity, so careful patient selection should be considered [17]. Those were mild and temporary in our group of patients. In our series, 70% of the cases had a high ICP above 21 cmH$_2$O, which can constitute a part of the pathophysiology. However, the smaller number without elevation of ICP were spared from a permanent CSF diversion.

Our 100% success rate of CSF leak control is consistent with previous reports. We believe that the high rate of success in this subset of patients, is basically related to the ability to control their ICP.

This approach is properly tailored to the individual patient, addressing both the elevated ICP and CSF leak in a single setting. Using this selective and specific protocol, a better diagnosis and control of the accompanying elevated ICP, when present, can be achieved. This avoids a second operative intervention, shortens the hospital stay, with an increase in the success rate. In the same time, the smaller number of patients with normal ICP can avoid further drainage.

5. Conclusions

We emphasize that management of elevated CSF in spontaneous CSF leak patients should be considered as an integral part of the control of the leak and prevent its recurrence.

In the cases with proved elevated ICP preoperatively by demographic, clinical, and radiological criteria as well as by measuring of CSF pressure at the end of the repair, permanent CSF diversion in the same setting should be considered. Further prospective case control studies are definitely needed to determine the need for long-term CSF diversion in that specific group of patients.

References

[1] Schlosser, R. and Bolger, W. (2003) Significance of Empty Sella in Cerebrospinal Fluid Leaks. *Otolaryngology—Head and Neck Surgery*, **128**, 32-38. http://dx.doi.org/10.1067/mhn.2003.43

[2] Wang, E.W., Vandergrift III, W.A. and Schlosser, R.J. (2011) Spontaneous CSF Leaks. *Otolaryngologic Clinics of North America*, **44**, 845-856. http://dx.doi.org/10.1016/j.otc.2011.06.018

[3] Woodworth, B.A., Prince, A., Chiu, A.G., Cohen, N.A., Schlosser, R.J., Bolger, W.E., Kennedy, D.W. and Palmer, J.N. (2008) Spontaneous CSF Leaks: A Paradigm for Definitive Repair and Management of Intracranial Hypertension. *Otolaryngology—Head and Neck Surgery*, **138**, 715-720. http://dx.doi.org/10.1016/j.otohns.2008.02.010

[4] Woodworth, B., Bolger, W. and Schlosser, R. (2006) Nasal Cerebrospinal Fluid Leaks and Encephaloceles. *Operative Techniques in Otolaryngology*, **17**, 111-116. http://dx.doi.org/10.1016/j.otot.2006.03.001

[5] Schlosser, R.J., Wilensky, E.M., Grady, M.S., Palmer, J.N., Kennedy, D.W. and Bolger, W.E. (2004) Cerebrospinal

Fluid Pressure Monitoring after Repair of Cerebrospinal Fluid Leaks. *Otolaryngology—Head and Neck Surgery*, **130**, 443-448. http://dx.doi.org/10.1016/j.otohns.2003.12.018

[6]   Schlosser, R.J. and Bolger, W.E. (2002) Management of Multiple Spontaneous Nasal Meningoencephaloceles. *Laryngoscope*, **112**, 980-985. http://dx.doi.org/10.1097/00005537-200206000-00008

[7]   Schlosser, R.J., Maloney-Wilensky, E., Grady, M.S., *et al.* (2003) Elevated Intracranial Pressures in Spontaneous Cerebrospinal Fluid Leaks. *American Journal of Rhinology*, **17**, 191-196.

[8]   Schlosser, R.J. and Bolger, W.E. (2004) Nasal Cerebrospinal Fluid Leaks: Critical Reviews and Surgical Considerations. *Laryngoscope*, **114**, 255-265. http://dx.doi.org/10.1097/00005537-200402000-00015

[9]   Schlosser, R.J. and Bolger, W.E. (2006) Spontaneous Cerebrospinal Fluid Leaks: A Variant of Benign Intracranial Hypertension. *Annals of Otology, Rhinology, and Laryngology*, **115**, 495-500. http://dx.doi.org/10.1177/000348940611500703

[10] Pérez, M.A., Bialer, O.Y., Bruce, B.B., Newman, N.J. and Biousse, V. (2013) Primary Spontaneous Cerebrospinal Fluid Leaks and Idiopathic Intracranial Hypertension. *Journal of Neuro-Ophthalmology*, **33**, 330-337. http://dx.doi.org/10.1097/WNO.0b013e318299c292

[11] Chaaban, M.R., Illing, E., Riley, K.O. and Woodworth, B.A. (2014) Spontaneous Cerebrospinal Fluid Leak Repair: A Five-Year Prospective Evaluation. *Laryngoscope*, **124**, 70-75. http://dx.doi.org/10.1002/lary.24160

[12] Woodworth, B.A. and Palmer, J.N. (2009) Spontaneous Cerebrospinal Fluid Leaks. *Current Opinion in Otolaryngology & Head & Neck Surgery*, **17**, 59-65. http://dx.doi.org/10.1097/MOO.0b013e3283200017

[13] Schlosser, R.J., Wilensky, E.M., Grady, M.S., Palmer, J.N., Kennedy, D.W. and Bolger, W.E. (2004) Cerebrospinal Fluid Pressure Monitoring after Repair of Cerebrospinal Fluid Leaks. *Otolaryngology—Head and Neck Surgery*, **130**, 443-448. http://dx.doi.org/10.1016/j.otohns.2003.12.018

[14] Schlosser, R.J., Woodworth, B.A., Wilensky, E.M., Sean Grady, M. and Bolger, W.E. (2006) Spontaneous Cerebrospinal Fluid Leaks: A Variant of Benign Intracranial Hypertension. *Annals of Otology, Rhinology & Laryngology*, **115**, 495-500. http://dx.doi.org/10.1177/000348940611500703

[15] Schlosser, R.J. and Bolger, W.E. (2006) Endoscopic Management of Cerebrospinal Fluid Rhinorrhea. *Otolaryngologic Clinics of North America*, **39**, 523-538.

[16] Banks, C., Palmer, J., Chiu, A., O'Malley Jr., B., Woodworth, B. and Kennedy, D. (2009) Endoscopic Closure of CSF Rhinorrhea: 193 Cases over 21 Years. *Otolaryngology—Head and Neck Surgery*, **140**, 826-833. http://dx.doi.org/10.1016/j.otohns.2008.12.060

[17] Carrau, R.L., Snyderman, C.H. and Kassam, A.B. (2005) The Management of Cerebrospinal Fluid Leaks in Patients at Risk for High-Pressure Hydrocephalus. *Laryngoscope*, **115**, 205-212. http://dx.doi.org/10.1097/01.mlg.0000154719.62668.70

[18] Zweig, J.L., Carrau, R.L., Celin, S.E., Schaitkin, B.M., Pollice, P.A., Snyderman, C.H., Kassam, A. and Hegazy, H. (2000) Endoscopic Repair of Cerebrospinal Fluid Leaks to the Sinonasal Tract: Predictors of Success. *Otolaryngology—Head and Neck Surgery*, **123**, 195-201. http://dx.doi.org/10.1067/mhn.2000.107452

[19] Goddard, J.C., Meyer, T., Nguyen, S. and Lambert, P.R. (2010) New Considerations in the Cause of Spontaneous Cerebrospinal Fluid Otorrhea. *Otology & Neurotology*, **31**, 940-945. http://dx.doi.org/10.1097/MAO.0b013e3181e8f36c

[20] Kutz Jr., J.W., Husain, I.A., Isaacson, B. and Roland, P.S. (2008) Management of Spontaneous Cerebrospinal Fluid Otorrhea. *Laryngoscope*, **118**, 2195-2199. http://dx.doi.org/10.1097/MLG.0b013e318182f833

[21] Silver, R.I., Moonis, G., Schlosser, R.J., Bolger, W.E. and Loevner, L.A. (2007) Radiographic Signs of Elevated Intracranial Pressure in Idiopathic Cerebrospinal Fluid Leaks: A Possible Presentation of Idiopathic Intracranial Hypertension. *American Journal of Rhinology*, **21**, 257-261. http://dx.doi.org/10.2500/ajr.2007.21.3026

[22] Schlosser, R.J. and Bolger, W.E. (2003) Spontaneous Nasal Cerebrospinal Fluid Leaks and Empty Sella Syndrome: A Clinical Association. *American Journal of Rhinology*, **17**, 91-96.

[23] Chaaban, M.R., Illing, E., Riley, K.O. and Woodworth, B.A. (2013) Acetazolamide for High Intracranial Pressure Cerebrospinal Fluid Leaks. *International Forum of Allergy & Rhinology*, **3**, 718-721. http://dx.doi.org/10.1002/alr.21188

[24] Caballero, N., Bhalla, V., Stankiewicz, J.A. and Welch, K.C. (2012) Effect of Lumbar Drain Placement on Recurrence of Cerebrospinal Rhinorrhea after Endoscopic Repair. *International Forum of Allergy & Rhinology*, **2**, 222-226. http://dx.doi.org/10.1002/alr.21023

[25] Virk, J.S., Elmiyeh, B. and Saleh, H.A. (2013) Endoscopic Management of Cerebrospinal Fluid Rhinorrhea: The Charing Cross Experience. *Journal of Neurological Surgery. Part B, Skull Base*, **74**, 61-67.

[26] Casiano, R. and Jassir, D. (1999) Endoscopic Cerebrospinal Fluid Rhinorrhea Repair: Is a Lumbar Drain Necessary? *Otolaryngology—Head and Neck Surgery*, **121**, 745-749. http://dx.doi.org/10.1053/hn.1999.v121.a98754

23

The Evolution of Laser in Laryngology

Asil Tahir

Department of Otolaryngology/Head & Neck Surgery, Leighton Hospital, Crewe, UK
Email: asiltahir@hotmail.com

Abstract

Technological breakthroughs in physics are often adapted and incorporated into the ever growing field of otolaryngology. When first discovered, "The Incredible Laser" had promised to be science's new "Aladdin's lamp", it can "light up the moon", "kill instantly", or "perform miracle surgery" [1]. Although not quite fulfilling these roles, laser technology has been a key element in the development of endolaryngeal surgery. This article looks at the invention of Laser and it's progression into an invaluable tool in the field of laryngeal surgery.

Keywords

Laser, History, Laryngology

1. The Discovery of Laser

Albert Einstein propelled the theoretical foundation for the development of this landmark invention in 1916 when he proposed that photons could stimulate emission of identical photons from excited atoms [1]. Stimulated emission is where a photon interacts with an excited molecule or atom and causes the emission of a second photon having the same frequency, phase, polarization and direction. This theory has been fundamental in the development of laser technology. In 1940, the Russian physicist Valentin Fabrikant proposed that stimulated emission in a gas discharge may amplify light under specific conditions [1].

However, it was not until after the end of World War II when research into laser technology benefitted greatly from corporate and government investments into technological progress during the cold war era. This coupled with the growth in numbers of physicists and engineers and growth in the economy created the foundations for the invention of the ruby laser in 1960 by Theodore Maiman [2]. Soon after Maiman built the first laser, his assistant joked that the laser was "a solution looking for a problem." This of course contained some truth to it, as the laser was not a device invented to fill specific application requirement. It was more a discovery than an invention, a way to generate coherent light that laser developers expected would find applications in broader areas, such as research or communications [1].

2. The Principles of Laser Surgery

The atoms of a laser exist within a medium which can be either solid, liquid or gas. This is encased within an optical resonant chamber in-between two mirrors. The process of laser emission begins with an external source of energy, such as a flash lamp or an electric arc, which is used to excite the atoms in the medium. The internal energy contributes to a cascade of stimulated emissions that create the amplified light energy. The three important properties to laser are the wavelength, coherence and directionality. The particular wavelength of laser energy will decide it's precision as a scalpel and the haemostatic properties. The laser energy must be intense, sharply focused, and absorbed almost entirely at the surface for precise dissection with minimal surrounding thermal injury and tissue damage [1] [3] [4].

Currently there are a large number of lasers available for the otolaryngologist to utilise. They have varying characteristics including different wavelengths, interactions with tissue, modes of transmission and delivery systems. These include the Carbon Dioxide (CO_2), neodymium:yttrium-aluminum-garnet (Nd:YAG) in contact and non-contact modes, argon, potassium titanyl phosphate (KTP), Pulsed Dyed Laser (PDL), argon dye, holmium:YAG, erbium:YAG and free electron lasers [3] [5].

Further to its growing use in laryngology, laser surgery has developed in other areas of otolaryngology. Tumours of the tongue, floor of the mouth, palate and tonsils can be resected with excellent control and haemostasis using the CO_2 laser. The Nd:YAG, CO_2, KTP, and diode lasers have all been used with good short-term results of nasal airway obstruction and recurrent epistaxis. In ear surgery the precision of argon, KTP, and CO_2 lasers through a microscope have been shown to be very effective in stapedotomy, ossicular fixation and tympanosclerosis [3] [6].

Laser surgery has advantages when compared to cold surgery on the larynx. It offers an unobstructed view of the operation field, ability to work at longer distances, minimises tissue manipulation, increased sterility, better haemostasis and is associated with fewer post operative complications. However, lasers require a large number of personnel to ensure effectiveness and safety. There is also a significant cost associated with the installation of equipment, maintenance and updating technical developments can be significantly more costly than using cold instruments. Laser heat can increase scarring and cause damage to adjacent tissue. Other potential limitations of laser include potential for endotracheal explosion, facial burns, mucosal burns, vocal fold webs, stenoses and glottic incompetence [3]-[5].

3. The Carbon Dioxide Laser

It was not until 1964, when Patel invented the first carbon dioxide (CO_2) laser, did it gain immediate popularity and rapidly developed as an important surgical tool in laryngology [7]. The CO_2 laser was the first to be used on the larynx due to its ideal tissue properties for surgery; water absorbs the 10,600 nm wavelength really well, its high focus limits soft tissue penetration and minimises collateral thermal damage whilst providing good haemostasis [8]. It was initially experimented on cadaveric larynx and dogs and only became medically effective with the development of coupling of the microscope and the development of the micromanipulators by Polanyi and Bredemeier to deliver precise energy to the larynx [9].

Hungarian born Geza Jako, often called father of Laser surgery and was Inventor over 120 instruments. He introduced both cold microlaryngeal instruments in 1962, and in 1972 Jako experimented with the CO_2 laser integrated with a microscope on 12 dogs as a precise haemostatic scalpel on laryngeal tissue. He selectively evaporated predetermined amounts of normal vocal cord tissue through a laryngoscope with good results. All the dogs received antibiotics to reduce risk of complications post anaesthesia. One dog had died prior to follow up laryngoscopy and three dogs had accidental radiation to the trachea. The dogs were killed with anaesthesia overdose after a 3 - 4 weeks follow up laryngoscopy revealing normal healing similar to that of a clean surgical wound repair. The larynges were taken for histology and showed distinct demarcation between tissue destruction and normal tissue with good healing and epitheliazation [10]. CO_2 laser was especially useful for the majority of surgeons as the delivery of joystick and pedal enhanced the manual dexterity of surgeon working at a distance under high magnification. He advocated that the CO_2 laser should be used synergistically with cold instruments and not as an alternative [3].

4. The Use of Laser on Patient's Larynges

The first use of laser in patients was in 1975 by Strong who used the CO_2 laser to successfully treat 11 patients with early T1 laryngeal Cancer [11]. He described inadequate exposure or extension of the carcinoma to the anterior commissure, arytenoid or subglottic areas was a contraindication to laser excision. The excised areas showed good precision and very good healing even in post radiation larynges. The post operative voice was also shown to be as good as the remaining larynx would allow [11].

Joining his colleagues Strong and Jako, Vaughan from Boston Massachusetts went on to investigate the useful application of using CO_2 lasers in laryngeal cancers. They showed that the laser is a useful adjunct in treating laryngeal tumours, not only through direct excision, but also by helping establish proper staging, diagnosing reoccurrence after radiation therapy, debunking tumour mass for airway establishment and prior to radiotherapy and chemotherapy. This was all possible with minimal morbidity, as a day case, with good organ preservation and without requiring tracheostomies. All of which worked out well for cost benefit [12]. They also went on to explore its use with various benign and malignant disorders-including carcinoma, stenosis, papilloma, nodules, polyps, cysts and amyloidosis [13]. Nonetheless, their novel approach was met with biting resistance.

Building on these results Steiner developed new endoscopes, instruments and new techniques to handle the larynx and improve oncologic effectiveness [14]. Between 1979 and 1986 he treated almost 900 patients aged 15 - 91 including over 500 patients with laryngeal carcinoma. He describes that in early stages of growth, transpolar microsurgical resection using CO_2 laser is curative. And also now with laser the possibility of treating advanced tumours with or without radiotherapy while preserving functionally important organs without the need for tracheostomy. However in whenever the carcinoma has spread beyond the larynx or into arytenoids the use of laser is very limited [14]. A more recent study on laser treatment presented by Wolfgang Steiner, MD, in 2005 showed that of 333 patients with T1a tumors, 89.3% had their lesions controlled after five years, and 97.6% of those had their larynx preserved [15].

5. Photoangiolytic Lasers

Although CO_2 has initially been the primary laser used in Laryngology, fiber based photoangiolytic lasers such as Pulsed Dyed Laser (PDL) and potassium-titanyl-phosphate (KTP) are now increasingly used on laryngeal pathologies. Unlike the CO_2 laser the PDL and KTP deliver energy through thin glass fibres better suited to treat subepithelial resection such as nodules, cysts and polyps [3].

In the 1980s Anderson and his colleagues began using PDL on benign laryngeal lesions. These lasers have been previously specifically useful at treating vascular lesions on skin dues to the its wavelength which targets the absorbance peak of oxyhaemaglobin [16]. These were shown to be significantly effective on papillomatosis and dysplasia. The epithelium was largely preserved during laser resection, which meant these lesions could be treated without the concern of scarring, synechia or webbing. This was especially useful for lesions affecting the anterior commissure, which was commonly associated with an increased morbidity with repeat resection using cold instruments or CO_2 laser.

PDL and KTP lasers have recently been used to treat laryngeal cancers by targeting their blood supply and also in the management of Reinke's oedema, which would conventionally require cold knife surgical intervention [17]. Although significantly more expensive that CO_2 lasers, PDL has the potential of being carried out in a clinical setting using a flexible endoscope under local anaesthetic. This approach is likely to expand rapidly due to a reduction in patient morbidity and the potential of improvement in health-care delivery [3].

6. The Future

Years of development have vastly improved laser performance and have been an important solution for a variety of problems, not only in laryngology, but also in scientific research, consumer products, telecommunications, engineering and a host of other applications.

In the treatment of laryngeal cancer, laser surgery has already demonstrated reliable tumour removal with fewer complications than open surgery in managing many glottic and supraglottic lesions. Currently, there are a variety of different lasers available for otolaryngologists to utilise with extended applications and variable wavelengths such as CO_2, Nd:YAG, argon, PDL, KTP and argon dye. New lasers, such as the use of thulium on endolaryngeal resections, show promising results offering improved haemostasis and effective tangential dissection. The increased volume of ambulatory and office-based laser surgery has an important role in reducing costs and will continue to gain increased interest in financially stretched healthcare systems around the world. The considerable amount of research that continues to develop the use of laser in otolaryngology inevitably means further advancements in its clinical application [3] [4].

Conflicts of Interest

I can confirm there is no financial or personal relationship with any people or organizations related to this report that could inappropriately influence this work.

References

[1]   Hecht, J. (2010) A Short History of Laser Development. *Applied Optics*, **49**, F99-F122.
      http://dx.doi.org/10.1364/AO.49.000F99

[2]   Maiman, T.H. (1960) Stimulated Optical Radiation in Ruby. *Nature*, **187**, 493-494. http://dx.doi.org/10.1038/187493a0

[3]   Zeitels, S.M. and Burns, J.A. (2006) Laser Applications in Laryngology: Past, Present, and Future. *Otolaryngologic Clinics of North America*, **39**, 159-172. http://dx.doi.org/10.1016/j.otc.2005.10.001

[4]   Yan, Y., *et al.* (2010) Use of Lasers in Laryngeal Surgery. *Journal of Voice*, **24**, 102-109.
      http://dx.doi.org/10.1016/j.jvoice.2008.09.006

[5]   Shapiro, J., Zeitels, S.M. and Fried, M.P. (1992) Laser Surgery for Laryngeal Cancer. *Operative Techniques in Otolaryngology—Head and Neck Surgery*, **3**, 84-92. http://dx.doi.org/10.1016/S1043-1810(10)80245-3

[6]   Ossoff, R.H., *et al.* (1994) Clinical Applications of Lasers in Otolaryngology—Head and Neck Surgery. *Lasers in Surgery and Medicine*, **15**, 217-248. http://dx.doi.org/10.1002/lsm.1900150302

[7]   Patel, C.K.N. (1964) Continuous-Wave Laser Action on Vibrational-Rotational Transitions of CO_2. *Physical Review*, **136**, A1187-A1193. http://dx.doi.org/10.1103/PhysRev.136.A1187

[8]   Rubinstein, M. and Armstrong, W.B. (2011) Transoral Laser Microsurgery for Laryngeal Cancer: A Primer and Review of Laser Dosimetry. *Lasers in Medical Science*, **26**, 113-124. http://dx.doi.org/10.1007/s10103-010-0834-5

[9]   Polanyi, T.G., Bredemeier, H.C. and Davis Jr., T.W. (1970) A CO_2 Laser for Surgical Research. *Medical & Biological Engineering*, **8**, 541-548. http://dx.doi.org/10.1007/BF02478228

[10] Jako, G.J. (1972) Laser Surgery of the Vocal Cords. An Experimental Study with Carbon Dioxide Lasers on Dogs. *Laryngoscope*, **82**, 2204-2216. http://dx.doi.org/10.1288/00005537-197212000-00009

[11] Strong, M.S. (1975) Laser Excision of Carcinoma of the Larynx. *Laryngoscope*, **85**, 1286-1289.
      http://dx.doi.org/10.1288/00005537-197508000-00003

[12] Vaughan, C.W. (1978) Transoral Laryngeal Surgery Using the CO_2 Laser: Laboratory Experiments and Clinical Experience. *Laryngoscope*, **88**, 1399-1420.

[13] Strong, M.S., *et al.* (1973) Laser Surgery in the Aerodigestive Tract. *American Journal of Surgery*, **126**, 529-533.
      http://dx.doi.org/10.1016/S0002-9610(73)80044-3

[14] Steiner, W. (1988) Experience in Endoscopic Laser Surgery of Malignant Tumours of the Upper Aero-Digestive Tract. *Advances in Oto-Rhino-Laryngology*, **39**, 135-144.

[15] Steiner, W., *et al.* (2004) Impact of Anterior Commissure Involvement on Local Control of Early Glottic Carcinoma Treated by Laser Microresection. *Laryngoscope*, **114**, 1485-1491.
      http://dx.doi.org/10.1097/00005537-200408000-00031

[16] Anderson, R.R., Jaenicke, K.F. and Parrish, J.A. (1983) Mechanisms of Selective Vascular Changes Caused by Dye Lasers. *Lasers in Surgery and Medicine*, **3**, 211-215. http://dx.doi.org/10.1002/lsm.1900030303

[17] Franco Jr., R.A., *et al.* (2003) 585-nm Pulsed Dye Laser Treatment of Glottal Dysplasia. *Annals of Otology, Rhinology Laryngology*, **112**, 751-758. http://dx.doi.org/10.1177/000348940311200902

24

Lipoma in Hard Palate—A Case Report

Prince Peter Dhas, Ravindran Ambika, Amirthagani Arumugam, Jagan Somasundaram

Department of ENT, Thanjavur Medical College, Thanjavur, India
Email: drprincembbs@gmail.com

Abstract

Lipoma is a benign neoplasm of the soft tissue that originates in mature adipocytes. Even though it is a very common tumor, it is relatively uncommon in oral cavity. It represents about 1% to 4% of all benign tumors in oral cavity (12). This article describes a case of a 39 years old male with an intraoral pedunculated mass in the right side of hard palate which was histopathologically proved as a simple lipoma.

Keywords

Hard Palate, Lipoma, Benign, Oral Cavity

1. Introduction

Lipomas are benign mesenchymal neoplasms composed of mature adipocytes usually surrounded by a thin fibrous capsule [1]. Lipomas can occur in any part of the human body, but the majority occur in trunk and neck [2]. They can present as a single swelling or multiple swellings. About 20% occur in the head and neck region and only 1% to 4% involve oral cavity [3] [4]. Half of oral lipomas are in the cheek and the remaining are found in the tongue, floor of the mouth, lips, palate, and gingival mucosa [5]. Lipomas are usually asymptomatic till they grow to a larger size and interfere with speech, mastication and swallowing [6]. Lipomas may occur sporadically or as one of the several inherited disorders such as familial multiple lipomatosis and benign symmetric lipomatosis [7].

Based on their histopathological aspects, lipomas can be characterized as classic lipoma, fibrolipoma, intramural lipoma, spindle cell lipoma, angiolipoma, sialolipoma, pleomorphic lipoma, myxoid lipoma and atypical lipoma. The malignant counterpart of the tumor is liposarcoma which is an another common soft tissue neoplasm but rare in oral cavity [8].

2. Case Report

A 39 years old male patient presented with a mass in the oral cavity. A small swelling appeared in the right side of the palate before 6 years which progressively increased in size. He had problems with speech and mastication.

He is a tobacco and betel nut chewer for 20 years. Physical examination revealed a soft pedunculated mass of size 6.5 × 3.5 cm arising from the right side of the hard palate at about 1 cm medial to right 2nd molar. It was covered with intact mucosa. With the aid of computed tomography, bony attachments/erosion was excluded. Also the mass failed to enhance with contrast. Complete surgical excision was done and the mass was subjected for histopathological examination. Macroscopically the resected mass was yellowish in colour. Microscopic appearance shows a well encapsulated tumor composed of muscle fat cells with vacuolated cytoplasm with intervening fibrous septae. There was no sarcomatous change. The wound healed well. The patient was followed up for 1 year without any recurrence (**Figures 1-6**).

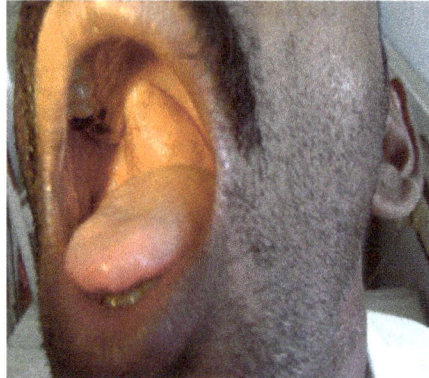

Figure 1. Showing mass in the hard palate.

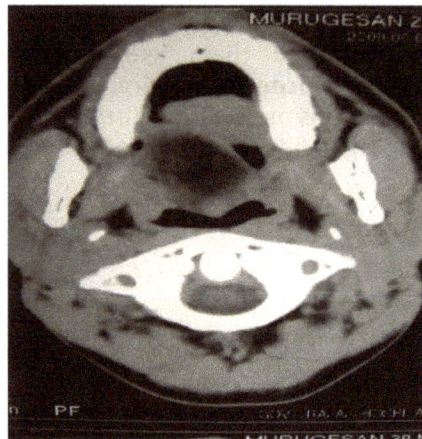

Figure 2. CT showing hypodense mass in hard palate.

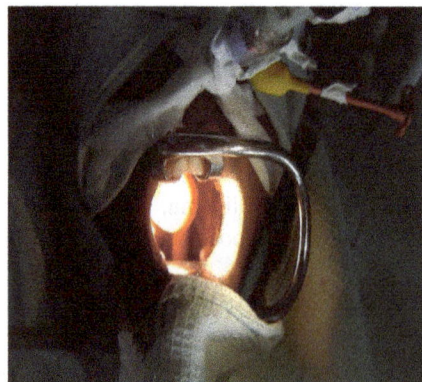

Figure 3. Preoperative picture.

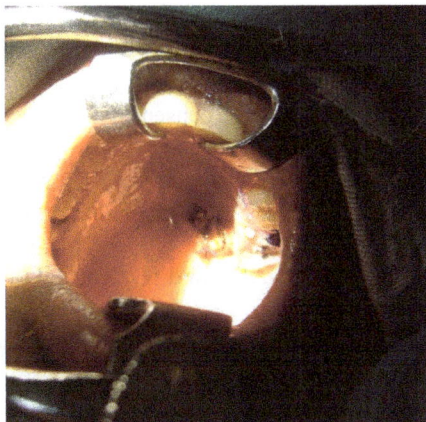

Figure 4. Post operative picture.

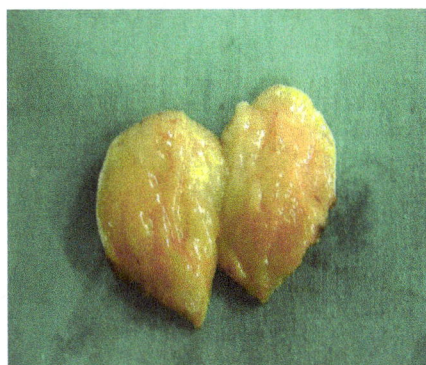

Figure 5. Cut section of excised mass.

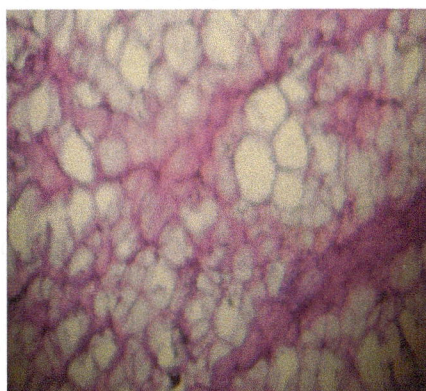

Figure 6. Microscopic picture showing mature adipocytes.

3. Discussion

The first oral lipoma was described by Roux in a review of alveolar masses in which he referred it as "Yellow Epulis" [9]. Lipoma is the commonest and most benign of all tumors. Intraoral region is a rare site for its development. The incidence does not differ with gender but a predilection for men has been reported [10]. The case we are presenting is very rare because of its site of attachment *i.e.* Hard palate. To the best of our knowledge only 2 cases of lipoma in hard palate mucosa has been reported (Hoceini *et al.*, 2010; Sushruth Nayak & Prachi Nayak) [11]. In a case series by Perez *et al.* on oral lipoma among 2270 cases of oral lesions in a period of 8 years, 6 cases were oral lipomas. Of the 4, 3 were reported to be in buccal mucosa, 1 in lower lip, 1 in tongue

[12].

Clinically oral lipomas generally present as mobile, painless submucosal nodules with a yellowish colour. In our patient it is a pedunculated mass which is a rare presentation.

The pathogenesis of lipoma still remains with lack of consensus. Various concepts such as obesity, hormonal influences, trauma and chronic irritation have been proposed [13].

Histopathologically our case is a classical lipoma which has been reported to be the commonest intraoral form in various literatures. Freital *et al.* (2009) reviewed 26 cases of intraoral lipomas and classic lipoma was the most common among them *i.e.* in 15 cases [14].

Surgical excision is the suggested treatment modality and if adequately resected, recurrence is rare. We followed the patient for 1 year without any recurrence.

4. Conclusion

We present this case for its rare site, size and presentation. A clinician must also recognize other differential diagnoses for such a mass which are to be excluded by radiological and histopathological examination to proceed with the correct treatment.

References

[1]   Fregnani, E.R., Pires, F.R., Falzoni, R., Lopes, M.A. and Vargas, P.A. (2003) Lipomas of the Oral Cavity: Clinical Findings, Histological Classification and Proliferative Activity of 46 Cases. *International Journal of Oral and Maxillofacial Surgery*, **32**, 49-53. http://dx.doi.org/10.1054/ijom.2002.0317

[2]   Rosai, J. (1989) Ackerman's Surgical Pathology. 7th Edition, The C.V. Mosby Co., St Louis, 1573-1579.

[3]   de Visscher, J.G. (1982) Lipomas and Fibrolipomas of the Oral Cavity. *Journal of Oral and Maxillofacial Surgery*, **10**, 177-181.

[4]   Gnepp, D.R. (2001) Diagnostic Surgical Pathology of the Head and Neck. WB Saunders, Philadelphia.

[5]   Vindenes, H. (1978) Lipomas of the Oral Cavity. *International Journal of Oral Surgery*, **7**, 162-166. http://dx.doi.org/10.1016/S0300-9785(78)80019-2

[6]   Keskin, G., Ustundag, E. and Ercin, C. (2002) Multiple Infiltrating Lipomas of the Tongue. *Journal of Laryngology Otology*, **116**, 395-397. http://dx.doi.org/10.1258/0022215021910906

[7]   Bradon, J.H., Blackwell, S.J., Mancoll, J.S.O., *et al.* (1999) Another Indication for Liposuction: Small Facial Lipomas. *Plastic and Reconstructive Surgery*, **103**, 1864-1867. http://dx.doi.org/10.1097/00006534-199906000-00008

[8]   Favia, G., Maiorano, E., Orsini, G. and Piattelli, A. (2001) Myxoid Liposarcoma of the Oral Cavity with Involvement of the Periodontal Tissues. *Journal of Clinical Periodontology*, **28**, 109-112. http://dx.doi.org/10.1034/j.1600-051x.2001.028002109.x

[9]   Manjunatha, B.S., Pateel, G.S. and Shah, V. (2010) Oralfibrolipoma—A Rare Histological Entity: Report of 3 Cases and Review of Literature. *Journal of Dentistry*, **7**, 226-231.

[10] Furlong, M.A., Fanburg-Smith, J.C. and Childers, E.L. (2004) Lipoma of the Oral and Maxillofacial Region: Site and Subclassification of 125 Cases. *Oral Surgery, Oral Medicine, Oral Pathology, Oral Radiology, and Endodontology*, **98**, 441-450. http://dx.doi.org/10.1016/j.tripleo.2004.02.071

[11] Nayak, S. and Nayak, P. (2011) Lipoma of Oral Mucosa: A Case Report. *Archieves of Orofacial Sciences*, **6**, 37-39.

[12] Bandéca, M.C., de Pádua, J.M., Nadalin, M.R., Ozório, J.E., Silva-Sousa, Y.T. and da Cruz Perez, D.E. (2007) Oral Soft Tissue Lipomas: A Case Series. *Journal of the Canadian Dental Association*, **73**, 431-434.

[13] Demir, Y. and Aktepe, F. (2002) Unusually Large Intraoral Submucosal Lipoma. *The Medical Journal of Kocatepe*, **3**, 61-65.

[14] Freitas, M.A., Freitas, V.S., Lima, A.A.S. and Pereira Jr., F.B. (2009) Intraoral Lipomas: A Study of 26 Cases in a Brazilian Population. *Quintessence International*, **40**, 79-85.

25

Lymphoepithelioma-Like Carcinoma of Parapharyngeal Space—A Case Report with Review of Literature

Produl Hazarika[1*], Seema Elina Punnoose[1], John Victor[1], Sreekala[2], Nirmali Dutta[3]

[1]Department of ENT, NMC Specialty Hospital, Abu Dhabi, UAE
[2]Department of Pathology, NMC Specialty Hospital, Abu Dhabi, UAE
[3]Department of Radiology, NMC Specialty Hospital, Abu Dhabi, UAE
Email: [*]produl_ent@rediffmail.com

Abstract

Extra-nasopharyngeal lymphoepithelioma-like carcinomas (LELC) are uncommon epithelial tumors. A few isolated case reports and series are available in literature involving the larynx, pharynx, salivary gland, lung etc., but involvement in the parapharyngeal space has not yet been reported. We aim to highlight one such case that has a clinical and radiological characteristic of a benign lesion whilst the histopathology reveals an infiltrating neoplasm. The typical clinical aggressiveness of a classical LELC of extra-nasopharyngeal lesion as described in literature is not present in our case. Also seen is an uncommon finding of abnormal branching of left external carotid artery. There is no standard treatment protocol for such a tumor; however, wide excision of this tumor in the parapharyngeal space via trans-cervical, trans-mandibular, trans-palatal approach has shown good and satisfactory tumor control of the primary site so far.

Keywords

Lymphoepithelioma-Like Carcinoma (LELC), Parapharyngeal Space, Trans-Cervical, Trans-Mandibular, Cells in Cords, Lymphoplasmacytoid

1. Introduction

Parapharyngeal space tumors are rare and comprise only 0.5% of all head and neck tumors and a vast majority of these are benign in nature [1]. Even more rare is a primary malignant tumor of parapharyngeal space. Our se-

---

[*]Corresponding author.

nior author [2] has published a series of 41 cases of parapharyngeal tumor where he found only 5 cases with malignant pathology. Herein reported is a rare case of lympho-epithelioma-like carcinoma (LELC) primarily arising from the parapharyngeal space having no clinical or radiological evidence of involvement of the nasopharynx. This neoplasm seems to have behaved in a fashion remniscent of nasopharyngeal carcinoma. However, predominant association of Ebstein Barr Virus in nasopharyngeal lymphoepithelioma is not seen commonly in LELC of extranasopharyngeal origin. A review of available English literature using search engines Medscape and Pubmed failed to show any previous report of LELC in parapharyngeal space. This case study of lymphoepithelioma-like carcinoma in the parapharyngeal space is peculiar and unusual. The preoperative diagnosis of this neoplasm was difficult and final definitive diagnosis was established only after immunohistochemistry and electron microscope studies. In the present case, the diagnosis is supported by histopathological studies and immunohistochemistry. There was no associated tumor involvement of nasopharynx or lung on clinical and radiological examination. The idea of presenting this case is to highlight its rare occurrence of this tumor in the parapharyngeal space, its diagnostic as well as management dilemmas along with the abnormal branching of external carotid artery. This could very well be the first reported case of primary lymphoepithelioma-like carcinoma found in the parapharyngeal space to the best of our knowledge.

2. Case Report

A 30 years old Indian male patient attended the ENT Clinic of NMC Specialty Hospital, Abu Dhabi, UAE on 7th October 2013 for his complaints of breathing difficulty, huskiness of voice and snoring during sleep of 6 months duration. There was no difficulty in swallowing but his initial symptoms of breathing difficulty aggravated in the last one month. Clinical examination revealed a globular, smooth and congested mass pushing the left side of soft palate and uvula downwards and medially causing narrowing of the oropharyngeal inlet. A rigid videolaryngoscopy showed the lower margin of the mass going beyond the left pharyngoepiglottic fold. The supraglottic larynx was pushed to the right side due to mass effect (**Figure 1**). A CT scan Neck with contrast was done on 10th October 2013 which revealed a well-defined elongated spindle shaped enhancing soft tissue mass in the left parapharyngeal space measuring 7.5 cm cranio-caudally, 3 cm antero-posteriorly and 4.5 cm transversely. The mass was extending from jugular foramen superiorly to the level of hyoid bone inferiorly. Medially, this mass was causing medial displacement of the visceral space with indentation on the left lateral wall of nasopharynx, oropharynx and hypopharynx (**Figure 2**). His hematological and biochemical investigations were within normal limits. We decided on an excision biopsy instead of FNAC and patient was posted for surgery on

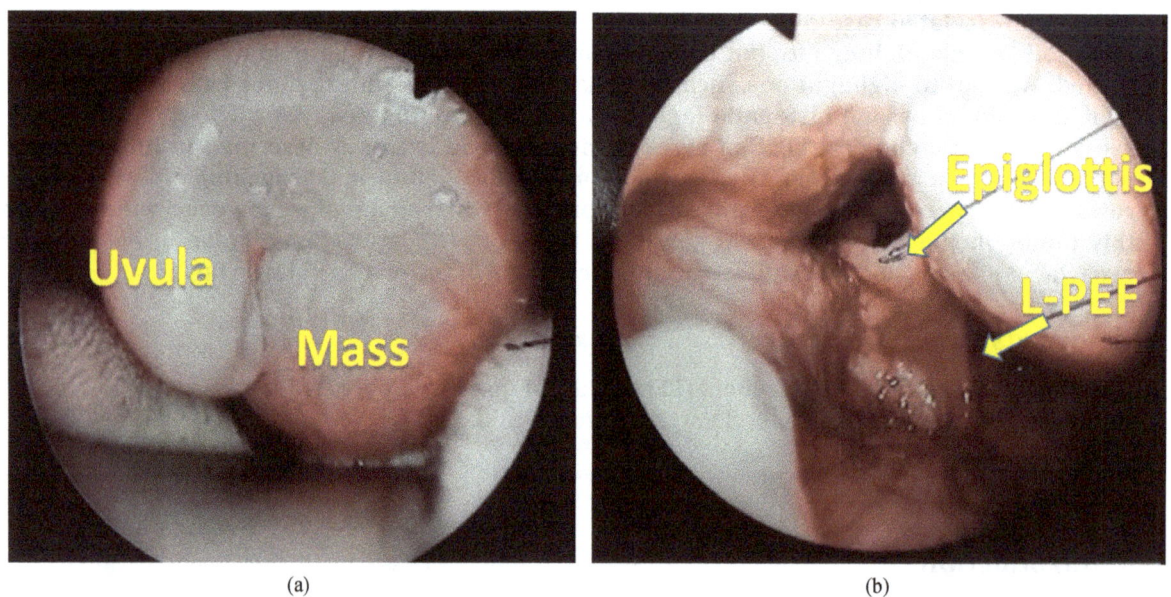

(a)   (b)

Figure 1. (a) Rigid videolaryngoscopy: the lower margin of the mass going beyond the left pharyngoepiglottic fold with mass effect pushing the supraglottic larynx to right side; (b) Globular, smooth and congested mass pushing the left side of soft palate and uvula downwards and medially with narrowing of the oropharyngeal inlet.

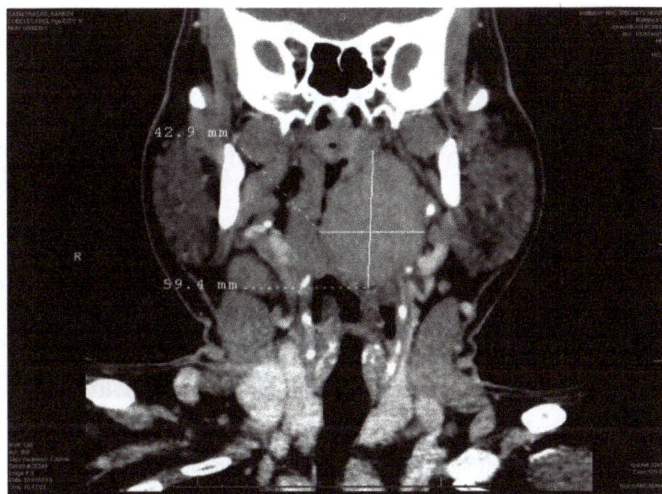

Figure 2. CT scan neck with contrast coronal cut: Well-defined elongated spindle shaped enhancing soft tissue mass in the left parapharyngeal space.

11th November 2013. Trans-cervical, trans-mandibular approach with lateral paramedian mandibulotomy was adopted for resection of the tumor. Intraoperatively, we encountered abnormal branching of left superior thyroid and left lingual artery from the left carotid bulb (**Figure 3(a)** and **Figure 3(b)**). The tumor was firmly adherent superiorly to the base of the skull and had to be removed in piecemeal at the superior pole in the area of attachment only and rest of the tumor was removed as a single well encapsulated tumor (**Figure 4**). A few level I and II cervical lymph glands were found on the left side which was removed and sent for histopathology along with the excised main mass. Histopathology showed a well encapsulated tissue with an infiltrating neoplasm of cells arranged in cords, nests and sheets in a dense lymphoplasmacytoid background. The cells had moderate to abundant eosinophilic cytoplasm with pleomorphic hyperchromatic nuclei having nucleoli. Dyskeratotic cells were also noted. The mitoses were frequent with apoptotic debris. The excised 5 cervical lymph glands were reactive in nature only. The histological diagnosis turned out to be lymphoepithelioma-like carcinoma of undifferentiated type. Due to the rarity of the lesion, the histopathological slide was further evaluated in the pathology department of Manipal University, India where the diagnosis was reconfirmed. Immunohistochemical analysis showed that the cells were positive for CK 5/6, PanCK and p63 and negative for CD3, CD20, S100 and CEA (**Figure 5(a)** and **Figure 5(b)**).

3. Discussion

Parapharyngeal tumours are mostly benign. Some published reports have commonly reported neurogenic tumours as being frequently seen. While various other authors in their series have reported salivary gland tumors as the most commonly encountered tumors in the parapharyngeal space. Malignant tumors are very rarely reported [2]-[4].

Lymphoepithelioma-like carcinoma (LELC) is a different histopathological entity having microscopic resemblance to nasopharyngeal lymphoepithelioma. This entity is a histological variant of malignant tumor arising from uncontrolled mitosis of the transformed cells originating in the epithelial tissue. However, LELC is believed to arise outside the nasopharynx yet resembling histologically with nasopharyngeal lymphoepithelioma [5].

LELC was first described in 1921 as a variant of squamous cell carcinoma. LELC grows either in nests or as a single infiltrating cell with cells round or oval vesicular nuclei, prominent nucleoli, indistinct cytoplasmic borders and numerous mitoses [6]. The cells are undifferentiated and non-keratinizing. It stains positive for epithelial marker such as cytokeratin and epithelial membrane antigen. Usually an inflammatory infiltrate rich in mature lymphocytes (predominantly CD8[+] and T cells) and occasionally eosinophils are seen, particularly obscuring the neoplastic epithelial component [7]. Conventionally, LELC is regarded as high grade based on poor histological differentiation.

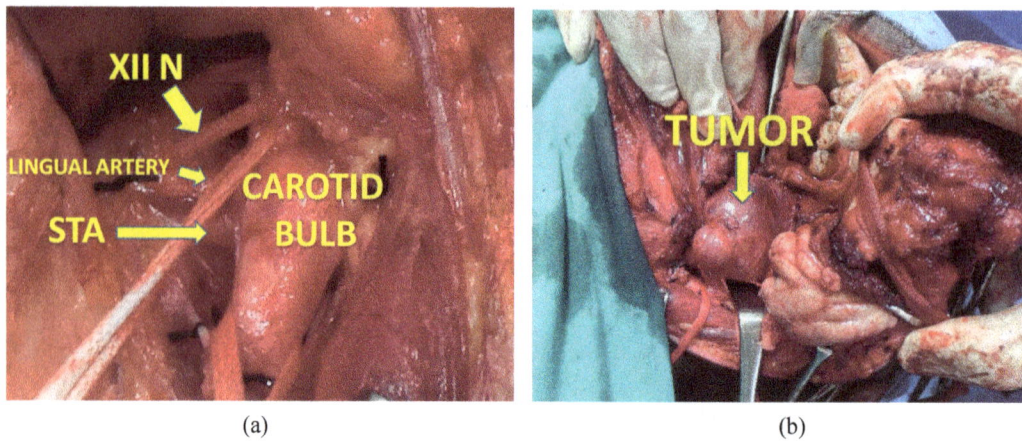

(a)   (b)

Figure 3. (a) An abnormal branching of left superior thyroid and left lingual artery from the left carotid bulb; (b) Intraoperative view of tumour exposed via transcervical transmandibular approach; the extent of the mass seen in the base of skull.

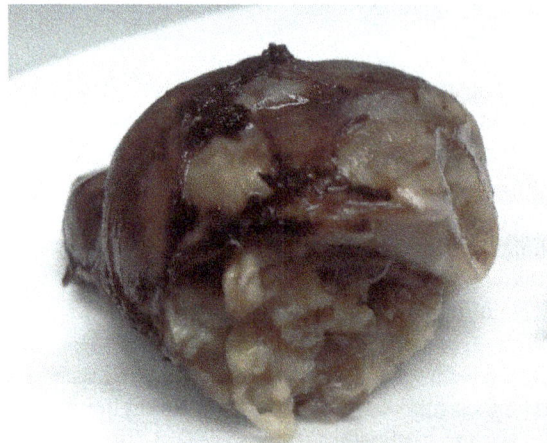

Figure 4. Post operative specimen showing single well encapsulated tumour removed from left parapharyngeal space.

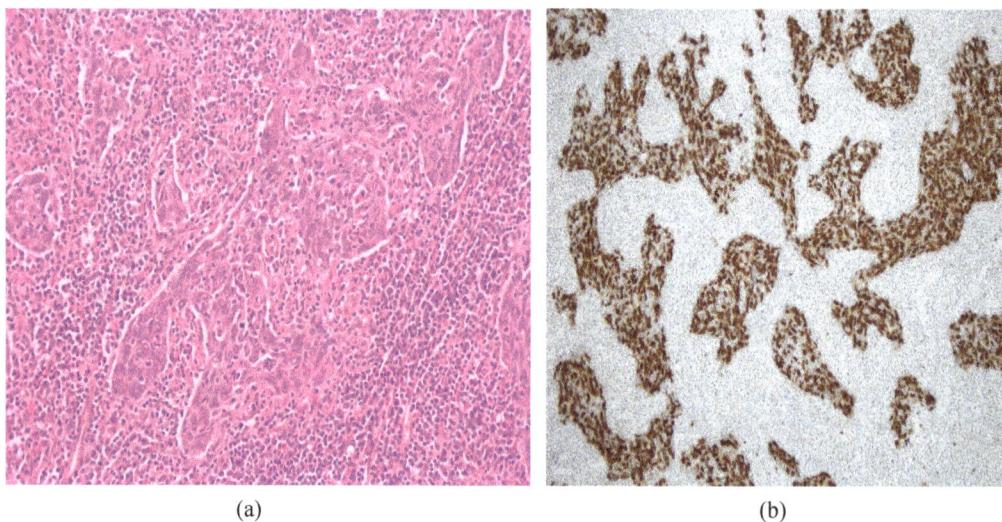

(a)   (b)

Figure 5. H & E 200×; LEC; islands and nests of tumor cells in a lymphoid background p63 positive in tumor cells.

LELC has a strong etiopathological association with EBV, mostly in South Eastern Asian population [8]. However, the connection between LELC and EBV is variable and may not always have any ethnic relevance. There have been reports of LELC arising from the pharynx or foregut derivatives in Asian population who are more prone for EBV than Caucasians [3]. The associations of EBV are more site specific and seen more in tumors arising from lung, stomach, thymus and salivary gland [9]. Circulating serum EBV DNA could be used as a tumor marker in the clinical management of LELCs. It is reported that patients with a pre-therapy serum EBV DNA more than 10,000 copies/ml had significantly worse survival rate [10]. Elevated levels 6 to 8 weeks after therapy were strongly associated with both progression free and overall survival [10] [11]. In our present case, circulating serum of EBV DNA was not done as our preoperative diagnosis was in favor of benign neurogenic tumor and hence was never thought of. *In-situ* hybridization (RNA-ISH) and polymerase chain reaction (PCR) for detection of Epstein Barr Virus genome in both epithelial and lymphoid population would have been more informative. Immunohistochemical studies done in our case shows cells were positive for tumor markers CK5/6, Pan CK and P63 and negative for CD3, CD20, S100 and CEA. These parameters are in favor of LELC.

Ma, Lin, Wang, *et al.* (2014) [12] reported sixty nine cases of lymphoepithelioma-like carcinoma from salivary gland but none of these are from the parapharyngeal space. CT scan neck and extensive sampling in histopathological studies in our case, failed to show any evidence of salivary gland tissue excluding the possibility of its origin from salivary gland. Extensive sampling was done from the post operative specimen after inking the surface. The lesion was well encapsulated and completely excised as shown in **Figure 4**.

Clinically, the most common symptom of a parapharyngeal tumour is a neck mass. Other symptoms include swallowing problems, feeling of obstruction and pain in the throat, unilateral tinnitus, trismus, dysarthia, glossopharyngeal neuralgia and cranial nerve palsies. Pain, trismus and cranial nerve palsies are often suggestive of malignancy. Our patient had initial symptoms of lump in the throat, huskiness of voice, mild breathing difficulty on exertion. No visible neck mass or gland was found. This could be because the tumor was arising high in the parapharyngeal space towards the skull base. However, the lump was seen on rigid laryngoscopy as a swelling in the left lateral pharyngeal wall pushing the supraglottic larynx towards the right side. The initial clinical impression in this case was favoring more towards benign tumors like schwanomma. LELC was the post operative histopathological diagnosis.

FNAC, MRI CT Scan Neck with or without contrast and Angiography are the common investigative tools used for parapharyngeal masses. In the present case, the classic CT angiographic findings pointed towards a benign tumor. Since the tumor was deep seated in the parapharyngeal space with a radiological evidence of benign character of tumor we decided excision biopsy as our ideal option rather than FNAC because of its high level of specificity.

Management of such tumors is difficult as there is no validated therapeutic management that exists for LELC. Surgical excision [6] has been reported as the best option in localized disease occasionally followed by radiotherapy [9]. Chemotherapy is not a conventional option. Taxanes, platinum derivatives and 5-fluorouracil combined with folinic acid are active drugs [13]. Surgical approaches for the excision of parapharyngeal tumors are numerous but trans-cervical approach is more popular because of its versatility. However, the surgical dilemma involved is in the selection of the appropriate approach while avoiding injury to the great vessels with preservation of functions of lower cranial nerves, with or without mandibulotomy and reduction of traction trauma to the soft tissues intraoperatively. In our present case, we found an unusual branching of left external carotid artery where the superior thyroid and lingual artery were branching from the left carotid bulb instead of the left external carotid artery. This kind of abnormal branching is rare but has been reported earlier [14]. So, meticulous dissection is also imperative to look out for any structural abnormality of vessels and nerves thus avoiding inadvertent injury.

LELC has generally been considered as highly radiosensitive and hence radiotherapy is to be considered especially for residual tumors, high grade tumors or tumors with only loco-regional metastasis. Prognosis depends on the stage and grading of the tumor. Our present case was treated with primary surgery. Radiotherapy will be a considered optiion if recurrence of the tumor is found in the follow up period. A repeat CT scan Neck done on 25th February 2014 showed no recurrence of the primary tumor in the parapharyngeal space and during his last visit on 3rd January 2015 to our outpatient department patient was asymptomatic and doing well. He is currently under our close watch and follow up.

4. Conclusion

Lymphoepithelioma like carcinoma has a close histopathological similarity with nasopharyngeal lymphoepithelioma and can arise primarily from extra nasopharyngeal sites like salivary gland, oropharynx, larynx, gastric mucosa, lung etc. However, LELC arising primarily from parapharyngeal space has not been reported in English literature. One such case is reported here because of its rarity and dilemma in management. Such diagnosis often requires immunohistopathology and electron microscopy for confirmation.

Acknowledgements

We, the authors acknowledge the immense help and support that we received from our NMC group medical director Dr. B. R. Shetty and Medical Director of NMC Specialty Hospital, Abu Dhabi Dr. C. R. Shetty without whom none of this would have been possible.

References

[1]   Panda, N., Gosh, S., Jain, A. and Vadhishta, R. (2004) Unusual Malignant Tumours of the Parapharyngeal Space—A Diagnostic Dilemma. *The Internet Journal of Otorhinolaryngology*, **4**, 1.

[2]   Hazarika, P., Dipak, R.N., Parul, P. and Kailesh, P. (2004) Surgical Access to Parapharyngeal Space Tumors: The Manipal Experience. *Medical Journal of Malaysia*, **59**, 323-329.

[3]   Carru, R.L., Myers, E.N. and Johnson, J.T. (1990) Management of Tumors Arising in Parapharyngeal Space. *Laryngoscope*, **100**, 583-489.

[4]   Pensak, M.L., Gluckman, J.L. and Shumrick, K.A. (1994) Parapharyngeal Space Tumors: An Algorithm for Evaluation and Management. *Laryngoscope*, **104**, 1170-1173. http://dx.doi.org/10.1288/00005537-199409000-00022

[5]   Aurilio, G., Ricci, V., Devita, F., Fasano, M., Fazio, N., Orditura, M., Funicelli, L., De Lusa, G., Lasevoli, D., Lovino, F., Ciardiello, F., Conzo, G., Nole, F. and Lamendolla, M.G. (2010) A Possible Connective Tissue Primary Lymphoepithelioma Like Carcinoma. *E-Cancer Medical Science*, **4**, 197.

[6]   Bildirici, K., Ak, G., Peker, B., Metintas, M., Alatas, F., Erginel, S. and Ucgun, I. (2005) Primary Lymphoepithelioma of Lung. *Tuberk Toraks*, **53**, 69-73.

[7]   Kobayashi, M., Ito, M., Sano, K., Honda, T. and Nakayama, J. (2004) Pulmonary Lymphoepithelioma-Like Carcinoma: Predominant Infiltration of Tumor-Associated Cytotoxic T Lymphocytes Might Represent the Enhanced Tumor Immunity. *Internal Medicine*, **43**, 323-326. http://dx.doi.org/10.2169/internalmedicine.43.323

[8]   Lezzone, J.C., Gaffey, M.J. and Weiss, L.M. (1995) The Role of Epstein-Barr-Virus in Lymphoepithelioma Like Carcinoma. *American Journal of Pathology*, **103**, 308-315.

[9]   Nagan, R.K., Yip, T.T., Cheng, W.W., Chan, J.K., Cho, W.C., Ma, V.W., Wan, K.K., Au, J.S. and Law, C.K. (2004) Clinical Role of Circulating Epstein Barr Virus DNA as a Tumor Marker in Lymphoepitheloma Like Carcinoma of the Lung. *Annals of the New York Academy of Sciences*, **1022**, 263-270. http://dx.doi.org/10.1196/annals.1318.041

[10] Griffin, B.E. and Xue, S.A. (1998) Epstein Barr Virus Infections and Their Association with Human Malignancy: Some Key Questions. *Annals of Medicine*, **30**, 294-259. http://dx.doi.org/10.3109/07853899809005852

[11] Sun, X.N., Xu, J., Yang, Q.C., Hu, J.B. and Wang, Q. (2006) Lymphoepithelioma Like Carcinoma of the Salivary Gland: A Case Report. *Chinese Medical Journal (English Edition)*, **119**, 1315-1317.

[12] Ma, H., Lin, Y., Wang, L., Rao, H., Xu, G., He, Y. and Liang, Y. (2014) Primary Lymphoepithelioma-Like Carcinoma of Salivary Gland: Sixty Nine Cases with Long Term Follow-Up. *Head & Neck*, **36**, 1305-1312.

[13] Chan, A.T., Teo, P.M., Lam, K.C., Chan, W.Y., Chow, T.H., Yim, A.P., Mok, T.S., Kwan, W.H., Leung, T.W. and Johnson, P.J. (1998) Multimodality Treatment of Primary Epithelioma Like Carcinoma of the Lung. *Cancer*, **83**, 925-929. http://dx.doi.org/10.1002/(SICI)1097-0142(19980901)83:5<925::AID-CNCR18>3.0.CO;2-X

[14] Gluncic, V., Pentanjek, Z., Marusic, A. and Gluncic, I. (2001) High Bifurcation of Common Carotid Artery, Anomalous Origin of Ascending Pharyngeal Artery and Anomalous Branching Pattern of External Carotid Artery. *Surgical and Radiologic Anatomy*, **23**, 123-125. http://dx.doi.org/10.1007/s00276-001-0123-x

26

Analysis of Changing Factors on Airborne Allergenic Pollens Distribution in Taiyuan Downtown, North China

Kejun Zhang, Binquan Wang*, Yanli Zhang, Nasha Cheng, Changsheng Wang, Chunming Zhang, Wei Gao, Ganggang Chen

Department of Otolaryngology, Head and Neck Surgery, First Hospital, Shanxi Medical University, Taiyuan, China
Email: zhangkejun54@126.com, *wbq_xy@sxent.org

Abstract

To study and analyse 2 surveys on airborne allergenic pollens distribution in Taiyuan Downtown, North China 30 years apart, the surveys focused on the phenomenon and the influence factors on types, counts, drift patterns, growth and decline rhythm and distribution features of airborne pollen with the same methods in the region in March 1977 to February 1978 and July 2008 to June 2009, respectively. The data of two airborne pollens surveys were treated with statistics, comparation and analysis, and the influence factors of pollen distribution in Taiyuan Downtown were explored. In the 2 surveys, 24 species and 35 species of pollen were collected in the region, respectively. Two pollen drift peaks were formed in spring and autumn in the two surveys. *Artemisia L.* is still the absolute dominant allergy airborne pollen. The types, counts, drift patterns and composition of pollen in air could be changed by the plants variation. Climate warming might affect pollen peak appearing time and lasting time, climate warming and Poplar & Willow contents changes in spring and autumn reversed the airborne pollen peak. It was found that *Humulus L.* had become the region's main allergic pollen. Invasive strong allergen ragweed was spread to the inland city Taiyuan. Allergists should focus on exotic invasive harmful plants in the region.

Keywords

Airborne Pollen, Identification of Pollen, Pollen Count, Seasonal Distribution of Airborne Pollen, Taiyuan

---

*Corresponding author.

1. Introduction

Hay fever caused by airborn pollens is worldwide common and frequently-occurring diseases, and belongs to the environmental diseases. Strictly speaking, there is the existence of patients suffering from hay fever wherever there are higher plants. More than 50 million people worldwide suffer from hay fever [1]. It was reported in 2005 that by more than 5000 samples of epidemiological survey, it was found that the incidence of hay fever and mild nasal allergy in survey area in China was as much as 17.8% [2]. It was reported in 2007 that 38203 persons in 11 cities in China were interviewed by telephone and the incidence of allergic rhinitis ranged between 8.7% - 24.1% in different cities [3]. An airborne pollen survey was conducted for a period of a year in 1970s in Taiyuan Downtown, North China [4] [5], so far in the past 30 years. With the process of urbanization in Taiyuan, urban strengthening virescence, vegetation variation and exotic invasive harmful plants, the airborne pollen types and counts may change. China is a vast territory country and different regions have different pollen distributions. There were at least 5 - 10 million pollen allergic patients in China and in recent years the incidence of pollinosis rate had a growth trend [1]. To re-survey the distribution of pollen and its influencing factors in the region will have an important significance on allergenic pollen prevention and treatment in North China. For this purpose, an airborne pollen re-survey and study was conducted with the same methods in the region in July 1, 2008 to June 30, 2009, and the re-survey result was compared with survey result in the same region in March 1977 to February 1978 [6]. It is believed that two pollen surveys 30 years apart in the same place should be the first in China. After the influencing factors on the two survey results on airborne pollen distribution in this region were analyzed and researched, the research findings would be reported as follows.

2. Materials and Methods

2.1. Preparation of Pollen Standard Slides

The 28 pollen standard slides were prepared according to the preparing method [7] developed by Beijing Union Medical College Hospital and used for identification of airborne pollens in the survey. The pollens were collected locally or provided by Allergy Department of Beijing Union Medical College Hospital.

2.2. Collection of Airborne Pollens

Ye's [1]-[8] airborne pollen fixed-point sampler was made with gravity sedimentation method according to national uniform standard [7]. The petrolatum alba and glycerol agar-basic fuchsin stain [7] were prepared and placed in the refrigerator for spare. The pollen sampler was placed on the roof of the 4 storey outpatient building of First Hospital of Shanxi Medical University and was maintained in the location basically the same as 30 years ago with a height (12 m) [5] and coordinate (longitude 112°30' [5], latitude 37°52' [5]). One slide was exposed daily to collect airborne pollens.

2.3. Counting and Identification Pollens

At the same time daily, the exposed slid was removed from and a new slide was placed on the sampler stand. The exposed slid t was stained with glycerol agar-basic fuchsin stain, covered with a 22 mm × 22 mm cover slip to dry, sealed and mounted under an optical microscope to carry pollen morphological identification. Refering "Color Atlas of Air-borne Pollens and Plants in China" edited by Bingshan Qiao [9] and according to the prepared pollen standard slides, pollen morphological identification was carried within 22 mm × 22 mm area to identify the pollen species and count the pollen number. The rare pollens to difficult to identify were photographed by a microscopic camera according to Hong Yaping's pollen Image-taking method [10]. The pollens pictures were sent to prf. Haijuan He, Beijing Union Medical College Hospital, for assistant to identify the pollen species.

2.4. Collection of Meteorological Data

The growth and decline of all living beings is influenced by meteorological factors [11] and so is the pollens. The pollens' growth and spread into the atmosphere is closely related to meteorological factors also. After the completion of the investigation, the Taiyuan Downtown's annual meteorological data of abovementioned two years were taken from the Meteorological Bureau of Shanxi Province respectively. Combining with survey data the influences of meteorological factors on airborne pollens' growth, decline and spread were comprehensively analyzed, and the relationship between meteorological factors and the spread of pollens were investigated.

2.5. Comparison of Two Pollen Survey Results

This survey result was analyzed and compared with the survey result of late 1970s in Taiyuan [6], so was the pollens distribution changes, pollens composition and its influencing factors of annual, spring and autumn and pollen spices collected and spices differences in 30 years.

2.6. Statistical Analysis Methods

The pollen species are qualitative data, and were described by the proportion and the detection rate. The atmospheric temperatures and the temperature differences are quantitative data, and were described by the mean data. Line graphs and bar charts were drawn to reflect the counts of pollen grains and the changing trends of average atmospheric temperatures with the month throughout the years.

3. Results

3.1. Annual Survey

3.1.1. Annual Survey Results

365 slides were exposed respectively throughout the year in the 2 airborne pollen surveys. 18,491 (belonging to 24 families and genera) survey and 17,192 (belonging to 35 families and genera) grains of pollens (respectively in 1970s and this surveys) were observed. 12 new families and genera were observed in this survey (according to counts of collected grains respectively: *Rumex L., Ginkgo biloba L., Plantaginaceae, Palmae, Cruciferae, Polygonaceae, Albizia Durazz, Urtica L., Luffa L., Ambrosia L., Xanthium L.* and *Cryptomeria D. Don*). The proportion of *Populus L.* and *Salix L.* pollens were significantly reduced in the annual and spring airborne pollen constitutes and exited the main Allergenic pollen rank: *Populus L.* pollen was reduced from 19.37% [6] and 37.06% [6] in 1977-1978 to 12.00% and 28.79% in 2008-2009, and *Salix L.* pollen from 18.00% [6], and 34.51% [6] to 3.16% and 7.02%, respectively. The annual airborne pollen counts, families and genera, the monthly distribution and the annual total of the two surveys were shown in **Tables 1-3**.

Table 1. The exposure slide results of the two surveys in 1977-1978 and 2008-2009 in Taiyuan Downtown.

Year	Exposed tablets (n)	Grains/year	The main allergenic pollens		Absolute dominant pollens		New families and genera	No appearing families and genera
			Species	%/year	Species	%/year		
1977-1978	365	18,491	*Artemisia L.* *Populus L.* *Salix L.* *Pinus L.* *Chenopodium L.* *Amaranthus L.*	76.72	*Artemisia L.*	26.20		
2008-2009	365	17,192	*Artemisia L.* *Populus L.* *Pinus L.* *Humulus L.*	73.32	*Artemisia L.*	38.37	12	1

Table 2. Month distributions of airborne pollens and annual totals in 1977-1978 and 2008-2009 in Taiyuan Downtown.

Year	Pollen species, families and genera	Month number of grains of pollen distribution (grains, %)												Total
		Jan	Feb	Mar	Apr	May	Jun	Jul	Aug	Sep	Oct	Nov	Dec	
1977-1978	24%	24	15	762	7183	1694	318	368	5922	2073	56	44	32	**18,491**
		0.13	0.08	4.12	38.85	9.16	1.72	1.99	32.03	11.21	0.30	0.24	0.17	**100.00**
2008-2009	35%	22	56	2477	1944	2755	451	356	3705	4811	317	73	225	**17,192**
		0.13	**0.33**	**14.41**	**11.31**	**16.02**	**2.62**	**2.07**	**21.55**	**27.98**	**1.84**	**0.43**	**1.31**	**100.00**

Table 3. The contrast of the two investigations of airborne pollens on *Populus L.* and *Salix L.* in Taiyuan in 1977-1978 and 2008-2009.

Year	Grains/year	Populus L.				Salix L.			
		Grains		%		Grains		%	
		Year	Spring	Year	Spring	Year	Spring	Year	Spring
1977-1978	18,491	3583	3572	19.38	37.06	3329	3326	18.00	34.51
2008-2009	17,192	2062	2062	11.99	28.79	543	543	3.16	7.02

3.1.2. Annual Pollen Spread Peak Distribution and Monthly Mean Temperatures

In this pollen survey, pollens were visible almost all year around in Taiyuan Downtown. The pollen species and content were in each season were different. There were 2 peaks of pollen spread in spring and autumn every year respectively. The peak in spring was higher than in autumn in 1977-1978 survey, and peak in autumn was higher than in spring in 2008-2009 survey. After the hoar frost descends, plants tended to wither and airborne pollen content in the air reduced to minimum values for the whole year. The monthly airborne pollen counts and spread curves of the two surveys were shown in **Table 2** and **Figure 1**, **Figure 2**. After the completion of investigation, the Taiyuan Downtown's monthly average temperatures and other meteorological data of above-mentioned two years were taken from the Meteorological Bureau of Shanxi Province respectively. The annual average temperature of this region was 10.23°C in 1977-1978 survey year and 11.72°C in 2008-2009 survey year. The annual average temperature was increased by 1.49°C in the past 30 years. The monthly average temperatures and pollen spread curves of the two surveys were shown in **Table 4** and **Figure 1**, **Figure 2**.

3.2. Spring and Autumn Surveys

3.2.1. Exposure Slides Results of Spring and Autumn

In 1977-1978 survey year, 22 families and genera were observed in the spring, and 8 in the autumn. In 2008-2009 survey year, in the spring, 30 families and genera were observed, *Pterocarya* was not collected, harmful species *Ambrosia L.* was collected, 9 new families and genera to the 1977-1978 survey year were collected, according to counts of collected grains respectively: *Ginkgo biloba L., Rumex L., Polygonaceae, Ricinus L., Ambrosia L., Palmae, Cryptomeria D. Don, Helianthus L., Cruciferae*; in the autumn, 20 families and genera were observed, *Ricinus L., Helianthus L., Fraxinus L.* were not collected, harmful species *Ambrosia L.* was collected, 15 new families and genera to the 1977-1978 survey year were collected, according to counts of collected grains respectively: *Rumex L., Plantaginaceae, Broussonetia L., Albizia Durazz, Palmae, Urtica L., Luffa L., Ambrosia L., Polygonaceae, Platanus L., Xanthium L., Cyperaceae, Cupressaceae, Picea Dietr.* The pollen contents and constituent ratio in spring and autumn of two surveys (exclusive of unknown pollens) shown in **Table 5** and **Table 6**.

3.2.2. Pollen Spread Peak Distribution in Spring and Autumn of 2 Survey Years

The last survey data showed that spring airborne pollen spread peak appeared in April., *Populus L., Salix L., Pinus L., Cupressaceae, Ulmus L.* and *Acer L.* (the collected pollen grains > 100, later the same) are six dominant pollens (accounted for 93.88% of the spring pollens). This survey data showed that spring airborne pollen spread duration lasted up to three months and three airborne pollen spread peaks appeared, respectively: 1) March peak with *Populus L., Ulmus L., Salix L.*, and *Cupressaceae* as main species; 2) April peak with *Populus L., Salix L., Betula L., Ailanthus Desf, Fraxinus L.* and *Quercus L.* as main species; and 3) May peak with *Pinus L., Ailanthus Desf, Picea Dietr* and *Chenopodium L. & Amaranthus L.* as main species (12 pollens accounted for 95.16% of spring pollens). Autumn airborne pollen spread of two surveys both appeared in August and September. There were five main pollens: *Artemisia L., Humulus L., Chenopodium L. & Amaranthus L., Gramineae* and *Ricinus L.* (accounted for 99.30% of autumn pollens) in 1977-1978 autumn peak. There were four main pollens: *Artemisia L., Humulus L., Chenopodium L. & Amaranthus L.* and *Gramineae* (accounted for 95.76% of autumn pollens) in 1977-1978 autumn peak. For airborne pollen spread peak values, spring peak was higher than autumn peak in 1977-1978 survey year; and spring peak was lower than autumn peak in 2009-2009 survey year. Autumn airborne pollen spread appeared dominant in august and clearly weak in September in 1977-1978 survey year; and dominant in August and September and even higher in September in 2008-2009 survey year. The airborne pollen spread peak values of spring and autumn of two survey years is show in **Figure 3** and **Figure 4**.

Table 4. The average temperatures and temperature difference in 1977-1978 and 2008-2009 survey years in Taiyuan Downtown.

Annual	Jan	Feb	Mar	Apr	May	Jun	Jul	Aug	Sep	Oct	Nov	Dec	Annual average temperature (˚C)
1977-1978	−4.7	−3.9	5.4	12.7	17.4	20.9	23.2	21.1	17.0	12.2	3.0	−1.6	**10.23**
2008-2009	−5.1	1.5	6.7	14.9	19.2	24.5	24.9	23.5	17.8	11.5	3.9	−2.7	**11.72**
Temperature difference	−1.4	5.4	1.3	2.2	1.8	3.6	1.7	2.4	0.8	−0.7	0.9	−1.1	1.49

Table 5. Pollen contents and constituent ratio in spring and autumn in 1977-1978 and in 2008-2009 in Taiyuan Downtown.

	1977-1978							2008-2009						
	Spring				Autumn			Spring				Autumn		
Month	Mar	Apr	May	Total	Aug	Sep	Total	Mar	Apr	May	Total	Aug	Sep	Total
Grains	762	7183	1694	9639	5922	2073	7995	2471	1939	2753	7163	3676	4782	8458
%	7.91	74.52	17.57	100.00	74.07	25.93	100.00	34.50	27.07	38.43	100.00	43.46	56.54	100.00

Table 6. Pollen contents, constituent ratio and families and genera in spring and autumn in 1977-1978 and in 2008-2009 in Taiyuan Downtown.

Year	Season	Pollens		Families and genera	New families and genera	No appearing families and genera
		Grains	%			
1977-1978	Spring	9639	52.13	22		
	Autumn	7995	41.67	8		
	Total	18,491	100	30		
2008-2009	Spring	7163	41.62	30	9	1
	Autumn	8458	49.20	20	15	3
	Total	17,192	100	50	24	4

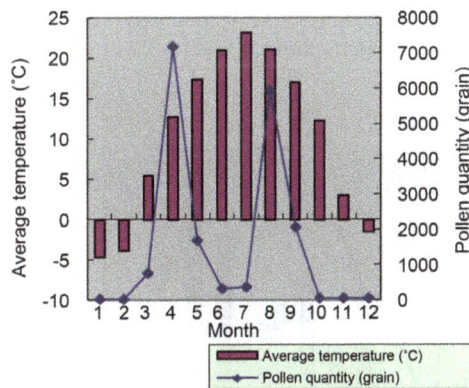

Figure 1. Average temperature and air pollen distribution in Taiyuan in 1977-1978.

The highest monthly average temperature was July (23.2˚C) and formed the peak top of monthly average temperature distribution curve in 1977-1978 survey year. The higher monthly average temperatures were June, July and August (24.5˚C, 24.9˚C and 23.5˚C respectively, mean 24.3˚C) and formed nearly a plateau duration last up to three months of monthly average temperature distribution curve in 2008-2009 survey year. The monthly average temperatures, average temperature distribution curves and relationship between the monthly average temperatures and the airborne pollen spread peak were shown in **Table 3** and **Figure 3** and **Figure 4**.

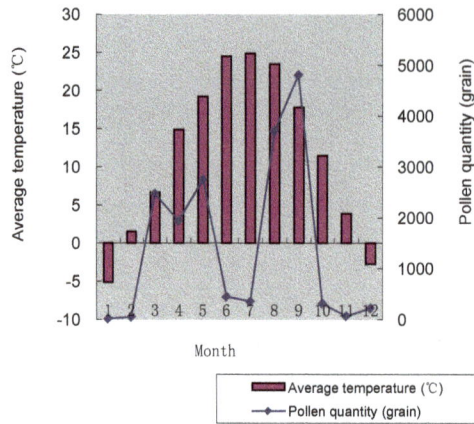

Figure 2. Average temperature and air pollen distribution in Taiyuan in 2008-2009.

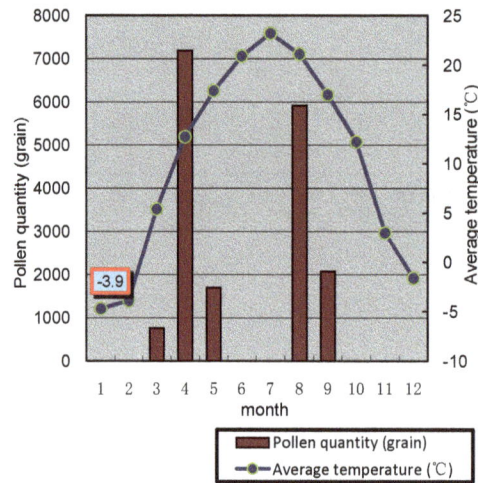

Figure 3. Airborne pollens of spring and autumn and monthly average temperature distributions in 1977-1978 in Taiyuan Downtown.

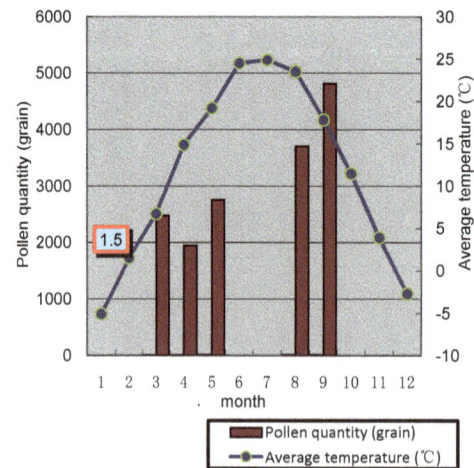

Figure 4. Airborne pollens of spring and autumn and monthly average temperature distributions in 2008-2009 in Taiyuan Downtown.

4. Discussion

4.1. The Relationships between Airborne Pollen Spread Duration with Climate in Two Surveys

Taiyuan City is located in the middle of the Yellow River basin of north China; has a temperate monsoon climate, have clear four seasons throughout the year, is no severe cold in winter and intense heat in summer, has an annual average temperature above 10°C; has a large plant species, a longer flowering duration and longer plant growing season. In the two surveys, the same location, the same fixed-point pollen sampling method were selected. The survey results showed that the airborne pollen spread were throughout the year and both formed two spread peaks in spring and autumn. Spring airborne pollen spread peaks duration: in 1977-1978 survey year, the spread peak appeared in April, lasted about one month, consist of *Populus L., Salix L., Pinus L., Cupressaceae, Ulmus L.* and *Acer L.*; in 2008-2009 survey year, the spread peaks appeared in march, April and May, lasted long for three months, formed "M" three peaks, respectively: 1) March peak with *Populus L., Ulmus L., Salix L.,* and *Cupressaceae* as main species; 2) April peak with *Populus L., Salix L., Betula L., Ailanthus Desf, Fraxinus L.* and *Quercus L.* as main species; and 3) May peak with *Pinus L., Ailanthus Desf, Picea Dietr* and *Chenopodium L. & Amaranthus L.* as main species. Autumn air spread pollen spread peaks duration: in two surveys the spread peak both appeared in August and September; in 1977-1978 survey year, the autumn peak appeared higher in August and Significantly weak in September; in 2008-2009 survey year, autumn peak appeared high in August and Significantly higher in September; in two surveys the spread peak both consist of *Artemisia L., Humulus L.* and *Chenopodium L. & Amaranthus L.* The air temperature gradually rose in March in 1977-1978 survey year and began to rise in February in 2008-2009 survey year. The air temperature gradually declined in October both in two survey years. The annual average temperature was 1.49°C higher in 2008-2009 survey year than 30 years ago. The average temperature in February was 5.4°C higher in 2008-2009 survey year than 30 years ago. The average temperatures in spring and autumn were higher in 2008-2009 survey year than the same duration 30 years ago, suggesting that warmer climate might be the main reason that the spring airborne pollen spread was peaked earlier and lasted long for up to 3 months, and autumn airborne pollen spread maintained strong for up to 2 months and was peaked later to September.

4.2. The Relationships between Airborne Pollen Families and Genera with Vegetation in Two Surveys

Nearly 30 years in Taiyuan Downtown, as the process of modernization, industrialization and urbanization, the green area of expanded, new plants were introduced, old plants were eradicated, the species of flowers, grasses and trees increased, airborne pollen contents increased, the annual collected airborne pollen species increased from 24 to 35, spring airborne pollen species increased from 22 to 30, and autumn airborne pollen species increased from 8 to 20. The dominant pollens were also varied in the 30 years. Before 1980s, willow catkins and poplar blowballs fluttered all over the sky in spring in Taiyuan Downtown. A large number of willows and poplars had been replaced by Sophora japonica, ginkgo, etc. The proportion of *Populus L.* and *Salix L.* pollens were significantly reduced in the annual and spring airborne pollen constitutes. This might be the main reason that the spring airborne pollen spread peak was exceeded by the autumn peak and the spring airborne pollen peak predominantly *Populus L.* and *Salix L.* pollens reason was significantly lower in 1977-1978 than 30 years ago. In 2008-2009 survey, the spring airborne pollen spread duration lasted for up to three months, the main pollens collected >100 grains were constituted by 6 species (*Populus L., Salix L., Pinus L., Cupressaceae, Ulmus L.* and *Acer L.*, respectively) in 1977-1978 and by 12 species (*Pinus L., Populus L., Ailanthus Desf, Salix L., Ulmus L., Betula L., Cupressaceae, Quercus L., Fraxinus L., Artemisia L., Chenopodium L. & Amaranthus L.* and *Picea Dietr*, respectively) in 2008-2009; the autumn airborne pollen spread duration lasted for up to two months, the main pollens collected >100 grains were constituted by 5 species (*Artemisia L., Humulus L., Chenopodium L. & Amaranthus L., Gramineae,* and *Ricinus L.*, respectively) in 1977-1978 and by 4 species (*Artemisia L., Humulus L., Chenopodium L. & Amaranthus L.* and *Gramineae*, respectively) in 2008-2009. The collected pollens were 12 species more than the last survey and *Ricinus L.* which was collected with a higher content in 1977-1978 survey was not detected in 2008-2009 survey. The above changes suggest that plants viriation would certainly change content of certain airborne pollens and strengthening virescence could change the constitute of airborne pollens.

5. Conclusion

Comparative analysis of spring and autumn data in two airborne pollen surveys in Taiyuan downtown is summarized as follows: 1) The spring airborne pollen species was increased from 22 in 1977-1978 to 30 in 2008-2009, and the autumn airborne pollen species was increased from 8 in 1977-1978 to 20 in 2008-2009. 2) The absolute dominant spring airborne pollens were *Populus L.* (37.06%) and *Salix L.* (34.51%) in 1977-1978, and *Pinus L.* (29.53%) and *Populus L.* (28.79%) in 2008-2009. The absolute dominant autumn airborne pollens in last and this surveys were both *Artemisia L.* (59.05% and 70.21%, respectively), and *Humulus L.* became the main autumn allergenic pollen. 3) Airborne pollen spread peak was higher in spring than in autumn in 1977-1978 survey, and in autumn than in spring in 2008-2009 survey. 4) Warmer climate might be the main reason that the spring airborne pollen spread was peaked earlier and lasted long for up to 3 months, and autumn airborne pollen spread maintained strong for up to 2 months and was peaked later to September. 5) Plants variation led to the fact that the annual percentage contents of *Populus L.* and *Salix L.* were significantly lower than 30 years ago, and the pollen spread peaks between spring and autumn were reversed; strengthening virescence could change the constitute of airborne pollens. 6) It is reported in 1977-1978 survey that exotic invasive harmful plant ragweed in North China was spread in inland city Taiyuan [4]. The hospitalized clinical allergen testing records of recent 20 years [12] were summarized and analyzed, and patients allergic to ragweed were found in the 1990s. The detection rate of ragweed pollen in hospitalized allergy patients was only 6.36% (28/440) in January 1994-December 1995 [12], and up to 31.24% (448/1434) 10 years later, in January 2004-December 2005 [12]. Allergists could not ignore the exotic invasive harmful allergenic pollen ragweed.

References

[1]   Ye, S.T. (1998) Allergology. Science Press, Beijing, 198-206.

[2]   He, G.W. (2005) The Mechanism Revealed on Traditional Chinese Medicine to Treat Hay Fever and Adjust Atopic Constitution. *China News of Traditional Chinese Medicine*.

[3]   Han, D.M., Zhang, L., Huang, D., *et al.* (2007) Self-Reported Prevalence of Allergic Rhinitis in Eleven Cities in China. *Chinese Journal of Otorhinolaryngology Head and Neck Surgery*, **42**, 378-384.

[4]   Li, W.-K. and Wang, C.-S. (1986) Survey of Air-Borne Allergy Pollens in North China: Contamination with Ragweed. *Allergy and Asthma Proceedings*, 7, 134-143. http://dx.doi.org/10.2500/108854186779047771

[5]   Allergy Group of Otolaryngology Department of the First Hospital of Shanxi Medical College (1983) Airborne Allergenic Pollen Distribution Investigation. *Shanxi Medicine Journal*, **12**, 272-273.

[6]   The Leading Group of China Airborne Allergenic Pollen Survey (1991) Airborne Allergenic Pollen Survey in China. Beijing Publishing House, Beijing, 40-42.

[7]   Qiao, B.S. (2002) Allergology Experiment Technique. 2nd Edition, China Union Medical University Press, Beijing, 176-182.

[8]   He, H.J., Wang, L.L. and Zhang, H.Y. (2008) Analysis of Airborne Pollens in Beijing Urban Area. *Chinese Journal of Allergy & Clinical Immunology*, **2**, 179-183.

[9]   Qiao, B.S. (2005) Color Atlas of Airborne Pollens and Plants in China. Peking Union Medical University Press, Beijing, 1-298.

[10] Hong, Y.P. (2007) A Simple Method of Preparing Thin of Fresh Pollen under Microscope. *Bulletin of Biology*, **42**, 56-57.

[11] Xie, H.X., Ma, L.L., Liu, Z.G., *et al.* (2006) Correlation between Airborne Pollen Dispersal and Seven Weather Factors. *Chinese Journal of Clinical Rehabilitation*, **10**, 56-58.

[12] Cai, H.J., Zhang, K.J., Wang, C.H., *et al.* (2008) Allergen Skin Test in the Diagnosis of Patients with Allergic Disease Value Research. *Journal of Chinese Basic Medicine*, **15**, 1601-1602.

27

A Comparative Study on Efficacy of Fludrocortisones versus Glucocorticoids and Vasodilators in the Treatment of Idiopathic Sensorineural Cochlear Hearing Loss

Daniel López-Campos[1], Daniel López-Aguado[2], Eugenia M. Campos-Bañales[2], José Luis de Serdio-Arias[3], Mar García-Sáinz[4]

[1]ENT Service, University Hospital of the Canary Islands, Tenerife, Spain
[2]Department of Otorhinolaryngology, La Laguna University, Tenerife, Spain
[3]ENT Service, University Hospital Nuestra Señora de Candelaria, Tenerife, Spain
[4]Pharmacology and Pharmacotherapy Service, University Hospital of the Canary Islands, Tenerife, Spain
Email: emcampos@ull.es

Abstract

Introduction and Objectives: The idiopathic sensorineural cochlear hearing loss is one of the most frequent human sensory deficits and there is no specific drug therapy for it. The possible hearing recovery is related with the reestablishment of normal ionic homeostasis of the endolymph controlled by the mineralocorticoid as could be demonstrate experimentally. The purpose of this clinical trial was to confirm the efficacy of mineralocorticoids to the recovery of hearing level in patients suffering idiopathic sensorineural hearing loss (SNHL) against the glucocorticoids and vasodilator drugs. **Material and Methods:** The research lasted three months and involved 90 patients allocated into four different groups: Placebo group, consisted of 20 patients (10 men and 10 women); the group consisting of 22 patients treated with glucocorticoid therapy (12 men and 10 female); the group treated with mineralocorticoid therapy encompassed 26 patients (13 males and 13 females) and the group of vasodilators formed by 22 patients (12 men and 10 women). The level of hearing loss was estimated by the tests Liminal Tone Audiometry (LTA) and Auditory Brainstem Response (ABR). **Results:** The main features in this research were overall better response in improving the hearing level with the mineralocorticoid therapy. This improvement in hearing levels was greater in women than in men, and a higher response was found in the left ear regardless of patient's gender. **Conclusions:** The hearing gain was significantly superior in the mineralocorticoids group followed by the glucocorticoids group whereas the response to vasodilators was lesser and with no statistical significance.

Keywords

Idiopathic Sensorineural Cochlear Hearing Loss (ISNCHL), Liminal Tonal Audiometry (LTA), Auditory Brainstem Response (ABR)

1. Introduction

Sensorineural hearing loss is a frequent human sensory deficit in the adult population and causes serious alteration to the hearing function in the patient due to underlying damage in the inner ear or in its neural pathways [1] [2].

The pathogenesis of SNH is multifactorial and includes both intrinsic causes (genetic predisposition, autoimmune, vascular…) and extrinsic causes (toxic, infectious, degenerative, traumatic and neoplastic). It is not possible to know exactly what causes damage to the inner ear, resulting in alterations to cochlear transduction and transmission of acoustic signals [1]-[3].

There is no specific drug therapy for sensorineural hearing loss [2] [3]. A majority of therapeutic approaches have focused on trials with therapies aimed at controlling its pathogenesis [4]-[9]. Recently a new hypothesis has related the decrease in hearing level in these pathologies to the imbalance of the ionic concentration of the inner ear, and the restoration of cochlear ion homeostasis, as the key concept to achieving hearing recovery [8].

About 25 years ago, it was known that there were corticoid receptors in the inner ear, in both glucocorticoid and mineralocorticoid forms [10] [11], and also at the Corti neuron and CNS [12]. Experimentally, it has been demonstrated that the mineralocorticoids are primarily involved in cochlear ionic regulation [13] [14].

Up to this moment, we know of its effects through some animal experiments which have been carried out by several researchers [13]-[15], but we do not know of any clinical studies about it.

The purpose of this paper, as a result of these experiments, is to defend the use of mineralocorticoid drugs to improve auditory level in adult patients with idiopathic sensorineural hearing loss.

2. Material and Methods

2.1. Financial Support

This clinical trial was funded by the Health Institute Carlos III after a call made for non-commercial clinical research projects on human drugs, and co-financed by the European Regional Development Fund (ERDF).

2.2. Sample Size

The study included a total of 90 patients who had been diagnosed of idiopathic bilateral sensorineural cochlear hearing loss (180 ears were studied).

2.3. Study and Patients

These 90 patients were divided into placebo group and treatment group and were treated during three months.

The patients came from two large university hospitals in "the autonomous region of *The Canaries*" who had been diagnosed of idiopathic sensorineural hearing loss. They were evaluated by the same health care professional, and regular monitoring was done by the same physician.

To take part in this study, it was required that patients were not taking vasodilators or steroids at that moment and at least in the three months prior to the start of the treatment. All patients were informed of the potential drawbacks of therapy and voluntarily consented to participate. All were studied again with gadolinium MRI to rule out pathology in the pontine angle.

The ages ranged between 19 and 71 years, 43 were women and 47 men (**Figure 1** and **Figure 2**). All these were suffering from sensorineural bilateral, but not symmetrical, hearing loss. 85.5% were older 50 years old (**Table 1**). The patients were matched for age, sex and auditory level hearing loss.

The design was single blind, taking as reference the placebo group.

2.3.1. Treatment Groups

Patients in the trial were distributed into 4 standard groups in a randomized fashion (**Figure 1** and **Figure 2**)

Females = 43

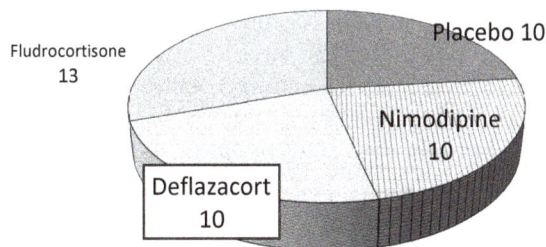

Figure 1. Distribution of female patients. According to treatment received.

Males = 47

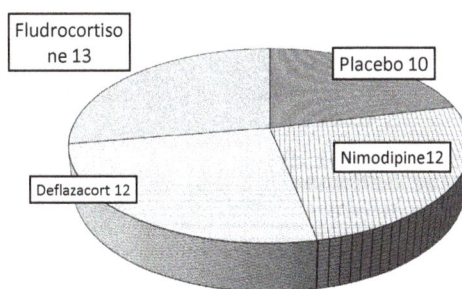

Figure 2. Distribution of male patients. According to treatment received.

Table 1. Percentage distribution of patients by age.

Age	Frequency	Percentage
19 - 41 years	13	14.44%
42 - 51 years	15	16.67%
52 - 74 years	62	68.89%
Total	90	100.00
Over 50 years	85.56%	

1) the placebo group, consisted of 20 patients, (10 of each sex), 2) another group of 22 patients were treated with glucocorticoids, deflazacort, (10 women and 12 men) at a dose 6 mg/12hours, 3) a group of 26 patients were treated with mineralocorticoids, fludrocortisone, (13 women and 13 men) at a dose 0.1 mg/12hours, and the last group 4) treated with vasodilators, nimodipine, was made up of 22 patients, (10 women and 12 men) at a dose 30 mg/every 8 hours.

Such therapy was individual and controlled for each patient, and the dose used was the minimal efficacy concentration among minimal margins of effectiveness, according to the literature consulted [8].

Results at the end of the trial were analyzed in relation to the studied ear, patient age, sex and drugs used.

2.3.2. Methodology

1) Basal hearing level evaluation

Initially all patients were evaluated using liminal tonal audiometry (LTA) and with the auditory brainstem response test (ABR) every 15 days during the first two months and at the end of the study.

The diagnosis of sensorineural hearing loss and the degree of hearing level was held according to the criteria adopted by the World Health Organization (WHO) [2].

Most had a liminal tone audiometry with greater decreases at high frequencies, the ABR showed no retrocochlear involvement, with no increment in the interval I/V, and a pattern of cochlear hearing loss. We used the disappearance of the wave V to compare gradation hearing in relation to the liminal tonal audiometry.

The gradation of hearing level of patients was estimated in the range of conversational frequencies as follows: mild losses: <35 dBs; moderate loss: >35 dBs and <50 dBs; moderate-severe: >50 dBs and <60 dBs; severe: >60 dBs and <75 dBs and profound: >75 dBs. The final measure result was based in the average between the measurement obtained using LTA (liminal tonal audiometry), only in the conversational frequencies, and that achieved by ABR (auditory brainstem response).

The efficacy of treatment was achieved comparatively for each drug and by crossing the results with the use of the different drugs.

3. Statistical Analysis

Univariate and bivariate descriptive statistics by gender, age, affected ear and degree of hearing loss were conducted.

The Bonferroni statistical method (multiple comparisons) was used to compare the efficacy between the different drugs.

4. Results

A total of 90 patients were studied, from 19 to 70 years of age. About 86% of them were older than 50 years of age (**Table 1**).

In all groups asymmetric hearing loss predominated (**Table 2**).

Table 2. Initial percentage classification of hearing level, in all patients.

Degrees of hearingloss	RE (N° ptes)	Percentage RE	LE (N° ptes)	Percentage LE
Patients of the placebo group				
Mild to moderate: 25 - 49 dBs	15	75.00%	6	30.00%
Moderate to severe: 50 - 59 dBs	5	25.00%	6	30.00%
Severe: 60 to 74 dBs	-	-	8	40.00%
Profound: >75 dBs	-	-	-	
Patients of the deflazacort group				
Mild to moderate: 25 - 49 dBs	10	45.00%	14	63.60%
Moderate to severe: 50 - 59 dBs	5	22.70%	3	13.60%
Severe: 60 to 74 dBs	5	22.70%	3	13.60%
Profound: >75 dBs	2	9.60	2	9.20%
Patients of the fludrocortisone group				
Mild to moderate: 25 - 49 dBs	16	61.50%	18	69.20%
Moderate to severe: 50 - 59 dBs	3	11.60%	3	11.60%
Severe: 60 to 74 dBs	7	26.90%	4	15.30%
Profound: >75 dBs	-	-	1	3.90%
Patients of the nimodipine group				
Mild to moderate: 25 - 49 dBs	12	54.50%	14	63.60%
Moderate to severe: 50 - 59 dBs	4	18.10%	2	9.30%
Severe: 60 to 74 dBs	4	18.10%	6	27.10%
Profound: >75 dBs	2	9.30%	-	-

RE = right ear; LE = left ear; N° ptes = n° patients; dBs = decibels.

Mainly the left ear exhibited a severe-deep hearing loss (27.35%) compared with the right ear (20.64%) while the right ear showed a high prevalence of hearing loss moderate-severe (78.35%) compared with the left ear (72.72%) (**Table 3**).

After treatment, the left ear had a higher increase in hearing (**Figure 3**) regardless of the sex of the patients (**Figure 4**). This increase was more evident in the fludrocortisone group (**Figure 5**, **Table 4**). There was a better response in women than in men, in all groups (**Figure 4**).

Table 3. Total percentage of binaural hearing loss, in all patients.

In the right ears	In the left ears
Mild to moderate = 59%. Moderate to severe = 19.35%. Severe = 15.92%. Profound = 4.72%	Mild to moderate = 56.6%. Moderate to severe = 16.12%. Severe = 24.0%. Profound = 3.27%

Table 4. Comparison of auditory gains by sex, ear and drug used Bonferroni method (multiple comparisons).

Drugs versus	Placebo RE	Deflazacort RE	Fludrocortisona RE	Placebo LE	Deflazacort LE	Fludrocortisone LE
			Males			
Deflazacort	6.74 P = 0.44			6.06 P = 0.00 P = 0.04		
Fludrocortisone	11.58 P = 0.00	4.77 P = 0.20		8.95 P = 0.27	2.88 P = 0.95	
Nimodipine	1.671 P = 1.00	−5.05 P = 0.15	−9.819 P = 0.000	4.120 P = 1.00	−1.944 P = 1.00	−4.8254 P = 0.07
			Females			
Deflazacort	10.34 P = 0. 10			8.09 P = 0.02		
Fludrocortisone	12.17 P = 0.02	1.83 P = 1.00		11.76 P = 0.000	3.68 P = 0.42	
Nimodipine	3.37 P = 1.00	−6.97 P = 0.40	−8.7 P = 0.11	2.47 P = 1.00	−5.61 P = 0.03	−9.27 P = 0.00

RE = right ear, LE = left ear, P = statistical significance.

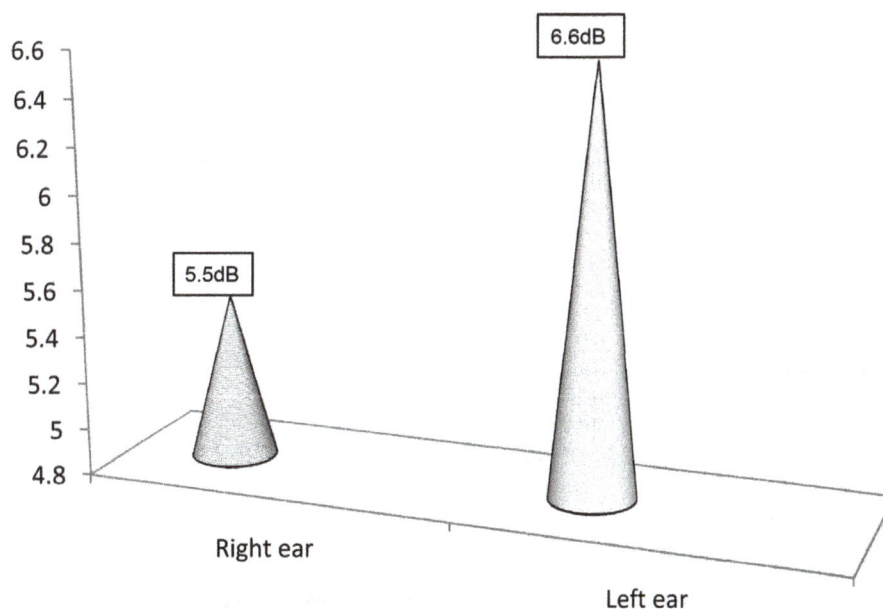

Figure 3. Average increase in hearing recovery, dB, in all ears at study end.

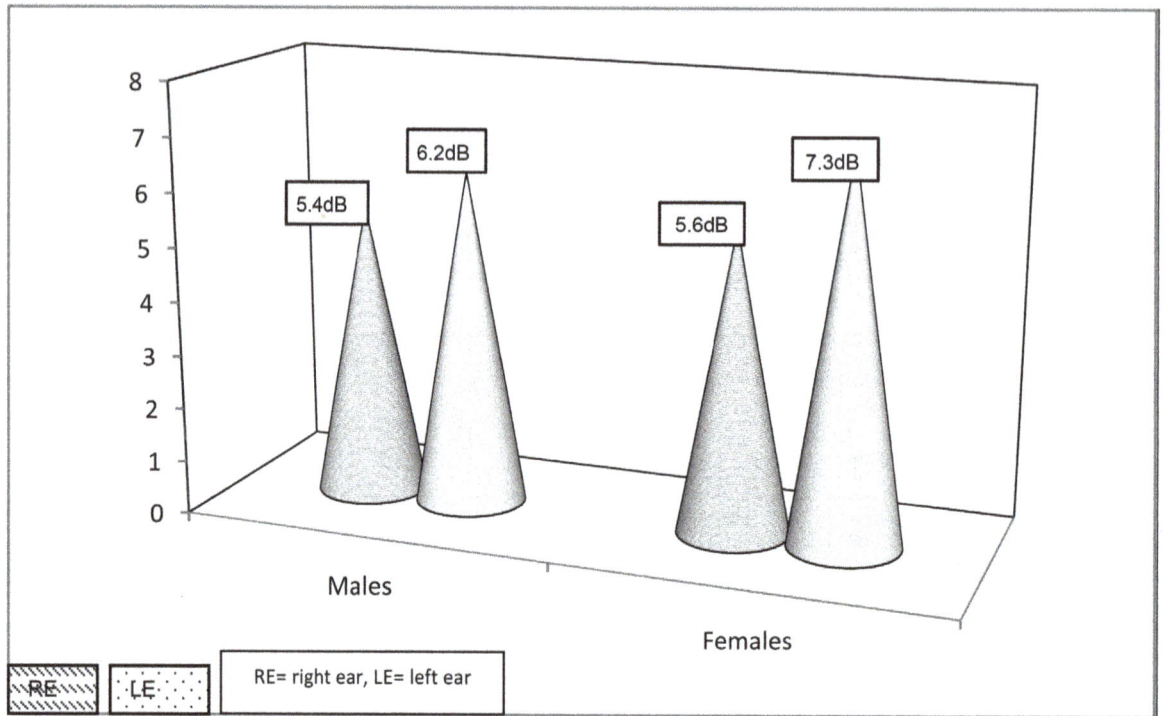

Figure 4. Average increase in binaural hearing recovery, dB, according to patient's sex.

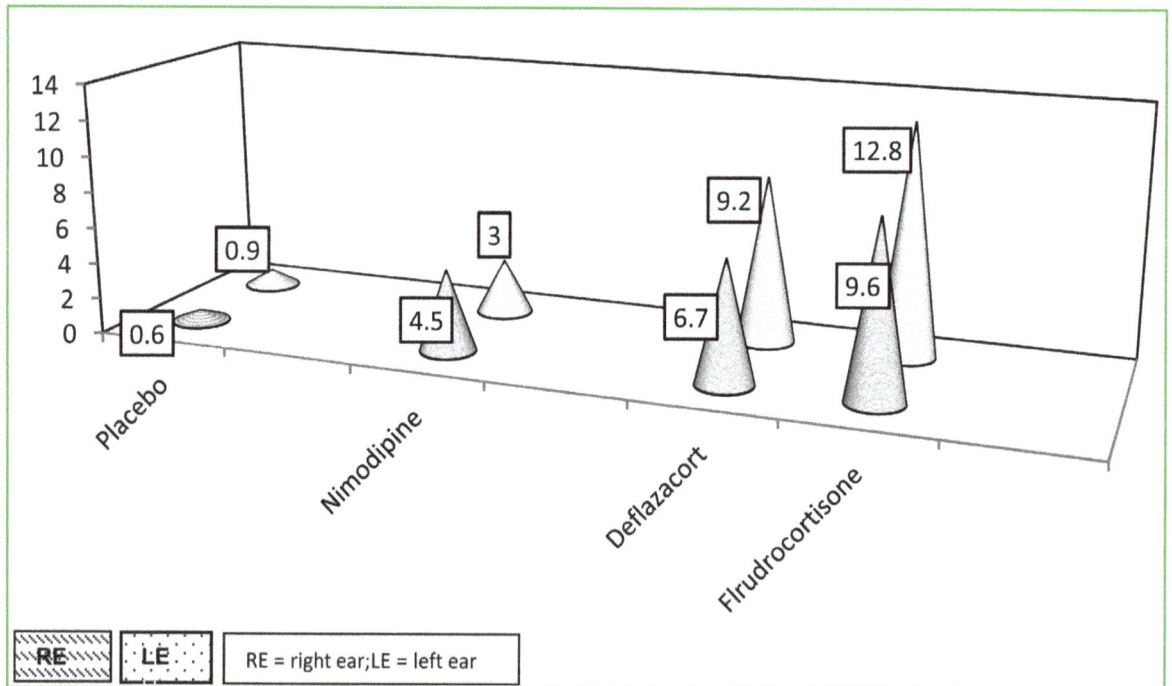

Figure 5. Average increase in hearing recovery, dB, for both ears, according to treatment group.

4.1. Characteristics by Group

4.1.1. Placebo Group

It comprised 20 people, 10 men and 10 women (**Figure 1** and **Figure 2**), who exhibited bilateral sensorineural hearing loss (**Table 2**).

Right ear: mild to moderate in 15 people (75%), and moderate to severe in 5 (25%). In the left ear: mild-moderate loss in 6 patients (30%), moderate-severe in 6 (30%) and severe in 8 (40%) The variations in the level of hearing at the end of the study were of 0.6 dBs for the right ear, and 0.9 dBs in the left one (**Figure 5**).

4.1.2. The Group of Patients Treated with Deflazacort

It was composed of 22 patients, 12 men and 10 women, with bilateral sensorineural hearing loss (**Table 2**).

In the right ear: mild to moderate loss in 10 patients (45%), moderate to severe in 5 patients (22.7%), severe in 5 (22.7%) and profound in 2 patients (9.6%). In the left ear: mild to moderate in 14 patients (63.6%), moderate to severe in 3 patient (13.6%), severe in 3 (13.6%) and profound in 2 patients (9.2%).

In these patients we found a gain of 6.7 dBs in the right ear and 9.2 dBs in the left ear (**Figure 5**).

4.1.3. Group Treated with Fludrocortisone

The group consists of 26 patients, 13 men and 13 women exhibiting bilateral sensorineural hearing loss (**Table 2**).

Right ear: mild to moderate in 16 cases (61.5%), moderate to severe in 3 cases (11.6%) and severe in 7 cases (26.9%).

In the left ear: mild-moderate loss in 18 patients (69.2%), moderate to severe in 3 cases (11.6%), severe in 4 (15.3%) and profound in 1 (3.9%).

We found an average hearing gain of about 9.6 dBs in the right ear, and 12.8 dBs in the left ear (**Figure 5**).

4.1.4. Group Treated with Nimodipine

Made up of 22 people, 12 men and 10 women, who were suffering binaural sensorineural hearing loss (**Table 2**).

In the right ear the loss was: mild to moderate in 12 patients (54.5%) moderate to severe in 4 patients (18.1%) severe in 4 patients (18.1%) and profound in 2 patients (9.3%). In the left ear the loss was: mild to moderate in 14 patients (63.6%), moderate to severe in 2 patients (9.3%) and severe in 6 (27.1%).

At the end of the study we found an average increase of 4.5 in dB for the right ear and 3.0 dB in the left one (**Figure 5**).

4.2. Final Valuation of the Results Achieved

The estimation of hearing gain achieved at the end of the study comparing with the initial hearing grade, was carried out individually for each ear (**Figure 3**), sex (**Figure 4**) and each one of the drugs used (**Figure 5**).

With the Bonferroni study we verified the efficacy of different drugs, achieved by multiple comparisons between them.

4.3. Valuation of the Side Effects

Overall there were no side effects, only small increments in blood pressure in 3 patients treated with deflazacort (13.6%) and 7 patients treated with fludrocortisones (26.8%). The blood pressure increase was normalized using a thiazidic diuretic drug.

5. Discussion

Hearing impairment is one of the six leading contributors to the burden of disease in industrialized countries, and it is one of the conditions that most severely impair the quality of life of those who suffer from it [2] [3].

There are two forms of hearing impairment: the conductive and the sensorineural one. The latter form resulting from either damage to the sensory cells of the inner ear-secondary to an impaired inner cochlear homeostasis-or from different diseases affecting the cochlear nerve (including its synapses) [2].

Idiopathic sensorineural hearing loss is predominant in middle-aged adults, and it is equally distributed by gender [1] [2], although, in this study, we found a non-significant higher prevalence in males (**Figure 1** and **Figure 2**).

Conductive hearing loss has various possibilities of treatment, whereas there is no specific drug therapy for sensorineural hearing loss, apart from symptomatic approaches with moderate efficacy [2]-[7].

One of the main reasons for the absence of specific tools to cure or prevent SNHL is the insufficient knowledge about the basic molecular mechanisms of normal and impaired adult hearing, thus therapeutic measures have focused on the recovery of hearing levels by trying to control its pathogenesis [1]-[9].

The hypothesis argued, in the case of sudden hearing loss, and in hearing loss secondary to acoustic trauma, is that it is caused by alterations to the hemodynamics of the cochlear level which end up ischemic injury, which could be controlled with vasodilators drugs [5] [6]. This therapy which we use, thinking that some of these factors could have pathogenetic implications, does not show to be effective for hearing recovery.

There is well documented evidence on the use of steroids in the treatment of pathologies of the inner ear [8] and has also been proved by different studies that demonstrate that there is a great amount of steroid receptors in the inner ear, not only in its neurons [12] but also in the Corti organ—here mainly concentrated in the cochlear stria vascularis [10] [11] whose mission is that of regulating the endolymphatic ionic balance.

It has been demonstrated by Trune *et al.* [13], in the autoimmune mouse, that mineralocorticoids are the key regulators of this balance [13] [14] and on this basis most researches advocate for glucocorticoids as the effective therapy for patients suffering from immune-mediate or inflammatory deafness processes, whereas mineralocorticoids should be used in the treatment of idiopathic or not well defined deafness [13]-[15].

Based on these findings, and with the evidence that the restoration of hearing with steroid treatment is due to increased stria sodium-potassium transport, to reestablish normal ionic balances in the endolymph, our study was aimed at demonstrating if it has any application in a clinical model.

This study aims to demonstrate the efficacy of mineralocorticoids in patients suffering from idiopathic cochlear hearing loss and to draw contrast with glucocorticoids and also with vasodilators drugs.

In all treated patients we observed a gain in binaural hearing, greater in the group treated with steroids than in the group treated with vasodilators, and it was much more significant with the mineralocorticoids (**Figure 5**, **Table 4**).

We found better response in women, and hearing recovery was greater in the left ear (**Figure 3** and **Figure 4**). We cannot give a justification for such results.

In all patients blood pressure side effects were easily regulated with thiazide treatment.

6. Conclusions

Mineralocorticoid therapy is effective in improving hearing function in patients with idiopathic HNS with cochlear BRA pattern.

Its use provides statistically significant results, higher than those observed with the use of glucocorticoids.
Vasodilator drugs lack these beneficial effects in the restoration of the hearing levels in these pathologies.
Side effects of steroids therapy can be easily controlled.

Acknowledgements and Economic Support

Funded through the Carlos III Health Institute agreement to carry out non-commercial clinical trials involving human drugs, co-financed by the European Regional Development Fund (ERDF).

Conflict of Interest

All authors of this study certify that there is no conflict of interest with any organization and that there is no financial or non-financial interest in the subject matter or materials discussed in this manuscript. This is an original study.

References

[1] Berretini, S., Ravecca, F., Forli, F., Sellari-Franceschini, S. and Piragine, F. (1998) Diagnostic and Therapeutic Approach to Progressive Sensorineural Hearing Loss. *Acta Otorhinolaryngologica Italica*, **18**, 87-94.

[2] Yamasoba, T., Lin, F.R., Someya, S., Kashio, A., Sakamoto, T. and Kondo, K. (2013) Current Concepts in Age-Related Hearing Loss: Epidemiology and Mechanistic Pathways. *Hearing Research*, **16**, 95-105.

[3] Zahnert, T. (2011) The Differential Diagnosis of Hearing Loss. *Deutsches Ärzteblatt international*, **108**, 433-444.

[4] Sekiya, T., Hatayama, T., Shimamura, N. and Suzuki, S. (2000) An *in Vivo* Quantificable Model of Cochlear Neuronal Degeneration Induced by Central Process Injury. *Experimental Neurology*, **161**, 409-502.
http://dx.doi.org/10.1006/exnr.1999.7280

[5] Fish, U., Nagahara, K. and Pollak, A. (1984) Sudden Hearing Loss Circulatory. *American Journal of Otolaryngology*,

5, 488-491.

[6]   Kansy, L., Ozkarakas, H., Efendi, H. and Okar, I. (2011) Protective Effects of Pentoxifylline and Nimodipine on Acoustic Trauma in Guinea Pig Cochlea. *Otology Neurotology*, **32**, 19-25.

[7]   Polon, Y.G., Humli, V., Andó, R., Aller, M., Horváth, T., Harnos, A., Tamás, L., Vizi, E.S. and Zelles, T. (2014) Protective Effect of Rasagiline in Aminoglycoside Ototoxicity. *Neuroscience*, **265**, 263-273. http://dx.doi.org/10.1016/j.neuroscience.2014.01.057

[8]   Trune, D.R. and Canlon, B. (2012) Corticosteroid Therapy for Hearing and Balance Disorders. *Anatomical Record*, **295**, 1928-1943. http://dx.doi.org/10.1002/ar.22576

[9]   Rita Fetoni, A., Bartolo, P., Eramo, S.L., Rolesi, R., Pacielo, F., *et al.* (2013) Noise-Induced Hearing Loss (NIHL) as a Target of Oxidative Stress-Mediated Damage: Cochlear and Cortical Responses Alter an Increase in Antioxidant Defense. *The Journal of Neuroscience*, **33**, 4011-4023. http://dx.doi.org/10.1523/JNEUROSCI.2282-12.2013

[10] Rarey, K.E. and Curtis, L.M. (1996) Receptors for Glucocorticoids in the Human Inner Ear. *Otolaryngology—Head and Neck Surgery*, **115**, 38-41. http://dx.doi.org/10.1016/S0194-5998(96)70133-X

[11] Sinha, P.K. and Pitovsky, D.Z. (1995) 3-H-Aldosterone Bingind Sites (Type I Receptors) in the Lateral Wall of the Cochlea: Distribution Assessment by Quantitative Auto Radiography. *Acta Oto-Laryngologica*, **115**, 643-647. http://dx.doi.org/10.3109/00016489509139380

[12] Jin, D.X., Lin, Z., Lei, D. and Bao, J. (2009) The Role of Glucocorticoids for Spiral Ganglion Neuron Survival. *Brain Research*, **1277**, 3-11. http://dx.doi.org/10.1016/j.brainres.2009.02.017

[13] Trune, D.R. and Kempton, J.B. (2001) Aldosterone and Prednisolone Control of Cochlear Function in MRL/MpJ-Fas(lpr) Autoimmune Mice. *Hearing Research*, **155**, 9-20. http://dx.doi.org/10.1016/S0378-5955(01)00240-4

[14] Trune, D.R., Kempton, J.B. and Gross, N.D. (2006) Mineralocorticoid Receptor Mediates Glucocorticoid Treatment Effects in the Autoimmune Mouse Ear. *Hearing Research*, **212**, 23-32. http://dx.doi.org/10.1016/j.heares.2005.10.006

[15] Trune, D.R., Kempton, J.B., Harrison, A.R. and Wobig, J.L. (2007) Glucocorticoid Impact on Cochlear Function and Systemic Side Effects in Autoimmune C3MRL-Fask or and Normal C3H-Hej Mice. *Hearing Research*, **226**, 209-212. http://dx.doi.org/10.1016/j.heares.2006.09.011

28

Prognostic and Predictive Protein Biomarkers in Laryngeal Squamous Cell Carcinoma—A Systematic Review

Matthew M. Kwok, Paul Goodyear

Department of Otolaryngology/Head and Neck Surgery, Western Health, Melbourne, Australia
Email: mattmkkwok@gmail.com

Abstract

Background: Despite recent advances in clinical management of laryngeal squamous cell carcinoma (LSCC), the overall 5-year survival continues to be poor. Consequently, biomarkers of treatment response will need to be identified. Proteomic strategies are one way to attempt to identify such biomarkers. Methods: The Medline, Embase and Cochrane Library databases were systematically searched until 1st March 2014 using the terms "larynx", "squamous cell carcinoma", "proteomic", and "biomarker". Articles which met inclusion criteria were assessed for the type of biomarker investigated, the proteomic technique used, and whether any validation had been performed. Results: Six studies identified biomarkers, including UCRP, ceramides, uPA, MT1-MMP, stratifin, transferrin, albumin, S100 calcium-binding protein A9, stathmin, enolase, PLAU, IGFBP7, MMP14, THBS1, and transthyretin. Transferrin was the only biomarker to appear in more than one study. Conclusions: Our review identified several potential biomarkers of outcome in LSCC. Well designed studies will need to further validate their use in the future.

Keywords

Laryngeal, Squamous Cell Carcinoma, Cancer, Proteomics, Biomarker

1. Introduction

Head and neck squamous cell carcinoma (HNSCC) is diagnosed in over 650,000 individuals annually worldwide and remains to be an important global health issue [1]. Laryngeal squamous cell carcinoma (LSCC) accounts for more than 150,000 of these cases, with an annual global mortality of approximately 83,000 individuals [1]. Although extensive research had been undertaken on LSCC in the past decade in an attempt to identify biomarkers of treatment response or outcome, there continued to be significant morbidity and mortality associated with this condition, to the extent that the overall 5-year survival had reduced between 1975 and 2010 in the USA [2]. The prognosis is especially poor for patients with metastatic disease, with a 5-year survival of less than 50% [3]. Consequently, a better understanding of biomarkers of outcome associated with LSCC may have clinical use in improved treatment stratification and prognostication and may even inform the development of future novel targeted therapies.

In recent years, biomarker development in other tumor types has resulted in treatment targeting and improved outcomes for biomarker derived subsets of patients. A notable example is the use of detection of the HER-2 receptor in breast cancer biopsy tissue [4].

There are three main clinical applications for biomarkers in cancer—in the diagnosis and characterization of tumors, as well as the potential development of novel targeted therapy against certain cancers.

As a diagnostic tool, molecular biomarkers may aid in the diagnosis of occult metastasis as well as the early detection of local and regional spread [5] [6]. Biomarkers, such as desmoglein 3 and Tissue-Specific Mir-205, have been shown to be associated with metastatic head and neck cancer and hence have the potential to be diagnostic biomarkers for this condition [7] [8].

In the characterization of tumors, they are used to better determine prognosis and treatment selection [5]. Epidermal growth factor receptor (EGFR) and p16 are well characterized biomarkers which are differentially expressed in a subset of LSCC [9] [10], and may play a role in the carcinogenesis of LSCC [11] [12]. Various targeted therapies against EGFR positive HNSCC have been developed, including anti-EGFR antibodies such as cetuximab, which improve overall survival without adverse effects on quality of life [13] [14].

Recent advances in proteomic technology and techniques have resulted in the discovery of new biomarkers in HNSCC [15], using various proteomic techniques. Protein separation techniques, such as 2-dimensional (2D) differential in-gel electrophoresis, have allowed large numbers of proteins to be sampled in a reproducible manner [16] [17]. Moreover, the differential expression of protein biomarkers identified using proteomic techniques such as matrix-assisted laser desorption/ionization (MALDI) time of flight (ToF) mass spectrometry (MS) [18], surface enhanced laser desorption/ionization (SELDI) ToF MS [19], laser capture [20], liquid chromatography mass spectrometry (LC-MS) [21], as well as newer techniques such as isobaric tag for relative and absolute quantitation (iTRAQ) [22] has led to a better understanding of the carcinogenesis of certain types of cancers [23] [24]. Various types of tissue samples may be used for proteomic analysis, which include fresh frozen, formalin-fixed paraffin embedded, and cell lines [25] [26]. Slight differences may exist among results obtained from different types of tissue samples [26]. Although previous reviews have evaluated studies utilizing proteomic techniques to characterize salivary cancer biomarkers [27] [28] and colorectal cancer biomarkers [29], no study has assessed the use of this technique in the identification of LSCC biomarkers.

This study aims to review the current literature to evaluate biomarkers in LSCC identified using proteomic techniques. In particular, this review will assess the type of biomarker and its potential use in LSCC, the proteomic technique used, and whether or not any validation of the biomarker has been performed.

2. Methods

A literature search for relevant articles was performed electronically by two independent reviewers—MK, a surgical HMO and PG, an otolaryngologist/head and neck surgeon. The Medline, Embase and Cochrane Library databases were searched using the following terms in combination: [laryngeal or larynx or glottis or glottis or supraglottic or supraglottis or subglottic or subglottis (all fields)] and ["squamous cell carcinoma" or SCC or cancer (all fields)] and [biomarker (all fields)] and [proteomic or proteome or electrophoresis or Maldi or "laser desorption ionization" or spectrometry (all fields)] in Medline; and (((("laryngeal or larynx or glottis or glottis or supraglottis or supraglottic or subglottis or subglottic") and "squamous cell carcinoma" or SCC or cancer) and biomarker) and (proteomic or proteome or electrophoresis or Maldi or "laser desorption ionization" or spectrometry)). mp. [mp = title, abstract, subject headings, heading word, drug trade name, original title, device manufacturer, drug manufacturer, device trade name, keyword] in Embase.

The search strategy is outlined in **Figure 1** and follows the PRISMA statement. All articles published from 1950 to 1st March 2014 in the above databases were searched for relevant articles. Full text articles retrieved

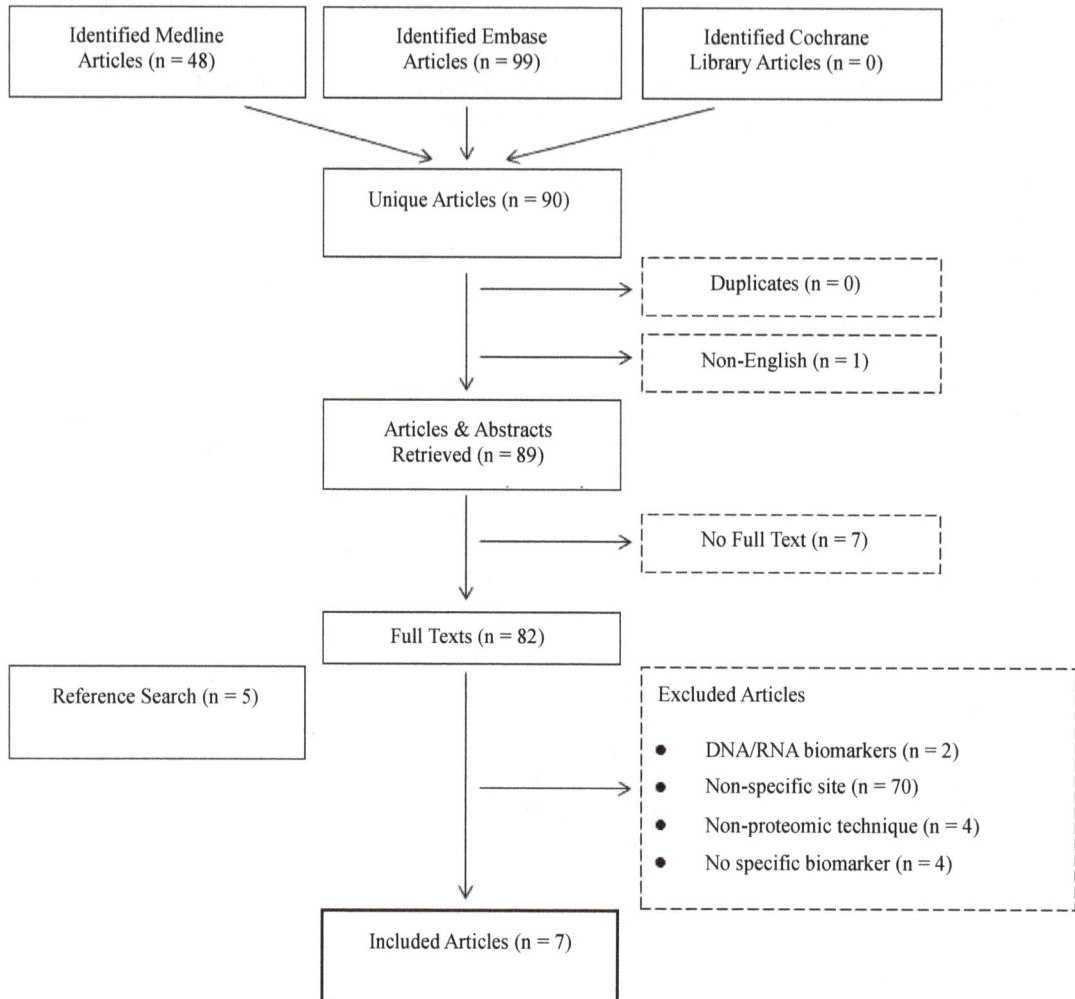

Figure 1. Systematic search strategy for studies included in this review.

were reviewed individually for eligibility into this study. Additionally, a manual search was performed on all reference lists of included articles.

Inclusion criteria were defined as articles which identify using a proteomic approach and/or validate biomarkers in laryngeal squamous cell carcinoma using immunohistochemical techniques on larger samples. Non-English articles, case reports, opinions, reviews and news articles were excluded from this study. Articles assessing DNA/RNA and those which did not identify specific biomarkers were also excluded.

Data retrieved from all unique articles identified include the date of publication, type of biomarker identified and its potential use in laryngeal SCC, proteomic technique used, source and tissue preparation, number of diseased and healthy subjects, and whether or not any validation of the biomarker had been performed. Due to the limited data available in the current literature, no statistical analysis could be performed.

3. Results

90 unique articles were identified in our search, with 7 meeting inclusion criteria for review in this study. The majority of excluded articles (n = 70) assessed head and neck SCC biomarkers on a non-specific anatomical site. **Table 1** outlines a summary of information retrieved from included studies.

Studies were published between 1996 and 2012, with 5 studies published in the last 10 years [23] [30]-[33]. A variety of proteomic techniques were identified, including liquid chromatography, mass spectrometry, electrospray ionization, matrix-assisted laser desorption/ionization, sodium dodecyl sulfate polyacrylamide gel electrophoresis, enzyme-linked immunosorbent assay and 2-dimensional electrophoresis.

Table 1. Summary of information obtained from included studies.

Authors	Year	Proteomic technique	Tissue source	n	Biomarkers identified	Validation
Chi *et al.*	2009	LC-MS/MS, LC-ESI-MALDI Tandem MS, MALDI-TOF	Oral cavity SCC cell lines—validated in laryngeal SCC	18	↑UCRP	Not in a separate population
Dowling *et al.*	2008	LC-MS, 2DE	Laryngeal SCC, salivary samples	4	↑S100 calcium binding protein A9, ↑beta fibrin, ↑transferrin, ↑immunoglobulin heavy chain constant region gamma, ↑cofilin, ↓transthyretin	S100 calcium binding protein validated by immunoblot analysis
Karahatay *et al.*	2007	LC/MS	Laryngeal SCC tissue	10	↑C16-, ↓C18-, ↑C24-, ↑C24:1-ceramides	Nil
Parolini *et al.*	1996	SDS-PAGE, ELISA	Laryngeal SCC tissue frozen or fixed in paraformaldehyde	70	↑uPA	uPA and mRNA expression using ISH
Sepiashvili *et al.*	2012	MS, 2DE	Laryngeal SCC cell lines	2	↑PLAU, ↑IGFBP7, ↑MMP14 and ↑THBS1	Validated using IHC and ELISA in 56 laryngeal SCC
Sewell *et al.*	2007	MALDI-TOF, MS, 2D-DIGE	Laryngeal SCC frozen tissue	2	↓stratifin, ↓S100 calcium-binding protein A9, ↓p21-ARC, ↓stathmin, and ↑enolase, ↑MAGE D3, ↑transferrin, ↑albumin, ↑tumor-associated calcium signal transducer	Nil
Yoshizaki *et al.*	1997	SDS-PAGE	Laryngeal SCC tissue fixed in formalin	9	↑MT1-MMP	Nil

LC: Liquid chromatography; MS: Mass spectrometry; ESI: Electrospray ionization; MALDI: Matrix-assisted laser desorption/ionization; TOF: Time of flight; SDS-PAGE: Sodium dodecyl sulfate polyacrylamide gel electrophoresis; ELISA: Enzyme-linked immunosorbent assay; 2D-DIGE: 2-dimensional difference gel electrophoresis; 2DE: 2-dimensional electrophoresis.

The number of samples in each study ranged between two to 70, 5 of the 6 studies having less than 50 samples. Laryngeal SCC samples were obtained from fresh tissue in four studies, saliva in one study and from cell lines in two studies. One study [30] validated biomarkers identified in oral cavity SCC using laryngeal SCC samples.

A number of laryngeal SCC biomarkers were identified in this review. These include ubiquitin cross-reactive protein (UCRP), C16-, C24-, C24:1-ceramides, urokinase plasminogen activator (uPA), membrane associated type 1 matrix metalloproteinase (MT1-MMP), stratifin, transferrin, albumin, tumor-associated calcium signal transducer, melanoma-associated antigen D3 (MAGE D3), S100 calcium-binding protein A9, p21-ARC, stathmin, enolase, plasminogen activator, urokinase (PLAU), insulin-like growth factor-binding protein 7 (IGFBP7), matrix metalloproteinase 14 (MMP14), Thrombospondin 1 (THBS1), beta fibrin, immunoglobulin heavy chain constant region gamma, cofilin, and transthyretin. A summary of the differential expression of laryngeal SCC biomarkers identified in this review are presented in **Table 2**. Transferrin was the only biomarker identified using proteomic techniques in more than one study. Only one study validated their identified biomarker using in a separate patient population [23] [31].

4. Discussion

LSCC remains to be associated with significant morbidity and mortality despite extensive research recently, being one of only two cancer types to have a reduction in 5 year survival over the last decades [1]-[3]. The lack of specific molecular biomarkers in the management of LSCC may contribute to these statistics [23]. A better understanding of biomarkers may therefore provide new management options in the diagnosis, characterization, and targeted therapy for LSCC [5]. Recent developments in biomarker research include p16 and EGFR, which are implicated in the carcinogenesis and targeted therapy for LSCC [9]-[14]. A review of LSCC biomarkers in 2004 by Almadori *et al.* [5] suggested the possible association of protein biomarkers S100A2 calcium binding protein and galectin-3 with the molecular characterization of LSCC.

Table 2. Differential expression of biomarkers identified.

Author	Up-regulated biomarkers	Down-regulated biomarkers
Chi *et al.* [30]	UCRP	
Dowling *et al.* [31]	S100 calcium binding protein Beta fibrin Transferrin Immunoglobulin heavy chain constant region gamma Cofilin	Transthyretin
Karahatay *et al.* [32]	C16- ceramide C24- ceramide C24:1- ceramide	C18- ceramide
Parolini *et al.* [35]	uPA	NA
Sepiashvili *et al.* [33]	PLAU IGFBP7 MMP14 THBS1	NA
Sewell *et al.* [23]	Enolase MAGE D3 Transferrin Albumin Tumor-associated calcium signal transducer	Stratifin S100 calcium-binding protein A9 p21-ARC Stathmin
Yoshizaki *et al.* [36]	MT1-MMP	NA

With the use of proteomic techniques such as 2DIGE and MALDI-TOF MS, it is now possible to sample large amount of proteins in the identification of potential cancer biomarkers [16]-[19]. This may aid in the process of identifying and validating biomarkers for LSCC. Although previous reviews had been conducted regarding the proteomic analysis of biomarkers associated with colorectal and endometrial cancer [29] [34], this is the first systematic review evaluating the use of proteomic techniques in the analysis of LSCC biomarkers.

This review has identified 25 proteins reported as differentially expressed by 7 studies [23] [30]-[33] [35] [36]. 2 of these proteins—S100 calcium binding protein A9 and transferrin were reported as differentially expressed by more than one study, with transferrin [23] [31] reported to be up-regulated in 2 studies, while the differential expression of S100 calcium binding protein A9 was inconsistently reported in 2 studies [23] [31]. A selection of identified proteins will be discussed below.

The S100 family is a subtype of calcium binding proteins consisting of at least 25 different proteins [37]. There is current evidence to suggest the role of S100 proteins in cancer cell differentiation [38], cell proliferation [39] [40], cell apoptosis [41] [42] and tumor metastasis [43] [44]. Members of the S100 family have been implicated in various types of cancers. For example, non-small cell lung cancer (NSCLC) had been associated with over-expression of S100A2, S100A8 and S100A9 [45]-[47], while S100A2 and S100A11 may be a prognostic marker for post-operative patients with pancreatic cancer [48] [49]. In HNSCC, patients with S100A2 positive LSCC had been shown to have better survival compared to S100A2 negative tumors [50]. S100A7 expression may also be implicated in the prognosis of HNSCC tumors [51]. Although serum S100 proteins may have potential implications in various types of cancers, there are still limited clinical applications for S100 proteins, with the only independent prognostic marker being serum S100B in melanoma [52] [53]. The differential reporting of S100 calcium binding protein by Dowling *et al.* and Sewell *et al.* as identified in this review may be secondary to the different sample sources (saliva and tumor tissue, respectively) and the use of control samples from the same patient by Dowling *et al.* [23] [31].

A number of biomarkers identified in this review may not have significance in the carcinogenesis of LSCC due to their non-specific nature in multiple disease processes, notably albumin and transferrin, which may be differentially expressed due to various physiological or pathological processes [54] [55]. Transthyretin has been shown to be a potential biomarker in pancreatic cancer [56] [57], but its association with multiple inflammatory disease processes may reduce its usefulness as a cancer biomarker [58]. Similarly, the use of fibrin and cofilin as LSCC biomarkers is limited by its non-specificity even though it is involved with various carcinogenic processes [59] [60].

Although Chi *et al.* identified the association of UCRP with LSCC, a protein previously shown to change tumor sensitivity to chemotherapy [61] [62], the lack of validation using proteomic techniques in LSCC samples highlights the need for further classification of this biomarker [30].

Stathmin over-expression is found in many types of cancers [63], and is involved in processes such as the regulation of cell migration [64] [65], which may have implications in the pathogenesis of LSCC. Likewise, IGFBP7 is differentially expressed in various cancers as a tumour suppressor protein [66] [67]. However, there is still insufficient evidence currently to demonstrate any significant associations between these proteins and LSCC.

Two biomarkers, uPA and MT1-MMP, were identified more than 10 years ago [32] [36]. uPA is a type of protease responsible for both proteolysis and fibrinolysis, processes which are required for tumor growth and metastasis [68]. Its expression is associated with various cancer types such as breast and colorectal tumors [69] [70]. It is the only biomarker identified in this review which had used a sample size of greater than 20. Moreover, recent studies have validated the over-expression of uPA in separate LSCC populations which suggests its potential as a biomarker in LSCC [71] [72]. MT1-MMP was also a novel biomarker and potential therapeutic target identified in the 1990s, but there had been limited studies regarding its use in LSCC since, with research focusing on other MMP subtypes such as MMP-2 and MMP-9 [73] [74].

Ceramides, a well-studied group of molecules, are involved in apoptotic cellular pathways [75]. They have been shown to assist in the induction of cell death by chemotherapeutic agents both in vivo and in situ [76] [77]. Karahatay *et al.* reported a lower level of C18-ceramide in patients with LSCC as well as an inverse relationship between ceramide levels and the risk of nodal metastasis [32]. Ceramides may therefore be an important prognostic marker in LSCC.

The small number of studies identified by this review limits the use of quantitative methods to analyse current LSCC biomarkers discovered by proteomic techniques, and may be a source of bias in this review. Although 25 different proteins were identified, only two were reported by more than one study. This highlights some of the pitfalls of using proteomic techniques in cancer biomarker research. Firstly, identified biomarkers require validation in a larger population with reproducible results [78]. Only one study validated the identified biomarker in a separate population and the vast majority of studies had sample sizes of less than 20. Secondly, using different proteomic techniques and technologies as well as different tissue preparations may produce varying results. There was great variability in the type of tissue analyzed and the proteomic technique used between studies. There was no standardized method of identifying LSCC biomarkers using proteomic techniques across the seven studies identified in this review. This highlights the need for further research in evaluating the molecular mechanisms for LSCC biomarkers by proteomic techniques, with the aim of developing novel diagnostic and therapeutic options for this condition.

5. Conclusion

Despite advances in biomarker research, LSCC remains to be associated with significant morbidity and mortality. This systematic review assessing LSCC biomarkers identified using proteomic techniques has found various differentially expressed protein biomarkers associated with LSCC, with no specific marker of clinical significance. Future studies may aim to further characterize these biomarkers to better understand their mechanism of action in LSCC, and validate their use in a clinical setting.

Acknowledgements

The authors would like to acknowledge S. Chan and T. Jones for their contribution towards this manuscript.

References

[1] Ferlay, J.S.I., Ervik, M., Dikshit, R., *et al.* (2013) Cancer Incidence and Mortality Worldwide: IARC CancerBase No. 11; GLOBOCAN 2012 v1.0 2013. International Agency for Research on Cancer, Lyon. http://globocan.iarc.fr

[2] Siegel, R., Ma, J., Zou, Z. and Jemal, A. (2014) Cancer Statistics, 2014. *CA: A Cancer Journal for Clinicians*, **64**, 9-29. http://dx.doi.org/10.3322/caac.21208

[3] Shah, J.P., Karnell, L.H., Hoffman, H.T., *et al.* (1997) Patterns of Care for Cancer of the Larynx in the United States. Archives of Otolaryngology—Head & Neck Surgery, **123**, 475-483. http://dx.doi.org/10.1001/archotol.1997.01900050021002

[4]   Mitri, Z., Constantine, T. and O'Regan, R. (2012) The HER2 Receptor in Breast Cancer: Pathophysiology, Clinical Use, and New Advances in Therapy. *Chemotherapy Research and Practice*, **2012**, Article ID: 743193. http://dx.doi.org/10.1155/2012/743193

[5]   Almadori, G., Bussu, F., Cadoni, G., Galli, J., Paludetti, G. and Maurizi, M. (2005) Molecular Markers in Laryngeal Squamous Cell Carcinoma: Towards an Integrated Clinicobiological Approach. *European Journal of Cancer*, **41**, 683-693.

[6]   Almadori, G., Bussu, F. and Paludettii, G. (2006) Predictive Factors of Neck Metastases in Laryngeal Squamous Cell Carcinoma. Towards an Integrated Clinico-Molecular Classification. *Acta Otorhinolaryngologica Italica*, **26**, 326-334.

[7]   Fletcher, A.M., Heaford, A.C. and Trask, D.K. (2008) Detection of Metastatic Head and Neck Squamous Cell Carcinoma Using the Relative Expression of Tissue-Specific Mir-205. *Translational Oncology*, **1**, 202-208. http://dx.doi.org/10.1593/tlo.08163

[8]   Patel, V., Martin, D., Malhotra, R., *et al.* (2013) DSG3 as a Biomarker for the Ultrasensitive Detection of Occult Lymph Node Metastasis in Oral Cancer Using Nanostructured Immunoarrays. *Oral Oncology*, **49**, 93-101. http://dx.doi.org/10.1016/j.oraloncology.2012.08.001

[9]   Grandis, J.R. and Tweardy, D.J. (1993) Elevated Levels of Transforming Growth Factor Alpha and Epidermal Growth Factor Receptor Messenger RNA Are Early Markers of Carcinogenesis in Head and Neck Cancer. *Cancer Research*, **53**, 3579-3584.

[10] Reed, A.L., Califano, J., Cairns, P., *et al.* (1996) High Frequency of p16 (CDKN2/MTS-1/INK4A) Inactivation in Head and Neck Squamous Cell Carcinoma. *Cancer Research*, **56**, 3630-3633.

[11] Combes, J.D. and Franceschi, S. (2014) Role of Human Papillomavirus in Non-Oropharyngeal Head and Neck Cancers. *Oral Oncology*, **50**, 370-379. http://dx.doi.org/10.1016/j.oraloncology.2013.11.004

[12] Gheit, T., Abedi-Ardekani, B., Carreira, C., Missad, C.G., Tommasino, M. and Torrente, M.C. (2014) Comprehensive Analysis of HPV Expression in Laryngeal Squamous Cell Carcinoma. *Journal of Medical Virology*, **86**, 642-646. http://dx.doi.org/10.1002/jmv.23866

[13] Bonner, J.A., Harari, P.M., Giralt, J., Azarnia, N., Shin, D.M., Cohen, R.B., *et al.* (2006) Radiotherapy plus Cetuximab for Squamous-Cell Carcinoma of the Head and Neck. *The New England Journal of Medicine*, **354**, 567-578. http://dx.doi.org/10.1056/NEJMoa053422

[14] Bonner, J.A., Harari, P.M., Giralt, J., Cohen, R.B., Jones, C.U., Sur, R.K., *et al.* (2010) Radiotherapy plus Cetuximab for Locoregionally Advanced Head and Neck Cancer: 5-Year Survival Data from a Phase 3 Randomized Trial, and Relation between Cetuximab-Induced Rash and Survival. *The Lancet Oncology*, **11**, 21-28. http://dx.doi.org/10.1016/S1470-2045(09)70311-0

[15] Rudert, F. (2000) Genomics and Proteomics Tools for the Clinic. *Current Opinion in Molecular Therapeutics*, **2**, 633-642.

[16] Celis, J.E. and Gromov, P. (1999) 2D Protein Electrophoresis: Can It Be Perfected? *Current Opinion in Biotechnology*, **10**, 16-21. http://dx.doi.org/10.1016/S0958-1669(99)80004-4

[17] Unlu, M. (1999) Difference Gel Electrophoresis. *Biochemical Society Transactions*, **27**, 547-549.

[18] Cheng, A.J., Chen, L.C., Chien, K.Y., Chen, Y.J., Chang, J.T.C., Wang, H.-M., *et al.* (2005) Oral Cancer Plasma Tumor Marker Identified with Bead-Based Affinity-Fractionated Proteomic Technology. *Clinical Chemistry*, **51**, 2236-2244. http://dx.doi.org/10.1373/clinchem.2005.052324

[19] Chapman, K. (2002) The Protein Chip Biomarker System from Ciphergen Biosystems: A Novel Proteomics Platform for Rapid Biomarker Discovery and Validation. *Biochemical Society Transactions*, **30**, 82-87. http://dx.doi.org/10.1042/BST0300082

[20] Craven, R.A. and Banks, R.E. (2001) Laser Capture Microdissection and Proteomics: Possibilities and Limitation. *Proteomics*, **1**, 1200-1204. http://dx.doi.org/10.1002/1615-9861(200110)1:10<1200::AID-PROT1200>3.0.CO;2-Q

[21] Qian, W.J., Jacobs, J.M., Liu, T., Camp II, D.G. and Smith, R.D. (2006) Advances and Challenges in Liquid Chromatography-Mass Spectrometry-Based Proteomics Profiling for Clinical Applications. *Molecular & Cellular Proteomics: MCP*, **5**, 1727-1744.

[22] Evans, C., Noirel, J., Ow, S.Y., *et al.* (2012) An Insight into iTRAQ: Where Do We Stand Now? *Analytical and Bioanalytical Chemistry*, **404**, 1011-1027. http://dx.doi.org/10.1007/s00216-012-5918-6

[23] Sewell, D.A., Yuan, C.X. and Robertson, E. (2007) Proteomic Signatures in Laryngeal Squamous Cell Carcinoma. *ORL: Journal for Oto-Rhino-Laryngology and Its Related Specialties*, **69**, 77-84. http://dx.doi.org/10.1159/000097406

[24] Conrads, T.P., Zhou, M., Petricoin 3rd, E.F., Liotta, L. and Veenstra, T.D. (2003) Cancer Diagnosis Using Proteomic Patterns. *Expert Review of Molecular Diagnostics*, **3**, 411-420. http://dx.doi.org/10.1586/14737159.3.4.411

[25] Schirle, M., Heurtier, M.A. and Kuster, B. (2013) Profiling Core Proteomes of Human Cell Lines by One-Dimensional PAGE and Liquid Chromatography-Tandem Mass Spectrometry. *Molecular & Cellular Proteomics: MCP*, **2**, 1297-1305.

[26] Tanca, A., Pagnozzi, D., Burrai, G.P., Polinas, M., Uzzau, S., Antuofermo, E. and Addis, M.F. (2012) Comparability of Differential Proteomics Data Generated from Paired Archival Fresh-Frozen and Formalin-Fixed Samples by GeLC-MS/MS and Spectral Counting. *Journal of Proteomics*, **77**, 561-576. http://dx.doi.org/10.1016/j.jprot.2012.09.033

[27] Streckfus, C.F. and Dubinsky, W.P. (2007) Proteomic Analysis of Saliva for Cancer Diagnosis. *Expert Review of Proteomics*, **4**, 329-332. http://dx.doi.org/10.1586/14789450.4.3.329

[28] Cheng, Y.S., Rees, T. and Wright, J. (2014) A Review of Research on Salivary Biomarkers for Oral Cancer Detection. *Clinical and Translational Medicine*, **3**, 3. http://dx.doi.org/10.1186/2001-1326-3-3

[29] Ma, Y., Zhang, P., Wang, F. and Qin, H. (2012) Searching for Consistently Reported Up- and Down-Regulated Biomarkers in Colorectal Cancer: A Systematic Review of Proteomic Studies. *Molecular Biology Reports*, **39**, 8483-8490. http://dx.doi.org/10.1007/s11033-012-1702-0

[30] Chi, L.M., Lee, C.W., Chang, K.P., Hao, S.-P., Lee, H.-M., Liang, Y., *et al.* (2009) Enhanced Interferon Signaling Pathway in Oral Cancer Revealed by Quantitative Proteome Analysis of Microdissected Specimens Using $^{16}O/^{18}O$ Labeling and Integrated Two-Dimensional LC-ESI-MALDI Tandem MS. *Molecular & Cellular Proteomics: MCP*, **8**, 1453-1474.

[31] Dowling, P., Wormald, R., Meleady, P., Henry, M., Curran, A. and Clynes, M. (2008) Analysis of the Saliva Proteome from Patients with Head and Neck Squamous Cell Carcinoma Reveals Differences in Abundance Levels of Proteins Associated with Tumour Progression and Metastasis. *Journal of Proteomics*, **71**, 168-175. http://dx.doi.org/10.1016/j.jprot.2008.04.004

[32] Karahatay, S., Thomas, K., Koybasi, S., Senkal, C.E., ElOjeimy, S., Liu, X., *et al.* (2007) Clinical Relevance of Ceramide Metabolism in the Pathogenesis of Human Head and Neck Squamous Cell Carcinoma (HNSCC): Attenuation of C_{18}-Ceramide in HNSCC Tumors Correlates with Lymphovascular Invasion and Nodal Metastasis. *Cancer Letters*, **256**, 101-111. http://dx.doi.org/10.1016/j.canlet.2007.06.003

[33] Sepiashvili, L., Hui, A., Ignatchenko, V., Shi, W., Su, S., Xu, W., *et al.* (2012) Potentially Novel Candidate Biomarkers for Head and Neck Squamous Cell Carcinoma Identified Using an Integrated Cell Line-Based Discovery Strategy. *Molecular & Cellular Proteomics: MCP*, **11**, 1404-1415.

[34] Galazis, N., Pang, Y.L., Galazi, M., Haoula, Z., Layfield, R. and Atiomo, W. (2013) Proteomic Biomarkers of Endometrial Cancer Risk in Women with Polycystic Ovary Syndrome: A Systematic Review and Biomarker Database Integration. *Gynecological Endocrinology: The Official Journal of the International Society of Gynecological Endocrinology*, **29**, 638-644.

[35] Parolini, S., Flagiello, D., Cinquetti, A., Gozzi, R., Cristini, S., Cappiello, J., *et al.* (1996) Up-Regulation of Urokinase-Type Plasminogen Activator in Squamous Cell Carcinoma of Human Larynx. *British Journal of Cancer*, **74**, 1168-1174. http://dx.doi.org/10.1038/bjc.1996.512

[36] Yoshizaki, T., Sato, H., Maruyama, Y., Murono, S., Furukawa, M., Park, C.-S. and Seiki, M. (1997) Increased Expression of Membrane Type 1-Matrix Metalloproteinase in Head and Neck Carcinoma. *Cancer*, **79**, 139-144. http://dx.doi.org/10.1002/(SICI)1097-0142(19970101)79:1<139::AID-CNCR20>3.0.CO;2-4

[37] Donato, R. (2001) S100: A Multigenic Family of Calcium-Modulated Proteins of the EF-Hand Type with Intracellular and Extracellular Functional Roles. *The International Journal of Biochemistry & Cell Biology*, **33**, 637-668. http://dx.doi.org/10.1016/S1357-2725(01)00046-2

[38] Cao, L.Y., Yin, Y., Li, H., Jiang, Y. and Zhang, H.F. (2009) Expression and Clinical Significance of S100A2 and p63 in Esophageal Carcinoma. *World Journal of Gastroenterology: WJG*, **15**, 4183-4188. http://dx.doi.org/10.3748/wjg.15.4183

[39] Fuentes, M.K., Nigavekar, S.S., Arumugam, T., Logsdon, C.D., Schmidt, A.M., Park, J.C. and Huang, E.H. (2007) RAGE Activation by S100P in Colon Cancer Stimulates Growth, Migration, and Cell Signaling Pathways. *Diseases of the Colon and Rectum*, **50**, 1230-1240. http://dx.doi.org/10.1007/s10350-006-0850-5

[40] Arumugam, T., Simeone, D.M., Van Golen, K. and Logsdon, C.D. (2005) S100P Promotes Pancreatic Cancer Growth, Survival, and Invasion. *Clinical Cancer Research: An Official Journal of the American Association for Cancer Research*, **11**, 5356-5364.

[41] Mahon, P.C., Baril, P., Bhakta, V., Chelala, C., Caulee, K., Harada, T. and Lemoine, N.R. (2007) S100A4 Contributes to the Suppression of BNIP3 Expression, Chemoresistance, and Inhibition of Apoptosis in Pancreatic Cancer. *Cancer Research*, **67**, 6786-6795. http://dx.doi.org/10.1158/0008-5472.CAN-07-0440

[42] Pedersen, K.B., Andersen, K., Fodstad, O. and Maelandsmo, G.M. (2004) Sensitization of Interferon-Gamma Induced

Apoptosis in Human Osteosarcoma Cells by Extracellular S100A4. *BMC Cancer*, **4**, 52.
http://dx.doi.org/10.1186/1471-2407-4-52

[43] Jenkinson, S.R., Barraclough, R., West, C.R. and Rudland, P.S. (2004) S100A4 Regulates Cell Motility and Invasion in an *in Vitro* Model for Breast Cancer Metastasis. *British Journal of Cancer*, **90**, 253-262.z
http://dx.doi.org/10.1038/sj.bjc.6601483

[44] Lo, J.F., Yu, C.C., Chiou, S.H., Huang, C.Y., Jan, C.I., Lin, S.C., *et al.* (2011) The Epithelial-Mesenchymal Transition Mediator S100A4 Maintains Cancer-Initiating Cells in Head and Neck Cancers. *Cancer Research*, **71**, 1912-1923.
http://dx.doi.org/10.1158/0008-5472.CAN-10-2350

[45] Kawai, H., Minamiya, Y. and Takahashi, N. (2011) Prognostic Impact of S100A9 Overexpression in Non-Small Cell Lung Cancer. *Tumour Biology: The Journal of the International Society for Oncodevelopmental Biology and Medicine*, **32**, 641-646.

[46] Smith, S.L., Gugger, M., Hoban, P., Ratschiller, D., Watson, S.G., Field, J.K., *et al.* (2004) S100A2 Is Strongly Expressed in Airway Basal Cells, Preoplastic Bronchial Lesions and Primary Non-Small Cell Lung Carcinomas. *British Journal of Cancer*, **91**, 1515-1524. http://dx.doi.org/10.1038/sj.bjc.6602188

[47] Wang, H., Zhang, Z., Li, R., Ang, K.K., Zhang, H., Caraway, N.P., *et al.* (2005) Overexpression of S100A2 Protein as a Prognostic Marker for Patients with Stage I Non Small Cell Lung Cancer. *International Journal of Cancer*, **116**, 285-290.

[48] Ohuchida, K., Mizumoto, K., Miyasaka, Y., Yu, J., Cui, L., Yamaguchi, H., *et al.* (2007) Over-Expression of S100A2 in Pancreatic Cancer Correlates with Progression and Poor Prognosis. *The Journal of Pathology*, **213**, 275-282.
http://dx.doi.org/10.1002/path.2250

[49] Xiao, M.B., Jiang, F., Ni, W.K., Chen, B.-Y., Lu, C.-H., Li, X.-Y. and Ni, R.-Z. (2012) High Expression of S100A11 in Pancreatic Adenocarcinoma Is an Unfavorable Prognostic Marker. *Medical Oncology*, **29**, 1886-1891.
http://dx.doi.org/10.1007/s12032-011-0058-y

[50] Almadori, G., Bussu, F., Galli, J., Rigante, M., Lauriola, L., Michetti, F., *et al.* (2009) Diminished Expression of S100A2, a Putative Tumour Suppressor, Is an Independent Predictive Factor of Neck Node Relapse in Laryngeal Squamous Cell Carcinoma. *Journal of Otolaryngology—Head & Neck Surgery*, **38**, 16-22.

[51] Tripathi, S.C., Matta, A., Kaur, J., Grigull, J., Chauhan, S.S., Thakar, A., *et al.* (2010) Nuclear S100A7 Is Associated with Poor Prognosis in Head and Neck Cancer. *PloS ONE*, **5**, e11939. http://dx.doi.org/10.1371/journal.pone.0011939

[52] Astrand, R., Unden, J. and Romner, B. (2013) Clinical Use of the Calcium-Binding S100B Protein. *Methods in Molecular Biology*, **963**, 373-384. http://dx.doi.org/10.1007/978-1-62703-230-8_23

[53] Hartman, K.G., McKnight, L.E., Liriano, M.A. and Weber, D.J. (2013) The Evolution of S100B Inhibitors for the Treatment of Malignant Melanoma. *Future Medicinal Chemistry*, **5**, 97-109. http://dx.doi.org/10.4155/fmc.12.191

[54] Szoke, D. and Panteghini, M. (2012) Diagnostic Value of Transferrin. Clinica Chimica Acta: International Journal of Clinical Chemistry, **413**, 1184-1189. http://dx.doi.org/10.1016/j.cca.2012.04.021

[55] Sethi, A., Sher, M., Akram, M.R., Karim, S., Khiljee, S., Sajjad, A., *et al.* (2013) Albumin as a Drug Delivery and Diagnostic Tool and Its Market Approved Products. *Acta Poloniae Pharmaceutica*, **70**, 597-600.

[56] Chen, J., Chen, L.J., Xia, Y.L., Zhou, H.-C., Yang, R.-B., Wu, W., *et al.* (2013) Identification and Verification of Transthyretin as a Potential Biomarker for Pancreatic Ductal Adenocarcinoma. *Journal of Cancer Research and Clinical Oncology*, **139**, 1117-1127. http://dx.doi.org/10.1007/s00432-013-1422-4

[57] Lv, S., Gao, J., Zhu, F., Li, Z.S., Gong, Y.F., Xu, G.M. and Ma, L. (2011) Transthyretin, Identified by Proteomics, Is Overabundant in Pancreatic Juice from Pancreatic Carcinoma and Originates from Pancreatic Islets. *Diagnostic Cytopathology*, **39**, 875-881. http://dx.doi.org/10.1002/dc.21484

[58] Fleming, C.E., Nunes, A.F. and Sousa, M.M. (2009) Transthyretin: More than Meets the Eye. *Progress in Neurobiology*, **89**, 266-276. http://dx.doi.org/10.1016/j.pneurobio.2009.07.007

[59] Mizuno, K. (2013) Signaling Mechanisms and Functional Roles of Cofilin Phosphorylation and Dephosphorylation. *Cellular Signalling*, **25**, 457-469. http://dx.doi.org/10.1016/j.cellsig.2012.11.001

[60] Fernandez, P.M., Patierno, S.R. and Rickles, F.R. (2004) Tissue Factor and Fibrin in Tumor Angiogenesis. *Seminars in Thrombosis and Hemostasis*, **30**, 31-44. http://dx.doi.org/10.1055/s-2004-822969

[61] Desai, S.D., Mao, Y., Sun, M., Li, T.K., Wu, J. and Liu, L.F. (2000) Ubiquitin, SUMO-1, and UCRP in Camptothecin Sensitivity and Resistance. *Annals of the New York Academy of Sciences*, **922**, 306-308.
http://dx.doi.org/10.1111/j.1749-6632.2000.tb07050.x

[62] Desai, S.D., Wood, L.M., Tsai, Y.C., Hsieh, T.-S., Marks, J.R., Scott, G.L., *et al.* (2008) ISG15 as a Novel Tumor Biomarker for Drug Sensitivity. *Molecular Cancer Therapeutics*, **7**, 1430-1439.
http://dx.doi.org/10.1158/1535-7163.MCT-07-2345

[63] Belletti, B. and Baldassarre, G. (2011) Stathmin: A Protein with Many Tasks. New Biomarker and Potential Target in Cancer. *Expert Opinion on Therapeutic Targets*, **15**, 1249-1266. http://dx.doi.org/10.1517/14728222.2011.620951

[64] Giampietro, C., Luzzati, F., Gambarotta, G., Giacobini, P., Boda, E., Fasolo, A. and Perroteau, I. (2005) Stathmin Expression Modulates Migratory Properties of GN-11 Neurons *in Vitro*. *Endocrinology*, **146**, 1825-1834. http://dx.doi.org/10.1210/en.2004-0972

[65] Jin, K., Mao, X.O., Cottrell, B., *et al.* (2004) Proteomic and Immunochemical Characterization of a Role for Stathmin in Adult Neurogenesis. *FASEB Journal: Official Publication of the Federation of American Societies for Experimental Biology*, **18**, 287-299.

[66] Chen, D., Yoo, B.K., Santhekadur, P.K., *et al.* (2011) Insulin-Like Growth Factor-Binding Protein-7 Functions as a Potential Tumor Suppressor in Hepatocellular Carcinoma. *Clinical Cancer Research: An Official Journal of the American Association for Cancer Research*, **17**, 6693-6701.

[67] Shersher, D.D., Vercillo, M.S., Fhied, C., Basu, S., Rouhi, O., Mahon, B., *et al.* (2011) Biomarkers of the Insulin-Like Growth Factor Pathway Predict Progression and Outcome in Lung Cancer. *The Annals of Thoracic Surgery*, **92**, 1805-1811; Discussion 1811. http://dx.doi.org/10.1016/j.athoracsur.2011.06.058

[68] Mignatti, P. and Rifkin, D.B. (1993) Biology and Biochemistry of Proteinases in Tumor Invasion. *Physiological Reviews*, **73**, 161-195.

[69] Duffy, M.J., Duggan, C., Mulcahy, H.E., McDermott, E.W. and O'Higgins, N.J. (1998) Urokinase Plasminogen Activator: A Prognostic Marker in Breast Cancer Including Patients with Axillary Node-Negative Disease. *Clinical Chemistry*, **44**, 1177-1183.

[70] Kim, T.D., Song, K.S., Li, G., Choi, H., Park, H.-D., Lim, K., *et al.* (2006) Activity and Expression of Urokinase-Type Plasminogen Activator and Matrix Metalloproteinases in Human Colorectal Cancer. *BMC Cancer*, **6**, 211. http://dx.doi.org/10.1186/1471-2407-6-211

[71] Wang, D. and Wang, T. (2005) Expressions and Clinical Significance of Urokinase-Type Activator (uPA) and uPA Receptor (uPAR) in Laryngeal Squamous Cell Carcinoma. *Journal of Clinical Otorhinolaryngology*, **19**, 529-531.

[72] Wu, H.Y., Shen, X.H., Ni, R.S., Qian, X.Y. and Gao, X. (2009) Expression of E-Cadherin and uPA and Their Prognostic Value in Carcinoma of Human Larynx. *Chinese Journal of Otorhinolaryngology Head and Neck Surgery*, **44**, 1024-1028.

[73] Gou, X., Chen, H., Jin, F., Wu, W., Li, Y., Long, J., *et al.* (2013) Expressions of CD147, MMP-2 and MMP-9 in Laryngeal Carcinoma and Its Correlation with Poor Prognosis. *Pathology Oncology Research: POR*, Published Online.

[74] Yang, L., Shang, X., Zhao, X., Lin, Y. and Liu, J. (2012) Correlation Study between OPN, CD44v6, MMP-9 and Distant Metastasis in Laryngeal Squamous Cell Carcinoma. *Journal of Clinical Otorhinolaryngology, Head, and Neck Surgery*, **26**, 989-992.

[75] Ogretmen, B. and Hannun, Y.A. (2004) Biologically Active Sphingolipids in Cancer Pathogenesis and Treatment. *Nature Reviews Cancer*, **4**, 604-616. http://dx.doi.org/10.1038/nrc1411

[76] Koybasi, S., Senkal, C.E., Sundararaj, K., Spassieva, S., Bielawski, J., Osta, W., *et al.* (2004) Defects in Cell Growth Regulation by C18:0-Ceramide and Longevity Assurance Gene 1 in Human Head and Neck Squamous Cell Carcinomas. *The Journal of Biological Chemistry*, **279**, 44311-44319. http://dx.doi.org/10.1074/jbc.M406920200

[77] Senkal, C.E., Ponnusamy, S., Rossi, M.J., Bialewski, J., Sinha, D., Jiang, J.C., *et al.* (2007) Role of Human Longevity Assurance Gene 1 and C_{18}-Ceramide in Chemotherapy-Induced Cell Death in Human Head and Neck Squamous Cell Carcinomas. *Molecular Cancer Therapeutics*, **6**, 712-722. http://dx.doi.org/10.1158/1535-7163.MCT-06-0558

[78] Issaq, H.J., Waybright, T.J. and Veenstra, T.D. (2011) Cancer Biomarker Discovery: Opportunities and Pitfalls in Analytical Methods. *Electrophoresis*, **32**, 967-975. http://dx.doi.org/10.1002/elps.201000588

29

Primary Tuberculosis of Tonsil in a Diabetic Patient—A Case Report

Nagula Parusharam[1], Kamreddy Ashok Reddy[1], Lokesh Rao Magar[2], Jadi Lingaiah[3]

[1]Department of E.N.T., Kakatiya Medical College, MGM Hospital, Warangal, India
[2]Department of Pathology, Kakatiya Medical College, MGM Hospital, Warangal, India
[3]Department of ENT & HNS, Chalmeda Anand Rao Institute of Medical Sciences, Karimnagar, India
Email: parashuramnagula@gmail.com, drjadi_ms@yahoo.com

Abstract

Though Tuberculosis is one of the most common causes of ill health and death worldwide, people with diabetes have 2 - 3 times higher risk of tuberculosis when compared with people without diabetes. Though tuberculosis can affect any part of the body, oral and oropharyngeal tuberculosis is rare, but reported. And it's association with diabetes mellitus because of the decreased host mechanism, is still rare, but reported. A 50-year-old female diabetic who was on insulin therapy came to OPD of MGM hospital, Kakatiya Medical College, Warangal with complaints of severe pain in throat for the last 6 months. On examination, right tonsil was enlarged with granular surface. Left tonsil and rest of the oropharynx were normal. Examination of chest was normal and there was no evidence of pulmonary tuberculosis. Punch biopsy revealed tuberculosis of tonsil. Isolated cases of primary tuberculosis of tonsil without evidence of pulmonary tuberculosis are rare. Presence of diabetes mellitus makes patients 2 - 3 times more vulnerable for tubercular infection.

Keywords

Tonsil, Primary Tuberculosis, Diabetes Mellitus

1. Introduction

Pulmonary tuberculosis (TB) is a common disease in India and also worldwide, but it is very rarely seen in oral cavity and orpharynx as primary tuberculosis. Isolated tuberculosis of tonsil without pulmonary involvement is a rare entity [1]. Nowadays, diabetes mellitus (DM) is also common in most parts of the world. Tuberculosis is 2 - 3 times more common in diabetes mellitus [2]. Non healing ulcer commonly points towards malignancy. In a non healing ulcer, if malignancy is not likely, then the most common differential diagnosis will be chronic granulomatous condition, of which TB is more common. After taking the consent from the patient to publish, we report such a case of primary tuberculosis of tonsil in a diabetic patient, mimicking ulcerated growth of tonsil.

2. Mini Literature Review

Both diabetes and tuberculosis are well recognized for their huge global burdens. Nearly one third of the world's population is infected with *M. tuberculosis* and about 10% is at risk of developing an active disease in their lifetime. At the same time, prevalence of diabetes is increasing alongside other noncommunicable diseases [3]. There are numerous studies from different regions of the world supporting this.

A country with one of the largest number of TB cases is India. In this highly endemic country, over 25% of TB patients were found to have diabetes and 24% pre-diabetes [4]. Altogether almost 50% of TB patients had some form of hyperglycemia. The risk factors for diabetes were similar to those in the general population such as increasing age, body mass index (BMI) category (18.5 - 22.9 kg/m^2), positive family history and sedentary occupation. Of interest, among TB patients with diabetes, almost 60% had been diagnosed with diabetes before. It is most likely that long-term diabetes has a negative effect on the immune response and may enhance TB morbidity. In another study from India, the number of TB patients needed to screen (NNS) to find one newly diagnosed diabetic case was 4 [5]. It was confirmed that nearly half of TB patients had diabetes, which was independently associated with male sex and age above 50 years. In another retrospective study from India, diabetes was found as the most frequent risk factor for pulmonary tuberculosis, far more common (30.9%) than classic risk factors for TB such as smoking (16.9%), alcoholism (12.6%), human immunodeficiency virus (HIV) (10.6%), malignancy (5.8%) as well as history of contact with TB (3.4%) and chronic corticosteroid therapy (2.9%) [6]. The strength of DM as a risk factor for TB appears to be equivalent to that of HIV infection. In a case-control study conducted in California, Pablos-Méndez *et al.* found that among Hispanics aged 25 - 54 the estimated risk due to DM was 25.2% whereas that due to HIV infection was 25.5% [7]. Higher risk for TB among diabetic patients was also confirmed in a Mexican study (prevalence of DM among TB patients: 39% in Texas and 36% in Mexico) [8]. Namely, diabetes contributed to TB five times more often than HIV infection (25% vs. 5%). It could be stated that the risk of TB due to DM seems to be smaller at the individual level compared with that of HIV infection (113-170-fold) [9]. However, it can also be said that at the population level the sheer numbers of diabetic patients are likely to have an equal or even greater effect. What is more, established risk factors for TB such as alcohol and drug abuse as well as HIV infection were found less frequently in the diabetic group [8] [10].

3. Case Report

A 50-year-old female of Asian race who was on treatment for Diabetes Mellitus came to OPD of Mahatma Gandhi Memorial Hospital, Kakatiya Medical College, Warangal, India with pain in throat and pain on swallowing. She also complained of ulcer in the throat for the past 6 months. There was no history of fever or cough. On examination right tonsil was enlarged (grade 3) and surface was granular in appearance (**Figure 1(a)** and **Figure 1(b)**). There were no acute signs of inflammation. Anterior and posterior pillars were normal. Left tonsil was normal. Posterior pharyngeal wall was normal. Indirect laryngoscopy was normal. There was no evidence of cervical lymphadenopathy. No history of weight loss. And family history was nil particular. And there was no history of milk intake as regular diet. On auscultation Lungs were clear.

4. Investigations

Routine investigations showed Hb%-12 gm%, TLC-10 500/mm^3, N-69%, L-25%, E-04%, M-02%, B-00%. RBC count-4 million/mm^3, ESR-90 mm 1st Hour, RBS-130 mg/dl. Complete Urine Examination-Normal, Blood Urea 27 mg%, S. Creatine 1 mg%, Mantoux Test-17 mm Positive after 48 Hrs. HIV 1 and 2-Negative and HBsAg-Negative, Chest X-Ray-Normal (**Figure 2**). Punch biopsy done under local anaesthesia and sent for histopathological examination. Histopathological examination reported as multiple sections studied shows structure of lymphoid tissue with marked number of lymphocytic infiltration, few granulomas noticed. Each granuloma consists of central caseous necrosis surrounded by epithelioid layer, lymphocytic layer, few Langhan's giant cells surrounded by a layer of fibroblasts, features suggestive of chronic inflammatory pathology *i.e.* chronic tuberculous

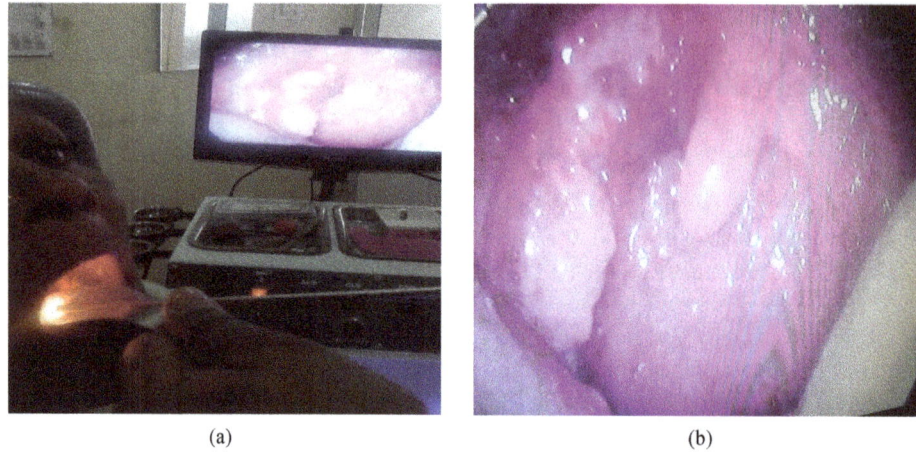

(a)   (b)

Figure 1. Endoscopic view of enlarged right tonsil with pale granular appearance.

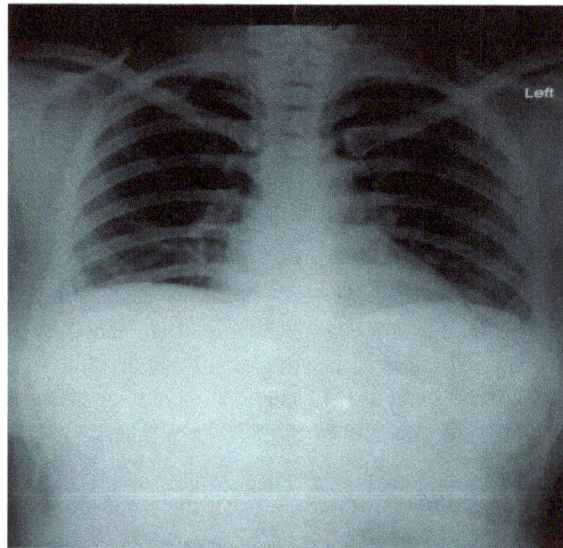

Figure 2. Normal X-ray chest.

tonsillitis (**Figure 3** and **Figure 4**).

Patient was started on Anti Tuberculous Treatment (ATT) with 4 drug regimen consisting of ETHAMBUTOL-500 mg + ISONIAZIDE-300 mg + PYRAZINAMIDE-750 mg + RIFAMPICICIN-450 mg for 2 months and ISONIAZIDE and RIFAMPICIN for 4 months. Patient responded well to the antituberculous treatment with tonsillar surface becoming normal without any granular appearance and symptoms disappeared completely after six months (**Figure 5**).

5. Discussion

Tuberculosis in humans is caused by mycobacterium tuberculosis and mycobacterium bovis. Though Tuberculosis can affect any part or organ of the body, pulmonary tuberculosis is most common which is about 75% of the cases, extra pulmonary tuberculosis being remaining 25% of overall morbidity of tuberculosis [11]. Among extra pulmonary tuberculosis, most commonly involved are lymph nodes. Other forms of extra pulmonary tuberculosis are like CNS, Genito urinary, abdominal, pericarditis, etc. Tuberculosis of oral cavity and tonsil is rare and usually secondary to pulmonary tuberculosis [12]. Primary tuberculosis affecting palatine tonsil is still extremely rare [13]. People with weak immune system as a result of chronic diseases such as diabetes mellitus and HIV are at high risk. People with diabetes mellitus have 2 - 3 times higher risk of tuberculosis when compared

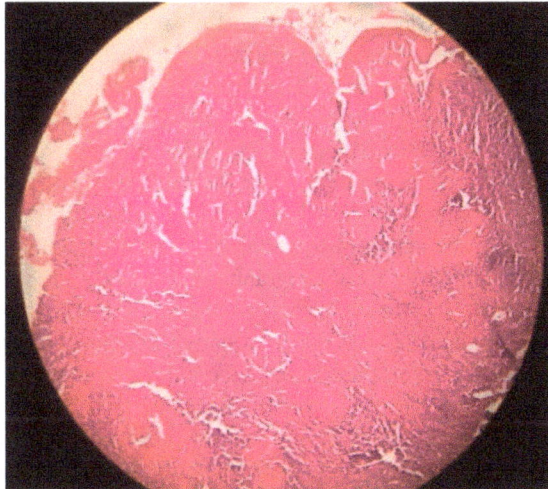

Figure 3. Microscopic appearance (4×).

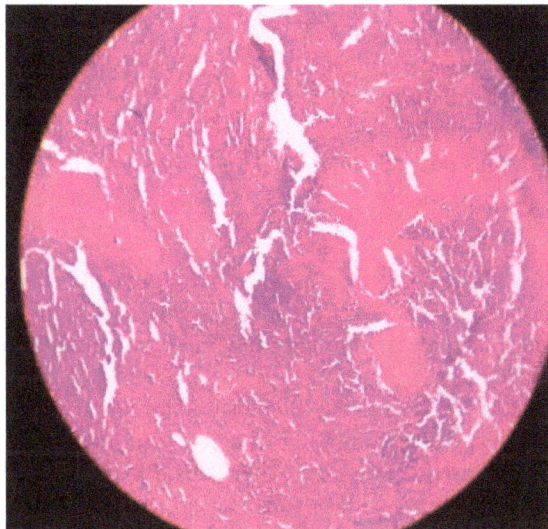

Figure 4. Microscopic appearance (20×).

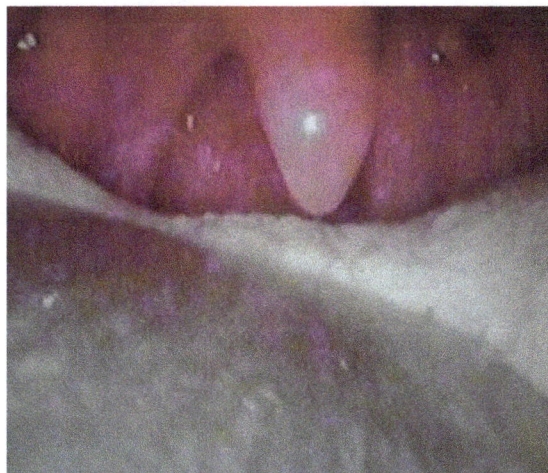

Figure 5. After 6 months of treatment right tonsil became normal. No granular surface.

to people without diabetes mellitus. About 10% of tuberculosis cases globally are linked to diabetes mellitus [2].

Oral and oropharyngeal tuberculosis is uncommon, may be primary or secondary. Incidence of tonsillar tuberculosis is less than 5% [14]. Tonsil may be primarily infected by contamination with material containing tubercle bacilli. These patients commonly present with sore throat. With availability of pasteurized milk, the incidence of TB has decreased as concluded by Miller in 1963 [15].

Tuberculosis of the tonsil is a rare disease because of the salivary act of antiseptic cleaning-mechanism [16] and epithelial covering of oropharyngeal mucosa has inhibitory effect on tubercule bacilli [17]. It has been documented that such infection may be acquired by inhalation and disease may be harboured in waldeyers ring [18]. Although tuberculosis tonsil is rare, tonsillar granulomata are commonly seen in patients with decreased immunity due to diabetes mellitus, HIV or chronic alcoholism. This patient was diabetic initially on oral anti-diabetic drugs but was not under control. Then she was started Insulin to bring her diabetes under control. Predisposing factors for primary oral and oropharyngeal tuberculosis are poor dental hygiene, periodontitis, leukoplakia. But this present case does not have these as predisposing factors.

Malignancy, syphilis, lymhpoma, taumatic ulcer, haematological disorders and other granulomatous conditions are differential diagnosis [19]. Arbols indicators [14] may help to think about this entity.

Arbols indicators are:

a) Pain on swallowing;

b) Obliteration of crypts;

c) Tonsillar enlargement without exudates;

d) Granular enlargement of tonsil.

The diagnosis is based on histopathological findings of tubercular Langhan's giant cells in a tonsillar tissue.

This case highlights the importance of being aware of association TB and DM the possibility of TB ulcer should be kept in mind in case of a non healing, non malignant looking ulcer in a diabetic patient.

6. Conclusions

It is concluded that tonsillar tuberculosis still exists and may be a diagnostic challenge to otolaryngologists. Tuberculosis of Tonsil is suspected in a patient if the tonsil is enlarged, with rough and granular surface with or without cervical lymph node enlargement, who is complaining of pain in throat and pain on swallowing. And more so if patient is also a diabetic.

In this case, only right tonsil is enlarged, the left tonsil being normal and there is no evidence of cervical lymph node enlargement, proper investigations and biopsy can confirm the diagnosis. Early detection and treatment are essential for cure. Decreased host immune mechanism like diabetes mellitus can predispose to tubercular infection and tonsillar granulomata with or without cervical lymphnode enlargement. Isolated unilateral tubercular infection of the tonsil without cervical lymphnode in a diabetic patient is rare, which encouraged us to report this case.

References

[1]   Kant, S., Verma, S.K. and Sanjay (2008) Isolated Tonsil Tuberculosis. *Lung India*, 25, 163-164.
       http://dx.doi.org/10.4103/0970-2113.45284

[2]   WHO (2011) www.who.int/tb/publications/2011

[3]   Skowroński, M., Zozulińska-Ziółkiewicz, D. and Barinow-Wojewódzki, A. (2014) Tuberculosis and Diabetes Mellitus—An Underappreciated Association. *Archives of Medical Science*, 10, 1019-1027.
       http://dx.doi.org/10.5114/aoms.2014.46220

[4]   Viswanathan, V., Kumpatla, S., Aravindalochanan, V., *et al.* (2012) Prevalence of Diabetes and Pre-Diabetes and Associated Risk Factors among Tuberculosis Patients in India. *PLoS ONE*, 7, e41367.
       http://dx.doi.org/10.1371/journal.pone.0041367

[5]   Balakrishnan, S., Vijayan, S., Nair, S., *et al.* (2012) High Diabetes Prevalence among Tuberculosis Cases in Kerala, India. *PLoS ONE*, 7, e46502. http://dx.doi.org/10.1371/journal.pone.0046502

[6]   Gupta, S., Shenoy, V., Mukhopadhyay, C., Bairy, I. and Muralidharan, S. (2011) Role of Risk Factors and Socio-Economic Status in Pulmonary Tuberculosis: A Search for the Root Cause in Patients in a Tertiary Care Hospital, South India. *Tropical Medicine & International Health*, 16, 74-78. http://dx.doi.org/10.1111/j.1365-3156.2010.02676.x

[7]   Pablos-Méndez, A., Blustein, J. and Knirsch, C. (1997) The Role of Diabetes Mellitus in the Higher Prevalence of Tu-

berculosis among Hispanics. *American Journal of Public Health*, **87**, 574-579.

[8]   Restrepo, B., Camerlin, A., Rahbar, M., *et al.* (2011) Cross-Sectional Assessment Reveals High Diabetes Prevalence among Newly-Diagnosed Tuberculosis Cases. *Bulletin of the World Health Organization*, **89**, 352-359. http://dx.doi.org/10.2471/BLT.10.085738

[9]   Corbett, E., Watt, C., Walker, N., *et al.* (2003) The Growing Burden of Tuberculosis: Global Trends and Interactions with the HIV Epidemic. *JAMA Internal Medicine*, **169**, 1009-1021. http://dx.doi.org/10.1001/archinte.163.9.1009

[10]   Restrepo, B., Fisher-Hoch, S., Smith, B., Jeon, S., Rahbar, M. and McCormick, J. (2008) Short Report: Mycobacterial Clearance from Sputum Is Delayed during the First Phase of Treatment in Patients with Diabetes. *The American Journal of Tropical Medicine and Hygiene*, **79**, 541-544.

[11]   Farer, L.S., Lowell, A.M. and Meader, M.P. (1992) Extra Pulmonary Tuberculosis in USA. *American Journal of Epidemiology*, **109**, 205-217.

[12]   Lathan, S.R. (1971) Tuberculosis of the Palate. *Journal of the American Medical Association*, **216**, 521. http://dx.doi.org/10.1001/jama.1971.03180290095030

[13]   Cleary, K. and Batsakis, J.G. (1955) Mycobacterial Disease of the Head and Neck: Current Perspective. *Annals of Otology: Rhinology and Laryngology*, **104**, 830-833. http://dx.doi.org/10.1177/000348949510401015

[14]   Balasubramanian, T. (2012) Tonsillar Tuberculosis: A Literature Review. Otolaryngology Online.

[15]   Miller, F.J., Seal, W. and Taylor, M.D. (1963) Tuberculosis in Children. J & A Churchill Ltd., London.

[16]   Verma, A., Mann, S.B.S. and Randotra, B. (1989) Primary Tuberculosis of the Tongue. *Ear, Nose and Throat Journal*, **68**, 719-720.

[17]   Rauch, D.M. and Freidman, E. (1978) Systemic Tuberculosis Initially Seen as an Oral Ulceration: Report of a Case. *Journal of Oral Surgery*, **36**, 384-389.

[18]   Selimoğlu, E., Sütbeyaz, Y., Çiftçioğlu, M.A., Parlak, M., Esrefoğlu, M. and Öztürk, A. (1995) Primary tonsillar tuberculosis: a case report. *The Journal of Laryngology & Otology*, **109**, 880-882. http://dx.doi.org/10.1017/S0022215100131573

[19]   Adiego, M.I., Millán, J., Royo, J., Dománguez, L., Castellote, M.A., Alfonso, J.I. and Vallés, H. (1994) Unusual Association of Secondary Tonsillar and Cerebral Tuberculosis. *Journal of Laryngology and Orology*, **108**, 348-349. http://dx.doi.org/10.1017/S0022215100126738

30

Tessier 30 Facial Cleft Associated with Complete Duplication of Tongue: A Rare Entity

Jayanto Tapadar[1], Preeti Tiwari[2*]

[1]Plastic Surgery, Smayan Hospital, Varanasi, India
[2]Trauma Centre, Institute of Medical Sciences, Banaras Hindu University, Varanasi, India
Email: tapadarjk@hotmail.com, *drtiwaripreeti@gmail.com

Abstract

Background: Median cleft of mandible and lower lip is a rare anomaly [1]. Only a few cases have been reported in literature with different variations till now. Herein we report a patient with Tessier 30 cleft associated with complete duplication of tongue. Aim: We herein report this rare variant as it posed special challenges for its management by virtue of its uniqueness, late presentation and limited affordability of patient for standard treatment. Case Report: A 12 years old female reported to us with a chief complaint of a midline gap in the lower lip and mandible since birth. On examination under anaesthesia, we found that tongue was not bifid. There was complete duplication of the tongue. The case was planned for staged repair of the defect. In the same sitting, a repair of the soft tissues in the midline was performed. Conclusion: There are no specific guidelines in literature for management of such cases. This makes all these cases worth for reporting in order to guide treating surgeons.

Keywords

Facial Cleft, Duplication of Tongue, Tessier 30 Cleft, Bifid Tongue

1. Introduction

Median cleft of mandible and lower lip is a rare anomaly [1]. Tessier published a detailed description of the classification of craniofacial clefts in 1976 [2]. Often serious asymmetry exists and multiple areas of the face are affected simultaneous. Further there is a continued restricted growth of affected tissues after birth. Because of this, the deformities at birth can become more obvious over the years. This results in a clear three-dimensional

---

*Corresponding author.

underdevelopment of hard and soft tissues of the orbit, maxilla, zygoma, nose and malar region. Couronne in 1819, first reported a case of midline mandibular cleft. Since then 66 cases have been reported worldwide till 2007 [3]. Only a few cases have been reported in literature with different variations till now. Herein we report a patient with Tessier 30 cleft associated with complete duplication of tongue.

2. Case Report

A 12 years old female reported to us with a chief complaint of a midline gap in the lower lip and mandible since birth (**Figure 1**). The child was psychologically depressed due to his appearance. The child was born as the first child to unrelated healthy parents at term by spontaneous vaginal delivery. There was no history of any relevant abnormalities in the family. His medical history was unremarkable, and she appeared as a healthy young girl of normal intelligence & neurocognitive development. On examination there was a midline cleft of mandible and lower lip. Further this was associated with bifid tongue. Orthopentomogram showed a bony defect in the midline of the mandible. Complete blood count and other haematological parameters were normal. After fitness for anaesthesia the patient was taken for examination under general anaesthesia. On examination under anaesthesia, we found that tongue was not bifid. There was complete duplication of the tongue (**Figure 2**). The case was planned for staged repair of the defect. In the same sitting a repair of the soft tissues in the midline was performed (**Figure 3** and **Figure 4**). No attempt was made to reconstruct the lower lip and tongue at this stage. The patient is currently being followed-up for assessment of the mandibular growth and midline union, assessment of dentition and planned for further management with secondary repair of the lower lip and repair of the duplicated tongue at a later stage.

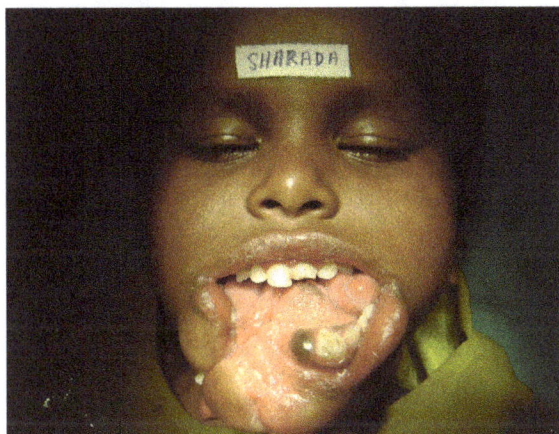

Figure 1. Tessier 30 cleft.

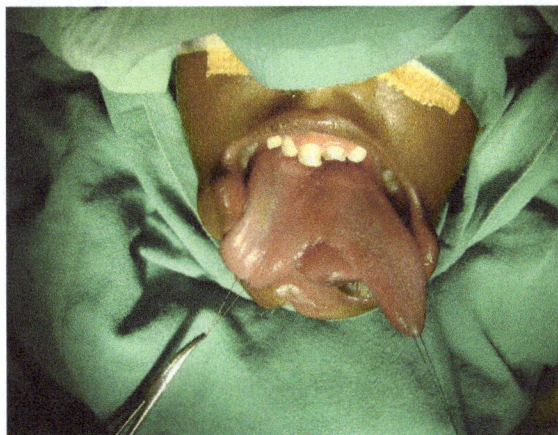

Figure 2. Examination under anesthesia showing complete duplication of tongue.

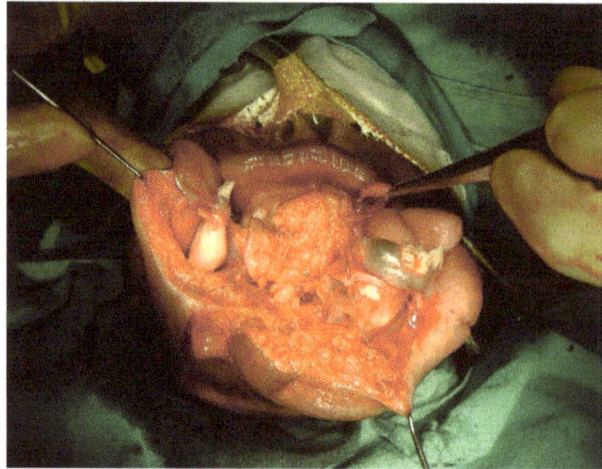

Figure 3. Intraop image of closure of cleft.

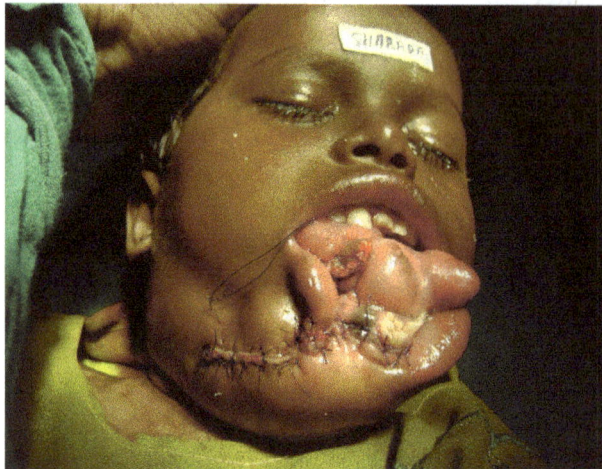

Figure 4. Immediate post op image after first stage of closure.

3. Discussion

Midline facial clefts are extremely rare congenital deformities. Their precise incidence in the population is unknown with reported incidence of [1]. Tessier described an anatomical classification system, in which number is assigned to each craniofacial cleft on the basis of its position relative to sagittal midline & the orbit [2]. The first report of midline mandibular cleft was reported by Couronne in 1819, since then 66 cases have been reported worldwide till 2007 [3]. The extent of cleft is variable and extent is variable. In the more severe forms, it may extend into the bony mandibular symphysis. In some cases, the neck structures like the hyoid bone, thyroid cartilage and even the strap muscles of the front of the neck may be involved. The anterior portion of the tongue may be bifid [4]. The extent of bifid tongue is also variable and is usually associated with ankyloglossia [5] [6]. The etiopathogenesis of atypical craniofacial clefts is still unclear. Typical cleft lip and palate result from a failure of union of the frontonasal process with the lateral maxillary prominences at about 3 - 5 weeks of gestation. Theories regarding the pathogenesis of these clefts include the failure in mesodermal migration and disruption of neural crest cell development along normal fusion planes in the developing facial skeleton. CT scans with three-dimensional reconstruction on the visible components of craniofacial clefts do not necessarily reflect the true extent of the cleft [6] [7]. The actual timing of corrections is often based on severity and nature of the deformity with consideration of functional problems, growth, and mental burden for the patient and wishes of patients and/or parents. However, previous conducted studies show that the intensity of the psychological burden for patients caused by the deformity is not directly related to the severity of the deformity. The case reported here had midline cleft of the lower lip with cleft of the mandible, associated with complete duplication of the tongue. There was no ankyloglossia and structures were completely duplicated upto posterior part. Although Britto *et al.* reported a case of double tongue with cleft palate, there has been no case report with Tessier 30 cleft with complete duplication of the tongue [7]. The case was taken up for staged repair. In the first stage, the two halves of the mandible were approximated. The treatment, as advocated by Armstrong and Waterhouse [8] is to tackle the condition in a staged manner. In the first stage, soft tissue correction including Z-plasty in chin, lip and neck is performed. In our case repair was performed after extensive midline mobilisation of soft tissues. Secondary repair of the lower lip to improve the cosmetic appearance and fusion of the two halves of the tongue will be taken up at subsequent stages.

Mandible reconstruction is done after 10 years of age to minimize damage to the developing tooth buds. However, earlier treatment may be indicated when the segments are hypermobile, causing respiratory or feeding difficulty [8].

4. Conclusion

The findings of this report demonstrate that this rare variant poses special challenges for its management by virtue of its uniqueness, late presentation and limited affordability of patient for standard treatment. There are no specific guidelines in literature for management of such cases. This makes all these cases worth for reporting in order to guide treating surgeons.

References

[1]   Kawamoto Jr., H.K. (1990) Rare Craniofacial Clefts. In: McCarthy, J.G., Ed., *Plastic Surgery*, Vol. 4, W.B. Saunders, Philadelphia, 2940.

[2]   Tessier, P. (1976) Anatomical Classification of Facial, Cranio-Facial and Latero-Facial Clefts. *Journal of Maxillofacial Surgery*, **4**, 69-70. http://dx.doi.org/10.1016/S0301-0503(76)80013-6

[3]   Senan, M., Padmakumar, G. and Jisha, K.T. (2007) Tessier Number 30. *Indian Journal of Plastic Surgery*, **40**, 57-60. http://dx.doi.org/10.4103/0970-0358.32666

[4]   Oostrom, C.A., Vermeij-Keers, C., Gilbert, P.M. and Van Der Meulen, J.C. (1996) Median Cleft of Lower Lip and Mandible: Case Reports, a New Embryologic Hypothesis and Subdivision. *Plastic & Reconstructive Surgery*, **97**, 313-320. http://dx.doi.org/10.1097/00006534-199602000-00006

[5]   Chidzonga, M.M., Lopez Perez, V.M. and Mzezewa, S. (1996) Treatment of Median Cleft of the Lower Lip, Mandible, and Bifid Tongue with Ankyloglossia: A Case Report. *International Journal of Oral and Maxillofacial Surgery*, **25**, 272-273. http://dx.doi.org/10.1016/S0901-5027(06)80054-8

[6]   Tiwari, V.K. (2000) Median Cleft of Lower Lip and Mandible: A Case Report. *Indian Journal of Plastic Surgery*, **33**, 98-100.

[7]   Britto, J.A., Ragoowansi, R.H. and Sommerlad, B.C. (2000) Double Tongue, Intraoral Anomalies and Cleft Palate—Case Reports and a Discussion of Developmental Pathology. *Cleft Palate-Craniofacial Journal*, **37**, 410-415. http://dx.doi.org/10.1597/1545-1569(2000)037<0410:DTIAAC>2.3.CO;2

[8]   Armstrong, A. and Waterhouse, N. (1996) Tessier 30 Median Mandibular Cleft: Case Report and Literature Review. *British Journal of Plastic Surgery*, **49**, 536-538. http://dx.doi.org/10.1016/S0007-1226(96)90130-7

31

Association between Hearing Loss and Vestibular Disorders: A Review of the Interference of Hearing in the Balance

Tatiana G. T. Santos[1], Alessandra Ramos Venosa[2], Andre Luiz Lopes Sampaio[2]

[1]University of Catholic Medical School, Brasilia, Brazil
[2]Department of Otolaryngology, University Hospital of Brasilia, Brasilia, Brazil
Email: tatiguthierre@hotmail.com

Abstract

Introduction: Dizziness is very prevalent and makes a great impact on people's life. Because of anatomical and functional similarities of hearing and vestibular systems, it is noted that there is a big relation between hearing loss and vestibular disorders. Depending on the age onset of hearing loss, it can cause even delay on motor development. Objective: To find literature that demonstrates the relation between hearing and balance. Confirming that hearing loss or even intervention to improve quality of hearing can interfere on vestibular system. Methodology: Revision of literature was carried out, preferring recent research only in English. Conclusion: Cochlea and vestibular systems have a close relationship; changes in one of them can cause big damage in the other. So, a complete evaluation of vestibular system is recommended before ear surgeries. Video Head Impulse Test is a new procedure able to evaluate high frequency movements of the head. It was an additional exam of vestibular status and came to help detect problems that were not diagnosed before. Efforts must be directed in order to protect the balance.

Keywords

Hearing Loss, Cochlear Implant, Vestibular Disorders, Dizziness and Vertigo

1. Introduction

Dizziness is among the most frequent symptoms in emergency room patients as demonstrated by Royl *et al.* in 2011 [1]. The management must be fast and effective due to similarities to central causes and to the great discomfort it causes to the patients. To make it possible, diagnostic tests must evolve.

The American Speech-Language-Hearing Association reports that the percentage of newborns with permanent hearing loss at birth is about 3% and that the number increases to 6% by the time children get old [2]. Almost 70% of children presenting with sensorineural hearing loss (SNHL) have vestibular system disturb, with 20% - 40% having severe bilateral vestibular loss. This population must be rehabilitated early in order to avoid motor and cognitional delayed development.

There are many causes of vestibular disorders. In this article, we will discuss about vestibular disorders related to: congenital hearing loss, age and surgical manipulation of the inner ear.

In adults, intervention must be quick to decrease long-term damages of auditory system and avoid interruption of their daily activities, increasing the patients' social interaction. The longer the time of hearing loss is, the higher the social impact of dizziness on the social life is. It can make patients change or quit work, reduce efficiency at work, disrupt in their social life, and suffer family difficulties, difficulties in travel, depression distress and anxiety, as reported by Beck in 2013 [3]. Seven years before Enticott had said that older patients seemed more susceptible to permanent injury after cochlear implantation surgery and it must be a great point of interest as the number of these patients submitted to that surgery was growing [4]. That group must be very well investigated previously the CI and followed after surgery as the electrical stimulation in that area can damage the vestibular system.

Although auditory and vestibular systems being distinct, they work just alike. So, there is a great relation among their functions. Once one is stimulated, the other suffers alteration as well.

2. Methodology

Revision of literature using Pubmed, Scopus and Web of Science and the keywords: hearing loss, cochlear implant, vestibular disorders, dizziness and vertigo. It was used only papers in English. It was selected 26 articles.

3. Results

There is a great association between vestibular and balance disorders with SNHL; however, most professionals do not routinely investigate for vestibular dysfunction among children with SNHL. The prevalence of vestibular and balance disorders in children is frequently underestimated, and it may range up to 15%. Estimates indicate that almost 70% of children presenting with SNHL have vestibular system disturb, with 20% - 40% having severe bilateral vestibular loss. This population will often have delayed motor development. They may evolve delayed development demonstrating poor head control beyond 6 weeks, delayed independent sitting beyond 9 months, and/or delayed walking beyond 18 months. If the clinician who examines those children inquires about motor milestones in case of presenting SNHL may do it correctly when, indeed, there is a true cause for concern, since SNHL relates to vestibular disturbs, that can cause motor delayed development [2].

Many identifiable etiologies of hearing loss have well-described associated vestibular impairments. They are in complete partition (type 1 to type 3), enlarged vestibular aqueduct syndrome, Usher Syndrome (the most important genetic diagnosis associated with vestibular impairment), meningitis, congenital CMV infection and children treated with ototoxic agents, such as aminoglycosides and chemotherapeutics. These children may present vestibular impairment progressive in nature, similar to the hearing loss. When progressive vestibular impairment occurs, these children may evolve with true vertigo, which can be severe and may last days or weeks. Vestibular impairment may occur associated with progression of hearing loss or independent of changes in hearing [2]. There is a suspicion that many of the children with cochlear nerve deficiency will also grow up with vestibular impairment on the ipsilateral side, and that is because of the relationship between auditory and vestibular systems [2]. Another study reveals that in the beginning of development, children depend on the visual system to maintain balance. Inoue et al. in 2013 evaluated that as they grow older, they progressively begin to use somatosensory and vestibular information until these systems reach full maturity around the age of 10 years. Children with profound hearing loss have dysfunction of the inferior as well as the superior vestibular nerve system and they show delayed acquisition of gross motor function [5].

In the same year, Cushing et al. said that children with SNHL may demonstrate associated vestibular impairment due to peripheral auditory and vestibular systems similarities. In a prospective and cross-sectional study were tested caloric, rotational stimuli responses of Horizontal canal and VEMP. One hundred fifty-three children with profound SNHL were tested; 119 had unilateral CI at time of testing, and 34 had no CI at the time of testing. Half of all children with profound SNHL presented vestibular end organ dysfunction. One third of the subjects displayed severe abnormalities. Vestibular end-organ dysfunction has great relation with etiology, meningitis and cochleovestibular anomalies have the highest rates of severe dysfunction. The ability to identify vestibular dysfunction in children with SNHL is very important because it allows prognostication of motor abilities and implementation of early therapy [6].

Ciuman made a review in 2011 describing that there are approximately 50 - 80 stereocillia and one kinocilium per vestibular hair cell. In contrast to vestibular system, the cochleacells does not have the kinocilium. The Glycocalyx and many others links keep all cells connected in both systems, despite of having different functions [7].

The auditory neuropathy is a disorder characterized by absent orseverely abnormal auditory brainstem responses withintact outer hair cell function, as seem in evoked otoacoustic emissions (OAE) and/or cochlearmicrophonics. Its etiology is multifactorial. The vestibular branch of the vestibulocochlear nerve, including the superior and the inferior vestibular nerves, is involved in maintaining a sense of equilibrium. The superior vestibular nerve and the semicircular canals can be assessed using electronystagmography (ENG): the inferior vestibular nerve and the saccule by the vestibular-evoked myogenic potentials. Sinha *et al.* two years later reviewed that the neuropathic condition in individuals with auditory neuropathy may additionally involve the vestibular nerve, and in most cases, the pathology is restricted to the peripheral vestibular system and does not affect the central oculomotor system [8].

Fujimoto *et al.* in 2014 published that approximately 40% of patients with idiopathic sudden hearing loss (ISHL) also suffer from vestibular symptoms which may occur at the onset of hearing loss or be delayed for hours or even days. Vertigo is more frequent in association with profound hearing loss and the recovery of hearing is worse in patients with vertigo than those without vertigo. The percentage of abnormal responses in patients with ISHL with vertigo was higher in the cVEMP test, followed by the oVEMP and caloric tests. These results suggest that the vestibular end organs closest to the cochlea tend to be preferentially affected in ISHL with vertigo [9].

Cochlear implant recipients usually complain of postoperative symptoms of dizziness. Although the auditory and vestibular systems are clearly distinct from one another, the mechanisms of neural transmission are identical. For this reason, the electrical stimulation through the cochlear implant may have an effect both on the auditory and vestibular systems. In a research it was described that 18% of 55 cochlear implant recipients saw connection between dizziness and the activation of the cochlear Implant. This gave grounds for supposing that the electricity spreads diffusely and could therefore stimulate the nerve endings of the vestibular nerve. Schwab *et al.* in 2010 found postoperatively that 33 patients (66%) had no vestibular symptoms, whereas 17 (34%) reported temporary symptoms of dizziness. Of these, eight patients (16%) had showed corresponding symptoms prior to surgery. Only a small percentage complained of sensations as paresthesia and irritation of the facial nerve during the activation of the cochlear implant [10].

Although this surgery is considered to be safe, balance disorder is a very frequent postoperative complaint in cochlear recipients. In 2013, Katsiari *et al* found that about one-third of them could experience a significant vestibular disturbance after surgery, independently of age, cause, or preoperative caloric result. Even cochlear implantation leading to measurable changes of the peripheral vestibular function, permanent vertigo is rare. Different etiologies can cause vertigo after the surgery: perilymphatic fistula induced by cochlear fenestration or a disruption of endolymphatic flow caused by the electrode itself, mechanical irritation of the membranous labyrinth or thelabyrinthitis triggered by aforeign body in the cochlea. Histopathological studies on temporal bones implanted have shown that cochlear implantation can damage the vestibular end organ. In summary, it is clear that electrical stimulation affect vestibular system function [10] [11].

Hui-Chi Tien *et al.* in 2002 evaluated that the overall incidence of vestibular end-organ damage after cochlear implantation was 54.5%, a higher estimative considering the literature based on history and/or functional tests. It must be considered the possibility of vestibular malfunction becaused by disease processes long before surgery. However, it can be consequence of trauma, associated infection, interruption of the endolymphatic system, hemorrhage, or vascular changes produced by insertion of implant electrodes. The saccule is the most frequent site of damage in the vestibular system, followed by the utricle and semicircular canals. It is safer to keep the electrode array in the scala tympani in order to minimize further vestibular damage. As the clinical incidence of balance disturbances after cochlear implantation is low, it demonstrates that damage of vestibular organs may occur and be asymptomatic [12].

During cochlear implant surgery planning, many items are considerate, one of which is the ear with poorer vestibular function. This requisite is important and normally selected as the site for implantation since surgery carries a low risk of iatrogenic labyrinthine injury. Hugh *et al.* in 2011 created an algorithm to help determine reasons to the choice of the better balance ear to implant. Reasons were divided into four categories: anatomical contraindications, attempting to attain binaural hearing, avoiding implantation of an ear with marked auditory deprivation, and patient preference. More studies are recommended and validation of that algorithm must be developed [13].

The study of incidence of vestibular dysfunction after cochlear implantation as well as its reasons is a big point of interest. It could help us to give better preoperative counseling and postoperative vestibular therapy to cochlear implant patients. Enticott *et al.* conducted a group in 2006 analyzing postoperative vestibular disturbance, defined as symptoms lasting for 1 week or longer after surgery [4]. The data in preoperative and postoperative vestibular function were measured from subjective assessments (Dizziness Handicap Inventory and Activity Balance Confidence questionnaires) and objective assessments (bithermal caloric tests). The information of the postoperative position of electrode was also classified as "loose", "regular", or "tight" fitting. About one third of patients reported vestibular disturbance, presenting poorer DHI, Activity Balance Confidence, and caloric results in the implanted ear after surgery. It seems that age, cause of hearing loss, and preoperative caloric result did not predict postoperative vestibular symptoms. Older patients had significantly poorer caloric results on the implanted side after surgery and that was not related to the intracochlear electrodes position or surgeons. They seem more susceptible to permanent injury after cochlear implantation (CI) surgery [7]. The number of adults who are potential candidates for cochlear implantation in the world is high and continue to increase. In research by Lin *et al.* in 2012 there is a negative association between the magnitude of the gain in speech scores and age at implantation, such that for every increasing year of age at CI the gain in speech scores was 1.3 percentage points less after adjusting for age at hearing loss onset. Individuals with higher pre-CI speech scores had significantly greater post-CI than those with lower pre-CI speech scores after adjusting for age at CI and age at hearing loss onset. In the future, research of CI in older patients should expand its evaluations to take into account the broad cognitive, social and physical outcomes that are likely detrimentally impacted by hearing loss [14].

Fina *et al.* in 2003 reported a group of 39% (29/75) of subjects with implants that were dizzy after implantation. It was more common in older patients, individuals with previous dizziness history, and those older at onset of the hearing loss. The majority of subjects experienced dizziness in a delayed episodic fashion. Dizziness had no relation to implant activation. There are some subjects characteristics that have higher probability of experiencing disturbing vestibular symptoms after cochlear implantation as preimplantation vestibular symptoms, especially Ménière's Disease; age at implantation greater than 59 years old; age at onset of hearing loss greater than 26 years old and preimplantation abnormal computerized dynamic posturography [15]. Specific surgical complications reported in the literature include an electrode dislocation, facial nerve lesion, apart from inflammation and bleeding, but also dizziness and taste disorders. Wagner *et al.* in 2010 evaluated whether there is a higher incidence of vestibular and taste disorders after bilateral as compared to unilateral cochlear implantation. They found that specific testing showed in one case (5%) a unilateral taste disorder after ipsilateral cochlear and that there is a higher risk for subjective vertigo after the second implantation. To increase patients' and medico legal safety in the procedure, the occurrence of unilateral and/or bilateral vestibular dysfunction and the potential risk of taste disorder should be included in the risk counseling before bilateral CI [16].

Other study by Steenerson *et al.* in 2001 evaluating vertigo after CI shows that imbalance was common preoperatively, positional vertigo was a common sequel postoperatively in the side of the implanted ear, responding well to vestibular therapy, and long-term intermittent vertigo or imbalance was rare in this group [17]. Vertigo and dizziness are among the risks after a CI surgery. It can occur soon after the surgery or after the implant activation. Bujang *et al.* in 2013 related that the postural stability of the experimental CI group have no significant difference with the normal control group in most tests situations, except in one specific test situation in which both the visual and somatosensory imputs was interrupted and modified. This study proposed that the exam that involves all the sensory measures is sensitive in evaluating the posture stability [18]. In 2001 Kubo *et al.* studied a group of 94 patients that presented the three types of dizziness after CI in 49% of the individuals [19]. This incidence is considerably higher than some previously reported, but is similar to the value reported by Ito in 1998 [20], in which 47% reported some kind of subjective dizziness. Those three types of dizziness occur immediately or soon after the surgery but lasting for a few weeks, lasting several months due to bilateral deficits in vestibular function and vertigo of delayed onset.

In relation to pain and dizziness after pediatrics CI, Birman *et al.* in 2015 documented that children tolerate this surgery well. They experience little postoperative pain only requiring paracetamolfor few days after discharge from the hospital. The ones submitted to the bilateral procedure usually require it for a longer time, few more days, as well as the younger patitens. Slight dizziness was reported by 8% of all children at 1 week after surgery. No child had marked dizziness or unsteadiness. Four children had large vestibular aqueducts on radiology scans, two (50%) of these children has slight unsteadiness at 1 week postoperatively [21].

Cochlear implantation has become more used recently to rehabilitate deaf born and postlingually deaf people. The acute, short-term dizziness after cochlear implantation seems to result primarily from a transient vestibular deficit of various origins. In contrast, chronic persisting dizziness after this surgery is largely based on a dysfunction of the saccular macula, which is an integral component of the otolith system. The data of Basta et al. in 2008 demonstrate that the saccular function can be profoundly influenced by cochlear implantation, and that surgical approaches trying to preserve saccular function are currently under development to prevent more damages. In the present original paper, they discuss also the possible coactivation of the inferior vestibular nerve by the electrical stimulation playing an additional role in the pathogenesis of the persisting postsurgical dizziness [22].

One year later Krause et al. evaluated patients with caloric and rotational chair vestibular function tests before and after CI surgery, which used the same approach. CI impairs the function of the horizontal semicircular canal (hSCC) but this alteration did not lead to vertigo complaints, so that no direct correlation could be established. Besides morphological changes, a CI also causes functional damage of vestibular parts of the labyrinth, but these findings did not lead to vertigo complaints. Other senses as visual afferents and central vestibular compensatory mechanisms play a role in order to the patient stay asymptomatic [23].

Vertigo and dizziness must always be a concern relating to complications after CI, even being usually a short-term symptom. With this in mind, Todt et al. in 2008 investigated the impact of different cochleostomy techniques on vestibular receptor integrity and vertigo after CI. They concluded that the round window approach for electrode insertion should be preferred to decrease the risk of vestibular dysfunction and vertigo [24].

In a study of Parmar et al. in 2012 they evaluated patients prior to CI surgery with preoperative bithermal caloric testing. One hundred seventy-seven patients were included, 148 in group A (CI in the ear with worse vestibular function) and 29 in group B (those implanted in the ear with better vestibular function). There was no significant difference in the frequency of dizziness before or after CI among groups, as well as the duration of dizziness postoperatively. This study has not searched for delayed onset dizziness, which has been documented in up to 40% of patients. The cause of such dizziness is often unknown, but up to 2% develop benign positional paroxysmal vertigo. As they used bithermal caloric testing, this means that the function of the utricle, saccule, and other semicircular canals was not tested. In addition, caloric testing may not entirely reflect the physiological function of the lateral canal as it mimics only low frequency stimulation [25].

Since cochlear surgical intervention is related to vestibular disturbs, it is extremely necessary doing the complete exam before intervention. As it works over a wide range of frequencies, it is important to test as many as possible. There is the caloric test, sensible to low frequencies (0.004 Hz) and the Rotary Chair Test to low to mid frequencies (0.01 - 1.28 Hz). The cVEMPs (cervical Vestibular evoked Myogenic Potentials) and oVEMPs (ocular Vestibular evoked Myogenic Potentials) have proven useful to evaluate the saccule and the inferior branch of the vestibular nerve, and the utricle and superior branch of the vestibular nerve, respectively. A new test is being implemented for high frequencies; the video head impulse test. This test relates to frequencies between 1 and 10 Hz.

Jutila et al in the same year determine change in vestibular function in patients receiving a unilateral cochlear implant by Motorized Head Impulse Test (MHIT) and other signs and symptoms. Horizontal high-frequency vestibuloocular reflex (VOR) was measured preoperatively and twice postoperatively with no significantly change. Quality of life score did not change significantly also. Late high-frequency loss of vestibular function or vestibular symptoms is rare but possible after cochlear implantation surgery, and must be considered in counseling especially in bilateral CI surgery [26].

4. Discussion

Anatomical, histologic and physiologic similarities between the cochlear and vestibular end organs explain the relation between hearing loss and vestibular disturbs. As both systems are related, in patients with hearing loss it is prior to proceed a complete study of balance in order to diagnose and prevent a worse vestibular problem.

In children with profound SNHL and consequent vestibular disorders may present delayed motor development.

As those systems are similar and anatomically just beside the vestibular end organs, close to the cochlea, they tend to be preferentially affected in ISHL with vertigo, as well as it happens with the electrical stimulation of vestibular system after cochlear implantation.

Cochlear implant surgery is becoming a popular procedure and it must be a concern the vestibular exam in advance in order to prevent equilibrium disorders after surgery. As vestibular system has a great frequency range, different kinds of exams must be applied to make a complete examination. Most of time, damages of vestibular organs may occur after surgery without symptoms and this must be understood.

Nowadays the number of adults and older patients being submitted to cochlear implant is growing, this way vestibular disturbs also increase, what must be related to surgical approach, previous disease and vestibular electrical stimulation for the cochlear implant.

Not all vestibular disorders have relationship with hearing loss, as we see in vestibular neuritis and vestibular migraine.

We started the analysis of the cochlear implant candidate patients' of HUB (Brasilia University Hospital).

All patients will answer dizziness handicap inventory (DHI) and perform vHIT before and after the surgery. All results will be analyzed and compared to literature. Until now, one patient had the complete evaluation and despite DHI became worse, vHIT continued normal. The second exam was performed 10 days after the cochlear implant.

In a previously analysis we can infer that some patients complain about dizziness after surgery. The fact of vHIT remained normal does not means that the vestibular system was not damaged. Other frequencies of movement that are not tested in vHIT could be injured, requiring a different kind of exam in order to evaluate other frequencies.

5. Conclusions

The inner ear contains organs responsible for hearing and balance. Cochlea and vestibular systems have a close relationship. So, disturb in one of them can cause a big damage in the other. Congenitally severe hearing loss can cause a great vestibular disturbance in children. Depending on the etiology of hearing loss, the vestibular disease can be extremely severe. Even the cochlear implant, because of either surgical approach or vestibular electrical stimulation by the implant, can cause vertigo after surgery.

Before a surgical manipulation in the inner ear, in order to promote better hearing, a complete exam of the vestibular system is required. Video Head Impulse Test is a new procedure able to evaluate high frequency movements of the head. That exam was an additional investigation of vestibular status, being able to detect problems that were not diagnosed before. Therefore, it came to improve evaluation of vestibular symptoms and investigation should be used regularly to prevent vertigo and other balance disorders after cochlear implant surgeries.

References

[1] Royl, G., Ploner, C.J. and Leithner, C. (2011) Dizziness in the Emergency Room: Diagnoses and Misdiagnoses. *European Neurology*, **66**, 256-263. http://dx.doi.org/10.1159/000331046

[2] Beck, D.L., Petrak, M., Madell, J.R. and Cushing, S.L. (2015) Update 2015: Pediatric Vestibular, Balance, and Hearing Disorders. *The Hearing Review*, **22**, 14.

[3] Yuri Agrawal, Y., Ward, B.K. and Minor, L.B. (2013) Vestibular Dysfunction: Prevalence, Impact and Need for Targeted Treatment. *Journal of Vestibular Research*, **23**, 113-117.

[4] Enticott, J.C., Tari, S., Koh, S.M., Dowell, R.C. and O'Leary, S.J. (2006) Cochlear Implant and Vestibular Function. *Otology & Neurotology*, **27**, 824-830. http://dx.doi.org/10.1097/01.mao.0000227903.47483.a6

[5] Inoue, A., Iwasaki, S., Ushio, M., Chihara, Y., Fujimoto, C., Egami, N. and Yamasoba, T. (2013) Effect of Vestibular Dysfunction on the Development of Gross Motor Function in Children with Profound Hearing Loss. *Audiology & Neurotology*, **18**, 143-151. http://dx.doi.org/10.1159/000346344

[6] Cushing, S.L., Gordon, K.A., Rutka, J.A., James, A.L. and Papsin, B.C. (2013) Vestibular End-Organ Dysfunction in Children with Sensorineural Hearing Loss and Cochlear Implants: An Expanded Cohort and Etiologic Assessment. *Otology & Neurotology*, **34**, 422-428.

[7]   Ciuman, R.R. (2011) Auditory and Vestibular Hair Cell Stereocilia: Relationship between Functionality and Inner Ear
       Disease. *The Journal of Laryngology & Otology*, **125**, 991-1003. http://dx.doi.org/10.1017/S0022215111001459

[8]   Sinha, S.K., Barman, A., Singh, N.K., Rajeshwari, G. and Sharanya, R. (2013) Vestibular Test Findings in Individuals
       with Auditory Neuropathy: Review. *The Journal of Laryngology & Otology*, **127**, 448-451.
       http://dx.doi.org/10.1017/S0022215113000406

[9]   Fujimoto, C., Egami, N., Kinoshita, M., Sugasawa, K., Yamasoba, T. and Iwasaki, S. (2014) Involvement of Vestibular
       Organs in Idiopathic Sudden Hearing Loss with Vertigo: An Analysis Using oVEMP and cVEMP Testing. *Clinical
       Neurophysiology*, **126**, 1388-2457.

[10]   Schwab, B., Durisin, M. and Kontorinis, G. (2010) Investigation of Balance Function Using Dynamic Posturography
       under Electrical—Acoustic Stimulation in Cochlear Implant Recipients. *International Journal of Otolaryngology*, **2010**,
       Article ID: 978594, 7 p.

[11]   Katsiari, E., Balatsouras, D.G., Sengas, J., Riga, M., Korres, G.S. and Xenelis, J. (2013) Influence of Cochlear Implan-
       tation on the Vestibular Function. *European Archives of Oto-Rhino-Laryngology*, **270**, 489-495.
       http://dx.doi.org/10.1007/s00405-012-1950-6

[12]   Tien, H.C. and Linthicum Jr., F.H. (2002) Histopathologic Changes in the Vestibule after Cochlear Implantation. *Oto-
       laryngology-Head and Neck Surgery*, **127**, 260-264. http://dx.doi.org/10.1067/mhn.2002.128555

[13]   Hugh, S.C., Shipp, D.B., Chen, J.M., Nedzelski, J.M. and Lin, V.Y.W. (2011) When Do We Choose the "Better Bal-
       ance" Ear for Cochlear Implants? *Cochlear Implants International*, **12**, 190-193.
       http://dx.doi.org/10.1179/1754762811Y.0000000006

[14]   Lin, F.R., Chien, W.W., Li, L., Niparko, J.K. and Francis, H.W. (2012) Cochlear Implantation in Older Adults. *Medi-
       cine (Baltimore)*, **91**, 229-241. http://dx.doi.org/10.1097/MD.0b013e31826b145a

[15]   Fina, M., Skinner, M., Goebel, J.A., Piccirillo, J.F. and Neely, J.G. (2003) Vestibular Dysfunction after Cochlear Im-
       plantation. *Otology & Neurotology*, **24**, 234-242. http://dx.doi.org/10.1097/00129492-200303000-00018

[16]   Wagner, J.H., Basta, D., Wagner, F., Seidl, R.O., Ernst, A. and Todt, I. (2010) Vestibular and Taste Disorders after Bi-
       lateral Cochlear Implantation. *European Archives of Oto-Rhino-Laryngology*, **267**, 1849-1854.
       http://dx.doi.org/10.1007/s00405-010-1320-1

[17]   Steenerson, R.L., Cronin, G.W. and Gary, L.B. (2001) Vertigo after Cochlear Implantation. *Otology & Neurotology*, **22**,
       842-843. http://dx.doi.org/10.1097/00129492-200111000-00021

[18]   Bujang, R., Wahat, N.H.A. and Umat, C. (2013) Posture Stability in Adult Cochlear Implant Recipients. *Journal of
       Medical Sciences*, **13**, 86-94.

[19]   Kubo, T., Yamamoto, K., Iwaki, T., Doi, K. and Tamura, M. (2001) Different Forms of Dizziness Occurring after
       Cochlear Implant. *European Archives of Oto-Rhino-Laryngology*, **258**, 9-12. http://dx.doi.org/10.1007/PL00007519

[20]   Ito, J. (1998) Influence of the Multichannel Cochlear Implant on Vestibular Function. *Otolaryngology-Head and Neck
       Surgery*, **118**, 900-902. http://dx.doi.org/10.1016/S0194-5998(98)70295-5

[21]   Birman, C.S., Gibson, W.P.R. and Elliott, E.J. (2015) Pediatric Cochlear Implantation: Associated with Minimal Post-
       operative Pain and Dizziness. *Otology & Neurotology*, **36**, 220-222.
       http://dx.doi.org/10.1097/MAO.0000000000000569

[22]   Basta, D., Todt, I., Goepel, F. and Ernst, A. (2008) Loss of Saccular Function after Cochlear Implantation: The Diag-
       nostic Impact of Intracochlear Electrically Elicited Vestibular Evoked Myogenic Potentials. *Audiology and Neuro-
       tology*, **13**, 187-192.

[23]   Krause, E., Louza, J.P.R., Hempel, J.M., Wechtenbruch, J., Rader, T. and Gürkov, R. (2009) Effect of Cochlear Im-
       plantation on Horizontal Semicircular Canal Function. *European Archives of Oto-Rhino-Laryngology*, **266**, 811-817.
       http://dx.doi.org/10.1007/s00405-008-0815-5

[24]   Todt, I., Basta, D. and Ernst, A. (2008) Does the Surgical Approach in Cochlear Implantation Influence the Occurrence
       of Postoperative Vertigo? *Otolaryngology-Head and Neck Surgery*, **138**, 8-12.
       http://dx.doi.org/10.1016/j.otohns.2007.09.003

[25]   Parmar, A., Savage, J., Wilkinson, A., Hajioff, D., Nunez, D.A. and Robinson, P. (2012) The Role of Vestibular Ca-
       loric Tests in Cochlear Implantation. *Otolaryngology-Head and Neck Surgery*, **147**, 127-131.
       http://dx.doi.org/10.1177/0194599812442059

[26]   Jutila, T., Aalto, H. and Hirvonen, T.P. (2012) Cochlear Implantation Rarely Alters Horizontal Vestibulo-Ocular Ref-
       lex in Motorized Head Impulse Test. *Otology & Neurotology*, **34**, 48-52.
       http://dx.doi.org/10.1097/MAO.0b013e318277a430

32

Hoarseness Due to Right Vocal Cord Paralysis Associated with Aortic Diverticulum from Right Aortic Arch— A Rare and Unusual Vascular Etiology of Right Vocal Cord Paralysis

Produl Hazarika[1]*, Seema E. Punnoose[1], Sanjay Arora[1], Ramagowdanapura Sadashivan Diesh[2], Raghavendra K. Itgampalli[3], Rohit Singh[4]

[1]Department of ENT, NMC Specialty Hospital, Abu Dhabi, UAE
[2]Department of Cardiothoracic Surgery, NMC Specialty Hospital, Abu Dhabi, UAE
[3]Department of Radiology, NMC Specialty Hospital, Abu Dhabi, UAE
[4]Department of ENT & Head-Neck Surgery, Kasturba Medical College, Manipal, India
Email: *produl_ent@rediffmail.com, seema1p@yahoo.com, sanjayaroraent@gmail.com, donusada@yahoo.co.in, raghavitgampalli@gmail.com, rohit.singh@gmail.com

Abstract

Right vocal cord paralysis in our present case was diagnosed on clinical and radiological examination which is precipitated by an anomalous right aortic arch with diverticulum. This is a very uncommon vascular etiology of hoarseness and is extremely rare. Because of this rarity, the practicing otolaryngologist may miss this finding while evaluating a case of idiopathic right vocal cord paralysis. Thus, the authors feel that idiopathic or unexplained right vocal cord paralysis should be routinely investigated with a CT or MRI of neck and chest with or without contrast to avoid such shortcomings. There is only one such case of right vocal cord paralysis by right aortic which has been reported earlier in literature.

Keywords

Hoarseness, Vocal Cord Paralysis, Right Aortic Arch, CT Scan Neck and Chest

---

*Corresponding author.

1. Introduction

Hoarseness due to unilateral or bilateral vocal cord paralysis is the common presenting symptom in laryngological practice. In fact, hoarseness is the first presenting symptom of various laryngeal diseases and fortunately most of the primary diseases of the larynx can be evaluated either by rigid or flexible laryngoscopy with or without biopsy and histopathology. However, neurogenic vocal cord paralysis causing hoarseness necessitates detailed evaluation as the cause of paralysis may be distal or proximal to the larynx. We herein present one such case of hoarseness with right vocal cord paralysis caused by very rarely seen right aortic arch with no cardiac or thoracic symptoms or complaints except mild essential hypertension. He did not have any visits to the cardiothoracic unit prior to our referral. Google and Pubmed search showed only one such case that had been reported earlier in KBB-Forum (2013)—A Turkish National Journal of Otolaryngology. This paper highlights the rarity of this condition and the need to include CT or MRI of neck and chest to evaluate idiopathic right vocal cord paralysis.

2. Case Report

Mr. A.R.P.A., 65 years old Indian male patient attended the ENT clinic of NMC Specialty Hospital, Abu Dhabi on 17th May 2011 for his complaints of nasal blocking, cough, fever, throat pain of one week duration associated with hoarseness since 7 years. Hoarseness had become progressively worse since last one week. He stated that he had undergone microlaryngoscopy and biopsy twice in the past on 15th & 31st May 2007 to rule out laryngeal pathology for hoarseness. He is a known hypertensive on antihypertensive medication since the last 5 years. Both his biopsy reports were negative for any specific pathology. He was diagnosed and treated for Acute Upper Respiratory Tract Infection in our clinic for symptoms of cough and change in voice with a follow up advice after 15 days for evaluation of hoarseness. He did not show up for follow up as advised. His next visit to our clinic was almost after three years on 23rd May 2014 and a video laryngoscopy revealed right vocal cord in the right paramedian position with restricted mobility and a phonatory gap. Right arytenoid was seen falling forward with no obvious growth to be seen in the larynx. CT scan of neck and upper chest with contrast was done on 5th June 2014. CT scan showed enlarged inferior recess of right pyriform sinus, medially displaced right aryepiglottic fold, anteromedial displacement of right arytenoid cartilage with features of right vocal cord paralysis (**Figure 1**). Visualized sections of thorax revealed right aortic arch with mirror image branching with small suspicious Kommerrell's diverticulum with a pressure effect over oesophagus and at tracheo-esophageal groove. A cardiothoracic consultation was sought due to the rarity of the aortic arch anomaly on 13th June 2014. A repeat CT scan with contrast of the whole chest was advised by the cardiothoracic surgeon on 28th June 2014. It revealed a right aortic arch with mirror image branching with aortic diverticulum measuring approximately 15 mm × 14 mm along medial border causing pressure effect over oesophagus at D2-D3 level and at tracheoesophageal groove (**Figure 2**). **Figure 3** shows volume rendered image of right aortic arch showing mirror image branching and **Figure 4** shows volume reduced image of thoracic aorta showing aortic diverticulum from medial wall of

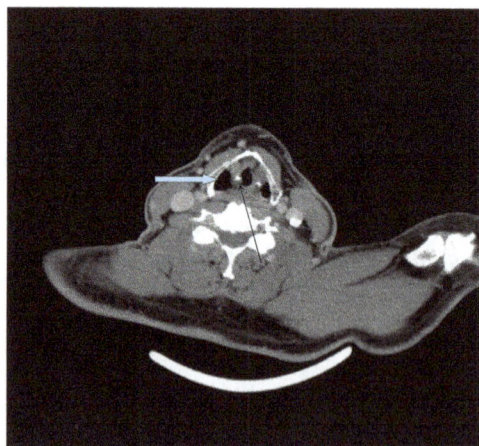

Figure 1. Axial CT contrast at the level of thyroid cartilage shows enlarged inferior recess of right pyriform fossa (block arrow) and anteromedial displacement of right arytenoids cartilage (thin arrow).

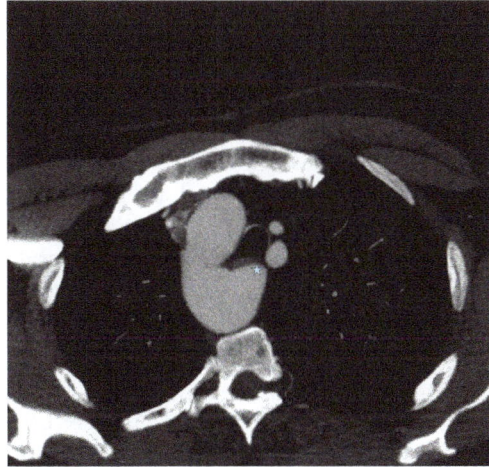

Figure 2. Axial contrast CT at the level of aortic arch shows Right sided aortic arch with an aortic diverticulum (asterix) along medial wall causing pressure effect over oesophagus/tracheosophageal groove.

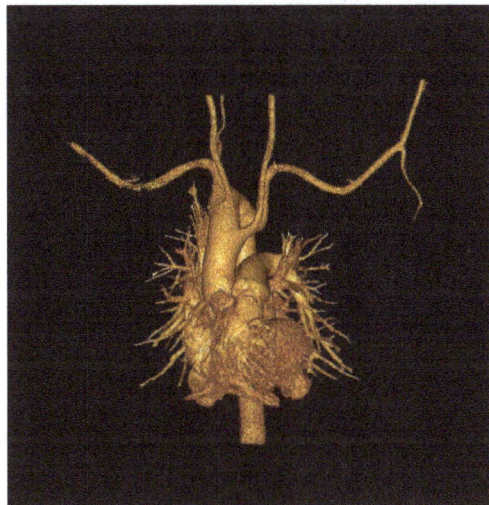

Figure 3. Volume rendered image of right aortic arch showing mirror image branching.

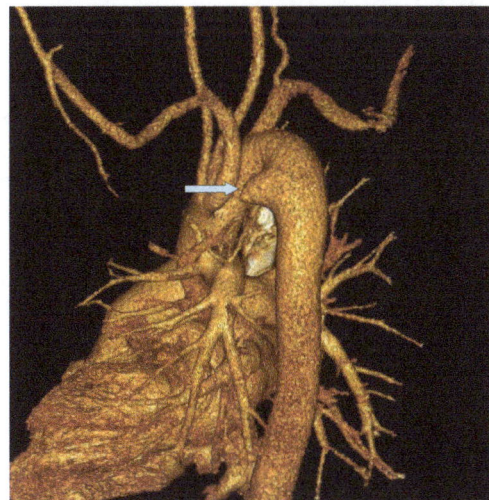

Figure 4. Volume reduced image of thoracic aorta showing aortic diverticulum (block arrow) from medial wall of aorta.

aorta. All these findings were discussed with the patient and our surgical colleague and a wait and watch policy was decided upon for the treatment of the diverticulum. For the symptom of hoarseness phonosurgical procedure was advised. An informed consent was also taken from the patient for the presentation.

3. Discussion

Neurogenic vocal cord paralysis may be unilateral or bilateral and can be caused by dysfunction of either the recurrent laryngeal nerve or the main vagus nerve trunk. Recurrent laryngeal nerve paralysis can be caused by various pathologies like inflammation, trauma, neurogenic or neuromuscular disease, neoplastic, viral, iatrogenic, idiopathic, vascular and cardiac diseases [1]. The recurrent laryngeal nerve paralysis associated with cardiovascular pathology is termed as cardiovocal syndrome or ortners syndrome [2]-[4]. The pathology of the cardiovocal syndrome generally includes aneurysm or cardiac dilatation causing compression injury mostly in left recurrent laryngeal nerve in the thorax. Left recurrent nerve palsy of cardiogenic origin has been well documented in the literature [5]. This is because left recurrent laryngeal nerve has a close relation to the left aortic arch. However, right recurrent laryngeal nerve injury causing right vocal cord paralysis due to right aortic arch without any other cardiac anomaly is extremely rare and so far only one such case has been reported in the literature [3]. This could have happened because of the abnormal origin of right recurrent laryngeal nerve from right vagus in thorax [6].

Anatomically, the left recurrent laryngeal nerve arises from left vagus at the level of left aortic arch, then hooks back posteriorly under the arch and ascends through superior mediastinum to reach the groove between the trachea and oesophagus. Left recurrent laryngeal nerve is more prone for paralysis than the right side because it pursues a longer intrathoracic course, coming into contact with the mediastinal surface of left lung, continuing along the mediastinal lymph nodes and finally looping around the aortic arch. Therefore, cardiac dilatation, aneurysm etc. can easily precipitate left vocal cord paralysis. However, right recurrent laryngeal nerve almost always springs off in the root of the neck and there is absolutely no chance of getting it affected in cardiac dilatation or aneurysm unless it has an abnormal origin from the right vagus in the thorax. Anatomical variations in the course of right recurrent laryngeal nerve are very common. But right recurrent nerve taking origin in the thorax instead of root of the neck is a very rare anomaly. Of the variation, the occurrence of non-recurrent laryngeal nerve is more common on the right side (0.6%) than on the left side (0.04%) [6] [7]. Variations are associated with the vascular anomalies such as an aberrant origin of the right subclavian artery from descending thoracic aorta or right sided aortic arch. When there is avascular anomaly of the right subclavian artery, right recurrent laryngeal nerve no longer recurs around the artery but proceeds from the vagus nerve in a more transverse direction to the larynx [4].

Right aortic arch is generally an asymptomatic congenital anomaly seen in 0.1% of the population [8]. Felson and Palayew (1963) mentioned mainly of two types of right aortic arch with their different branching patterns [9]. First one is the origin of brachiocephalic vessels from the arch in a mirror image fashion where the first branch is left innominate artery followed by right common carotid artery and then the right subclavian artery. The second type will have left common carotid artery as the first branch followed by right common carotid, right subclavian and then an aberrant left subclavian artery from the descending aorta via a diverticulum [10]. Right carotid arch with mirror image branching is almost always associated with congenital cardiac anomalies like Fallot's tetralogy with or without pulmonary atresia or truncusarteriosus. It is extremely rare to find a case like ours where there is right aortic arch with mirror image branching with no congenital cardiac anomalies but having right vocal cord paralysis. CT finding in the present case showed aortic diverticulum along the medial border causing pressure effect over oesophagus at D2-D3 level and tracheoesophageal groove. It is reported in the literature that right recurrent laryngeal nerve very rarely takes origin in the thorax in association with vascular anomalies like aberrant origin of right subclavian artery from descending thoracic aorta or right subclavian artery.

Right vocal cord palsy in our present case may be due to the compression injury of the nerve in the tracheoesophageal groove by the aortic diverticulum but not by any inflammation or any growth infiltration. Therefore, repeated microlaryngoscopy and biopsy failed to show any local pathology in larynx. This form of right vocal cord palsy is extremely rare and only one case has been reported previously. The possibility of this pathology has naturally been missed in previous laryngological examinations due to such an uncommon etiology of the vocal cord paralysis. So, the authors feel that an unexplained right vocal cord palsy should be further evaluated by performing a CT or MRI of neck and chest. This type of vocal cord paralysis perhaps should be considered as an ideal indication for phonosurgery, if acceptable to the patient after the management of his primary cause of hoarseness. A successful phonosurgical procedure will improve the voice quality and thus carries good prognosis. The cardiothoracic team of experts have recommended endovascular stenting of aorta to prevent an increase in size of diverticulum and rupture.

Acknowledgements

We, the authors acknowledge the immense help and support that we received from our NMC group medical director Dr. B. R. Shetty and Medical Director of NMC Specialty Hospital, Abu Dhabi Dr. C. R. Shetty. Also we are grateful to the Department of ENT & Head-Neck Surgery of Kasturba Medical College of Manipal University, India for helping us in preparation of this manuscript.

References

[1] Titche, L.L. (1976) Causes of Recurrent Laryngeal Nerve Paralysis. *Archives of Otolaryngology*, **102**, 259-261. http://dx.doi.org/10.1001/archotol.1976.00780100045002

[2] Omer, K., Hakan, B., Umit, A., Ozeyir, Y., Turan, I. and Burak, A. (2013) Recurrent Vocal Cord Paralysis Associated with Right Aortic Arch. *KBB-Forum*, **12**.

[3] Annema, J.T., Brahim, J.J. and Rabe, K.F. (2004) A Rare Case of Ortners Syndrome (Cardiovocal Hoarseness). *Thorax*, **59**, 636-637. http://dx.doi.org/10.1136/thx.2003.020503

[4] Zaki, S.A., Asif, S. and Shanbag, P. (2010) Ortner Syndrome in Infants. *Indian Pediatrics*, **47**, 351-353. http://dx.doi.org/10.1007/s13312-010-0053-y

[5] Song, S.W., Jun, B.C., Cho, K.J., Lee, S., Kim, Y.J. and Park, S.H. (2011) CT Evaluation of Vocal Cord Paralysis Due to Thoracic Diseases: A 10 Years Retrospective Study. *Yonsei Medical Journal*, **52**, 831-837. http://dx.doi.org/10.3349/ymj.2011.52.5.831

[6] Moosman, D.A. and DeWeese, M.S. (1968) The External Laryngeal Nerve as Related to Thyroidectomy. *Surgery, Gynecology Obstetrics*, **127**, 1101.

[7] Aniruddha, S. (2012) A Case Report of Abnormal Origin of Right Recurrent Laryngeal Nerve from Right Vagus in Thorax. *IJCRI*, **3**, 4-7. http://dx.doi.org/10.5348/ijcri-2012-03-97-CR-2

[8] Ballotta, E., Mion, E. and Bardini, R. (2003) Right Sided Aortic Arch and Aberrant Left Subclavianartery. *Journal of Cardiovascular Surgery* (*Torino*), **44**, 783-784.

[9] Felson, W. and Palayew, M.J. (1963) Two Types of Right Aortic Arch. *Radiology*, **81**, 745-759. http://dx.doi.org/10.1148/81.5.745

[10] McElhinney, D.B., Hoydu, A.K., Gaynor, J.W., Spray, T.L., Goldmuntz, E. and Weinberg, P.M. (2001) Patterns of Right Aortic Arch and Mirror-Image Branching of the Brachiocephalic Vessels without Associated Anomalies. *Pediatric Cardiology*, **22**, 285-291. http://dx.doi.org/10.1007/s002460010231

33

Preoperative Diagnosis of Thyroglossal Duct Cancer: A Case Report and Literature Review

Ai Suzuki[1,2], Kazumasa Suzuki[2], Yoshiaki Mori[2], Yoshifumi Fujita[2], Takashi Hatano[2], Nobuhiko Oridate[3]

[1]Department of Otorhinolaryngology, Yokosuka City Hospital, Yokosuka, Japan
[2]Department of Otorhinolaryngology, Yokosuka Kyosai Hospital, Yokosuka, Japan
[3]Department of Otorhinolaryngology—Head and Neck Surgery, Yokohama City University School of Medicine, Yokosuka, Japan
Email: aisuzu@jadecom.jp

Abstract

Objective: To clarify the preoperative diagnostic rate and elucidate the morphological features of thyroglossal duct cancer through a literature search on cases reported in Japan. Methods: A search of a medical database (Japan Medical Abstracts Society) identified 40 studies on thyroglossal duct cancer in Japanese patients between 1976 and 2014. A total of 47 cases, including the present case, are summarized herein. Patient characteristics, preoperative diagnosis, and morphological features were reviewed and analyzed. Morphological features of the internal portions in the cystic lesions were classified using the previously reported Yokosuka Kyosai Hospital criteria for ultrasonography findings of thyroid cystic tumors. Results: Preoperative diagnosis was described for 43 of the 47 cases. Malignancy was suspected in 18 (41.9%) of the 43 cases on the basis of fine needle aspiration (FNA) cytology (presence of suspected papillary carcinoma cells) and imaging studies (presence of calcifications), 12 and 6 cases, respectively. Preoperative FNA was performed in 24 cases with a correct diagnosis obtained in only 12 (50%) cases. Morphological features were evaluated by preoperative imaging studies and/or postoperative histopathology. We found 6 cases (15%) with solid lesions, 32 cases (80%) with cystic lesions containing a solid part, and 2 cases (5%) with solo cystic lesions, respectively. Calcification was observed in 28 (72.5%) cases. We further examined the internal morphology of 32 cases with cystic lesions according to the criteria for ultrasonography findings of thyroid cystic tumors described in Methods. Of the 32 cases, 25 (62.5%) and 7 (17.5%) were classified as "eccentric acute angle type (Ea)" and "multiseptate type (M)", respectively. The boundary between the solid part and the cystic part was irregular in all 7 "M" cases. No "eccentric and blunt angle type (Eb)" or "concentric type (C)" lesions were observed. Conclusions: The preoperative diagnostic rate for thyroglossal duct cancer using FNA is low, and it is important that diagnosis be performed in conjunction with imaging findings. The presence of solid parts or calcified lesions classified as "Ea" or "M with irregular boundaries" on the basis of imaging findings

is suggestive of malignancy.

Keywords

Thyroglossal Duct Cancer, Thyroglossal Duct Cyst, Preoperative Diagnosis

1. Introduction

Thyroglossal duct cysts are thought to arise from remnants of the thyroglossal duct, and develop together with the growth of the thyroid gland. Despite rare, cancer is known to be comorbid with thyroglossal duct cysts, with a reported frequency of 1% - 2% [1]-[3]. As the clinical presentation of thyroglossal duct carcinomas is often similar to that of benign cysts, a preoperative diagnosis is difficult to obtain. In fact, there are many reports of cancer being histopathologically diagnosed for the first time from a resected specimen [4]-[7]. We experienced such a case of thyroglossal duct cancer. The aim of this study was to perform a literature search on cases reported in Japan to clarify the preoperative diagnostic rate and elucidate the morphological features of thyroglossal duct cancer. We further examined the internal morphology of cystic lesions, according to previously reported criteria for ultrasonography findings of thyroid cystic tumors [8].

2. Patients and Methods

A search of a medical database (Japan Medical Abstracts Society) identified 40 studies on thyroglossal duct cancer published by Japanese researchers between 1976 and 2014. A total of 47 cases, including the present case, are summarized in **Table 1** [3]-[7] [9]-[43]. Patient characteristics, preoperative diagnosis, and morphological features were reviewed and analyzed.

Morphological features of the internal portions of the cystic lesions were classified using the Yokosuka Kyosai Hospital criteria for the ultrasonography findings of thyroid cystic tumors [8]. Briefly, thyroid gland carcinomas are divided into solid and cystic tumors. Solid tumors are tumors without any cystic part. Cystic tumors include tumors in which a cystic part is observed by ultrasonography studies and are classified as follows. Cases in which the solid part is eccentrically located on the tumor wall are referred to as "eccentric type (E)". This type is further divided into cases in which the angle made by the solid part and the tumor wall is less than 90 degrees, "eccentric acute angle type (Ea)", and those for which the angle is more than 90 degrees, "eccentric and blunt angle type (Eb)". Cases in which the cystic part is in the center of the tumor are referred to as "concentric type (C)", and cases with multiple septa are classified as "multiseptate type (M)" (**Table 2**).

3. Results

3.1. Case Report

A 48-year-old woman presented to the Yokosuka Kyosai Hospital with a neck mass that had persisted for one month. She was otherwise asymptomatic. She did not have thyroid disease or radioiodine exposure previously. A smooth rubbery mass of 2 cm in diameter was located on the right ala of the thyroid cartilage. The mass was not tender and its vertical mobility on deglutition was not limited. Ultrasonography of the neck showed a well-defined hypoechoic lesion with posterior enhancement (**Figure 1**), but no cervical lymphadenopathy. The thyroid gland did not contain a nodule and seemed completely normal. A Computed tomography (CT) scan showed a 25 × 18 × 15 mm cystic mass on the thyroid cartilage, containing a 5 × 4 × 6 mm solid part with microcalcifications (**Figure 2**). Fine needle aspiration (FNA) was performed and approximately 2 ml of thin light-yellow fluid was obtained. Cytology did not provide a diagnosis in spite of the presence of some epithelial cells with irregular nuclei. FNA was not repeated because we thought the diagnosis was thyroglossal cyst. Routine blood investigations including free T3, free T4 and TSH were within normal limits.

Under a preoperative diagnosis of thyroglossal duct cyst, an excision of the mass using the method described by Sistrunk was planned. The tumor mass was enucleated with no evident thyroglossal duct in the direction of the hyoid bone. Pathological examination revealed a papillary thyroid carcinoma in a small papillary excrescence within the cystic lumen of the mass. Normal epithelium and ectoic thyroid tissue without malignancy were

Table 1. Thyroglossal duct cancer cases reported in the Japanese literature.

Case	Age	Sex	Morphology of tumor	Calc.	FNA cytology	Preoperative diagnosis	LNM	Thyroid ca.	Histology	Year reported	Author
1	66	F	Ea	-	/	/	+	-	P	1976	Nagamine
2	38	F	Solid	-	/	Benign	-	-	P	1977	Izuo
3	23	F	/	+	/	Benign	-	-	P	1977	Inuyama
4	43	M	M Irreg	+	/	Benign	-	-	P	1979	Marubayashi
5	56	F	Ea	-	/	Benign	-	-	P	1981	Kinosita
6	48	F	M Irreg	+	/	Benign	-	-	P		
7	25	F	/	/	/	Benign	/	/	P		
8	25	F	/	/	Malignant	Malignant	+	/	P	1983	Hanamatsu
9	38	M	/	/	/	Benign	/	/	P		
10	30	F	Ea	-	Malignant	Malignant	+	-	P	1985	Tanaka
11	55	M	Ea	/	/	/	-	-	P	1986	Hirabuki
12	37	M	Cyst	+	/	Benign	+	-	P	1986	Nagasawa
13	35	F	/	+	/	Benign	-	-	P	1988	Takahasi
14	24	F	M Irreg	+	/	Benign	-	-	P	1989	Ymasoba
15	67	F	Ea	+	/	Malignant	-	-	P	1989	Mituyama
16	61	F	Ea	-	Benign	Benign	-	-	P	1990	Takeuti
17	22	M	Ea	+	/	Benign	-	-	P	1991	Kobayashi
18	17	F	M Irreg	+	/	Benign	-	-	P	1993	Hurukawa
19	42	M	Ea	+	Benign	Benign	-	-	P	1993	Takeuti
20	58	F	Ea	+	Malignant	Malignant	-	-	P	1994	Hoshino
21	37	F	Ea	-	Benign	Benign	-	-	P	1995	Taketani
22	67	F	M Irreg	+	Malignant	Malignant	+	-	P	1995	Hoshida
23	28	F	Ea	+	/	Benign	-	-	P	1995	Masuda
24	64	F	M Irreg	+	Malignant	Malignant	+	-	P	1996	Ohtsuki
25	33	M	/	+	/	/	-	+	P	1997	Imai
26	70	F	Solid	-	Malignant	Malignant	-	-	P	1998	Kitajiri
27	17	M	Ea	+	Benign	Malignant	-	-	P	1998	Simamoto
28	55	F	Ea	+	Benign	Malignant	-	+	P	1999	Yamamoto
29	47	F	Ea	+	Benign	Malignant	-	-	P	2000	Ikejiri
30	77	M	Ea	+	Benign	Malignant	-	-	P	2001	Kusunoki
31	26	F	Ea	+	Benign	Benign	-	-	P	2002	Ohtsuki
32	20	M	Ea	+	/	Benign	-	-	P	2004	Okabayashi
33	81	M	Solid	-	Malignant	Malignant	-	-	P	2005	Hori
34	43	M	Ea	+	/	Benign	-	-	P	2005	Sakabe
35	54	M	M Irreg	+	Malignant	Malignant	-	-	P	2006	Umiyama
36	32	F	Ea	+	Malignant	Malignant	-	-	P	2008	Kajikawa
37	63	M	Ea	+	/	Benign	+	+	P		
38	59	F	Ea	+	Benign	Benign	+	+	P	2008	Sato
39	36	M	Ea	/	Malignant	Malignant	+	+	P		
40	63	M	Cyst	-	Malignant	Malignant	-	-	P		
41	59	M	Solid	/	Benign	Benign	/	/	P	2008	Sakamoto
42	48	M	Ea	+	Benign	Malignant	/	/	P	2010	Kadokawa
43	30	F	Solid	-	Malignant	Malignant	-	-	P	2013	Uemura
44	38	F	Ea	+	Insufficient	Benign	-	-	P	2013	Present case
45	43	F	/	/	/	Benign	-	+	F	1982	Suzuki
46	75	F	Solid	-	/	Benign	-	-	F	1996	Otsuka
47	50	F	/	/	/	/	/	/	S	1992	Simizu

/: Not described; Calc.: Calcification; LNM: Lymph node metastasis; Thyroid ca.: Thyroid carcinoma; Ea: Eccentric and acute angle type; M Ireg: Multiseptate type case and that showed irregular boundaries between the solid part and the cystic part; P: Papillary adenocarcinoma; F: Follicular carcinoma; S: Squamous cell carcinoma.

Table 2. The typing of ultrasonography findings of thyroid cystic tumors.

Eccentric type		Concentric type	Multiseptate type
Cases in which the solid part is eccentrically located on the tumor wall.		Cases in which the cystic part is in the center of the tumor.	Cases with multiple septa.
Acute angle	Blunt angle		

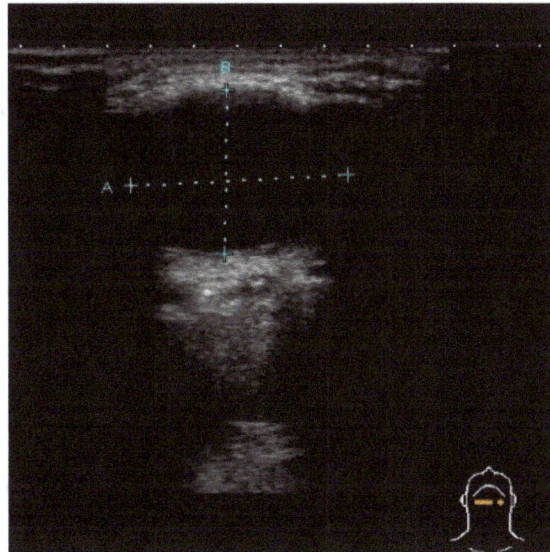

Figure 1. Ultrasonography of the neck.

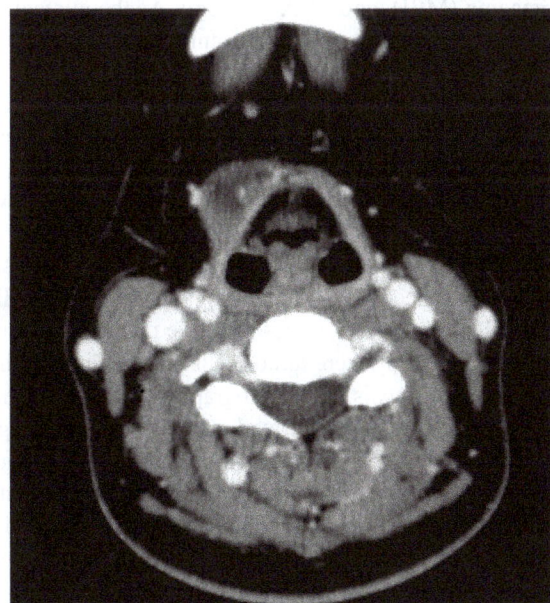

Figure 2. Computed tomography. A 5 × 4 × 6 mm solid part and microcalcifications (arrow) were observed on the head of the tumor.

also identified within the cyst. The surgical margin was negative. Additional surgery was not undertaken because of the negative surgical margin and absence of a thyroid nodule. The patient remained disease-free for two years and nine months after the surgery.

3.2. Previously Reported Cases of Thyroglossal Duct Cancer in Japan

The studies reported 18 male and 29 female patients, with ages ranging from 17 to 81 years (median: 43 years). There were 44 cases of papillary carcinoma, two cases of follicular carcinoma, and one case of squamous cell carcinoma. Lymph node involvement was observed in 9 (21.4%) of the 42 cases with description of lymph node involvement, and carcinoma in the thyroid gland was found in 6 (14.6%) of 41 cases with description of comorbidity. Preoperative diagnosis was reported in 43 of the 47 cases. Malignancy was suspected in 18 (41.9%) of these 43 cases on the basis of FNA cytology (presence of suspected papillary carcinoma cells) and imaging studies (presence of calcifications) in 12 and 6 cases, respectively. Preoperative FNA was performed in 24 cases, with a correct diagnosis obtained in only 12 (50%) cases.

3.3. Morphological Features of the Internal Portions of the Cystic Lesions for Cases Previously Reported in Japan

As the diagnostic accuracy of FNA cytology for thyroglossal duct cancer is not as high as that for papillary thyroid carcinoma, we speculated that preoperative imaging findings would be important for the preoperative diagnosis of thyroglossal duct cancer. We, therefore, investigated the morphological features of the internal portions of the cystic lesions. In 40 of the above 47 cases (including the present case), these features could be evaluated by the preoperative imaging studies and/or postoperative histopathology. We found 6 cases (15%) with solid lesions, 32 cases (80%) with cystic lesions containing a solid part, and 2 cases (5%) with solo cystic lesions. Calcification was observed in 28 (72.5%) cases. We further examined the internal morphology of the 32 cases with cystic lesions according to the criteria for ultrasonography findings of thyroid cystic tumors described in Methods 8). Of the 32 cases, 25 (62.5%) and 7 (17.5%) were classified as "Ea" and "M", respectively. The boundary between the solid part and the cystic part was irregular in all 7 "M" cases. No "Eb" or "C" lesions were observed.

4. Discussion

Pre-operative evaluation of lesions suspected of being thyroglossal duct cysts consists of ultrasonography, CT scans, magnetic resonance imaging (MRI), and FNA cytology. As the clinical presentation of thyroglossal duct carcinoma is often similar to that of benign cysts, these examinations have been indicated for patients with thyroglossal duct carcinomas well.

However, a preoperative diagnosis is difficult to obtain even after these examinations and the diagnosis of malignancy is often obtained postoperatively from histopathology reports. In this study population, malignancy was suspected in only 18 (41.9%) of the 43 cases for which a preoperative diagnosis was given. This low preoperative diagnostic rate for thyroglossal duct cancer is primarily due to the low correct diagnostic rate of FNA cytology.

It has been reported that the diagnostic rate of FNA cytology for this disease is 50% - 60%, which is lower than that for ordinary thyroid gland cancer [4]. FNA cytology can be readily diagnostic as long as enough material is obtained, and FNA cytology has led to a pre-operative diagnosis of malignancy in 50% of our patient cohort. On the other hand, in cystic lesions where tumor cells are confined to the wall, it may be difficult to obtain enough cells to reach a correct diagnosis. Ultrasonography guided FNA may be useful in such cases. Repeating FNA after the cystic contents have been aspirated may also be more diagnostic.

We speculated that preoperative imaging findings are important in increasing the preoperative diagnostic rate for thyroglossal duct cancer and, therefore, investigated the morphological features of this disease. It has been reported that the identification of calcified lesions or solid parts in imaging findings is suggestive of malignancy [4] [7]. In our series of patients, calcifications and lesions containing solid parts were observed in 28 (72.5%) and 38 (95%) cases, respectively. On the other hand, it has been reported that either solid parts or calcified lesions were absent in benign thyroglossal duct cysts examined by ultrasonography [44]-[46].

However, not all cases of thyroglossal duct cyst necessarily present with typical ultrasonography findings (*i.e.*, thin walls and no internal echoes). There are cases in which the cysts exhibit various kinds of internal echoes or wall thickening due to intracystic inflammation or proteins discharged from the epithelial cells of the cyst wall [44]-[46]. In some of these cases, partial thickening of the wall of more than 5 mm was observed [44] and this wall thickening might have been mistaken for a solid part.

In this study, we further examined the internal morphology of 32 cases with cystic lesions, according to the criteria for ultrasonography findings of thyroid cystic tumors described in Methods [8]. In our previous report summarizing the ultrasonography findings of operations for thyroid cystic tumors in Yokosuka Kyosai Hospital [8], we found a significant number of "Ea" malignant tumors. In addition, malignancy was also suggested in "Eb" lesions in which the solid part accounted for over 50% of the tumor mass, and in "M" lesions that showed irregular boundaries between the solid part and the cystic part. In this series of patients, all 32 cases with cystic lesions containing a solid part were classified as either "Ea" (25/32) or "M with irregular boundaries" between the solid part and the cystic part (7/32).

An incorrect diagnosis is thought likely to occur when a thickened wall is mistaken for a solid part, particularly in thyroglossal duct cysts with a partial thickened wall of more than 5 mm [44], which might be classified as "Eb" or "C" according to the criteria used. Therefore, we concluded that only a finding of "Ea" or "M with irregular boundaries" should be considered suggestive of malignancy in thyroglossal duct cysts.

We observed 2 cases in which the cysts did not contain solid part (Case 12 and 40). [16] [37] Preoperative diagnosis of thyroglossal duct cyst was obtained from ultrasonography examination for Case 12 and from MRI for Case 40. The existence of intracystic papillary cancer and normal thyroid gland tissue are described in both sets of postoperative histopathological results, suggesting the possibility that small solid lesions could be missed in the preoperative imaging examinations. This possibility was estimated to be 5% in this study.

5. Conclusion

The preoperative diagnostic rate for thyroglossal duct cancer using FNA is low, and it is important that diagnosis be performed in conjunction with imaging findings. The presence of solid parts or calcified lesions in lesions that are classified as "Ea" or "M with irregular boundaries" on the basis of imaging findings is suggestive of malignancy.

References

[1] Keeling, J.H. and Ochsner, A. (1959) Carcinoma in Thyroglossal Duct Remnants. Review of Literature and Report of 2 Cases. *Cancer*, **12**, 596-600.
http://dx.doi.org/10.1002/1097-0142(195905/06)12:3<596::AID-CNCR2820120319>3.0.CO;2-2

[2] Livolsi, V.A., Perzin, K.H. and Savetsky, L. (1974) Carcinoma Arising in Median Ectopic Thyroid (Including Thyroglossal Duct Tissue). *Cancer*, **34**, 1303-1315.
http://dx.doi.org/10.1002/1097-0142(197410)34:4<1303::AID-CNCR2820340442>3.0.CO;2-S

[3] Nagamine, N., Miyazaki, Y. and Syo, Y. (1976) A Case of a Carcinoma Arising from a Thyroglossal Duct Remnant: Report of a Case with a Review of the Literature. *Japanese Journal of Cancer Clinics*, **22**, 793-797.

[4] Shimamoto, K., Sugimoto, T., Noguchi, Y., Negishi, T., Haraguchi, H. and Komatsuzaki, A. (1998) A Case of Carcinoma Arising in a Thyroglossal Duct Remnant. *Practica Otologica*, **91**, 937-944.
http://dx.doi.org/10.5631/jibirin.91.937

[5] Yamamoto, K., Haji, T. and Tanaka, A. (1999) The Case of a Carcinoma Arising from a Thyroglossal Duct Remnant with a Thyroid Papillary Carcinoma. *Practica Otologica*, **92**, 773-777. http://dx.doi.org/10.5631/jibirin.92.773

[6] Kusunoki, T., Okita, A., Nishida, S., Tanaka, Y. and Murata, K. (2001) A Case of Carcinoma Arising from a Thyroglossal Duct Remnant with Difficulty Discrimination. *Practica Otologica*, **94**, 173-178.
http://dx.doi.org/10.5631/jibirin.94.173

[7] Sakabe, A., Udaka, T., Hiraki, N., Wakasugi, T., Kitamura, T. and Tokui, N. (2005) A Case of Papillary Carcinoma Arising from Thyroglossal Duct Cyst. *Practica Otologica*, **98**, 61-65. http://dx.doi.org/10.5631/jibirin.98.61

[8] Komatsu, A., Suzuki, K. and Fujita, Y. (2013) Preoperation Diagnosis of Cystic Thyroid Nodules. *Head and Neck Cancer (in Japanese)*, **39**, 77-82. http://dx.doi.org/10.5981/jjhnc.39.77

[9] Izuo, M., Kawai, T., Kusaba, T., Satoh, K., Kaneko, H., Hosono, O., Satoh, H., Ishida, T. and Azuma, Y. (1977) Report of a Case of a Carcinoma Arising from a Thyroglossal Duct Remnant with a Review of the Literature. *Japanese Journal of Cancer Clinics*, **23**, 546-549.

[10] Inuyama, S., Takahashi, K., Ozu, R., Kawashiro, N. and Inuyama, Y. (1977) Papillary Adenocarcinoma Arising from

the Remnants of the Thyroglossal Duct. *Otorhinolaryngology*, **49**, 653-657.

[11] Marubayashi, S., Aoki, Y., Tanaka, I., Dohi, K., Kodama, M. and Ezaki, H. (1979) A Case of a Carcinoma Arising from a Thyroglossal Duct Remnant. *Japanese Journal of Cancer Clinics*, **25**, 1333-1335.

[12] Kinoshita, Y., Kamata, H., Kurozu, T., Honma, Y., Kobayashi, S., Shimura, K. and Komori, A. (1981) Carcinoma Arising in Thyroglossal Duct Remnant: Report of Two Cases with a Review of the Literature. *Journal of Oral and Maxillofacial Surgery*, **27**, 117-124.

[13] Hanamatsu, M., Kaneda, I., Ogawa, H., Takahashi, S. and Kurihara, H. (1983) The Three Cases of Papillary Carcinoma Arising from Thyroglossal Duct Cyst. *Journal of Clinical Surgery*, **38**, 1253-1256.

[14] Tanaka, H., Okuno, M., Ohkita, H., Yamashita, T., Umeyama, K. and Sugano, S. (1985) A Case Report of Papillary Carcinoma Arising on a Thyroglossal Duct Remnant and a Review of the Literature. *Journal of the Japanese Practical Surgeon Society*, **46**, 346-353. http://dx.doi.org/10.3919/ringe1963.46.346

[15] Hirabuki, N., Maruyama, T., Arisawa, J., Mitomo, M., Kuroda, C., Taya, N. and Yamashita, K. (1986) Papillary Carcinoma Arising from Thyroglossal Duct Remnant. *Clinical Radiology*, **31**, 531-533.

[16] Nagasawa, A., Yajin, K., Shirane, M., Ohuchi, Y., Takano, A. and Hirata, S. (1986) Papillary Adenocarcinoma of a Thyroglossal Duct Cyst. *Practica Oto-Rhino-Laryngologica*, **79**, 1117-1125. http://dx.doi.org/10.5631/jibirin.79.1117

[17] Takahashi, M., Noguchi, I., Sato, Y., Ando, T., Hayama, S., Kurokawa, H., Kaneko, T., Yanada, Y., Ichihara, Y. and Usuki, S. (1988) A Case Report of Papillary Carcinoma Arising from a Thyroglossal Duct Cyst. *Japanese Journal of Oral and Maxillofacial Surgery*, **34**, 43-44.

[18] Yamasoba, T., Tanaka, T. and Takahashi, A. (1989) A Case Report of Papillary Carcinoma Arising from a Thyroglossal Duct Remnant. *Otolaryngology-Head and Neck Surgery* (*Tokyo*), **61**, 455-460.

[19] Mitsuyama, S., Nakamura, Y., Toyoshima, S. and Ito, J. (1989) A Case Report of Papillary Carcinoma Arising from a Thyroglossal Duct Remnant. *Surgical Diagnosis & Treatment*, **31**, 1537-1542.

[20] Takeuchi, K., Mukawa, K., Kato, R., Koitabashi, H., Nishida, Y. and Nagamachi, Y. (1990) A Case Report of Papillary Carcinoma Arising from a Thyroglossal Duct Remnant. *Surgical Diagnosis & Treatment*, **32**, 865-869.

[21] Kobayashi, T., Murakami, S., Takasuka, N., Furuya, K., Tao, S. and Kitani, S. (1991) Papillary Adenocarcinoma of the Thyroglossal Duct. *Ehime Medical Journal*, **10**, 110-115.

[22] Furukawa, T., Kitahara, S., Ikeda, M., Terahata, S., Tabe, T., Ogura, M. and Inouye, T. (1993) Papillary Carcinoma in a Remnant of the Thyroglossal Duct. *Nihon Kikan Shokudoka Gakkai Kaiho*, **44**, 239-243. http://dx.doi.org/10.2468/jbes.44.239

[23] Takeuchi, S., Kawata, I., Takeda, J., Arisawa, Y., Kashima, K., Kosai, M., Kondo, A. and Tadhibana, F. (1993) A Case of Carcinoma Arising from the Thyroglossal Duct Remnant. *Practica Oto-Rhino-Laryngologica*, **Supple 61**, 225-229. http://dx.doi.org/10.5631/jibirinsuppl1986.1993.Supplement61_225

[24] Hoshino, N., Sugiuchi, T., Okamoto, Y., Zusho, H. and Eguchi, M. (1994) Carcinoma Arising in Thyroglossal Duct Remnant: A Case Report and Review of the Literature. *Oto-Rhino-Laryngology, Tokyo*, **37**, 649-655.

[25] Taketani, S., Yoshikawa, K., Hashimoto, T., Yamaguchi, T., Dousei, T., Moriguchi, A., Taniguchi, M., Ueda, H., Utsumi, A., Suhara, H., *et al.* (1995) A Case Report of Ectopic Thyroid Cancer Originated from the Thyroglossal Duct Remnant. *Journal of the Japanese Practical Surgeon Society*, **56**, 948-952. http://dx.doi.org/10.3919/ringe1963.56.948

[26] Hoshida, Y., Haratome, S., Yamashita, N., Murakami, I., Miyake, K., Miyata, K. and Yoshino, T. (1995) A Case Thyroglossal Duct Carcinoma Diagnosed by Fine Needle Aspiration Cytology. *Journal of the Japanese Society of Clinical Cytology*, **34**, 692-697.

[27] Masuda, M., Makishima, T., Toriya, Y., Toyoshima, S. and Komiyama, S. (1995) A Case of Papillary Carcinoma Arising in Thyroglossal Duct Cyst. *Otologia Fukuoka*, **41**, 752-756.

[28] Ohtsuki, Y., Manabe, S., Iwata, J., Sonobe, H., Okada, Y., Sudo, S. and Ohmori, K. (1996) A Case of Thyroglossal Duct Cyst Combined with Papillary Carcinoma. *Journal of the Japanese Society of Clinical Cytology*, **35**, 451-455. http://dx.doi.org/10.5795/jjscc.35.451

[29] Imai, Y., Takahashi, K., Yoshihara, T. and Ishi, T. (1997) A Case Report of Papillary Carcinoma Arising from a Thyroglossal Duct Remnant. *Otolaryngology-Head and Neck Surgery* (*Tokyo*), **69**, 318-321.

[30] Kitajiri, S., Kaneko, K., Shoji, K., Kojima, H. and Asato, R. (1998) A Papillary Carcinoma Arising from the Thyroglossal Duct Remnant; A Case Report. *Practica Oto-Rhino-Laryngologica*, **91**, 715-719. http://dx.doi.org/10.5631/jibirin.91.715

[31] Ikejiri, K., Takeshita, M., Saitsu, H., Yakabe, S., Nonaka, M., Saku, M. and Yoshida, K. (2000) Papillary Thyroid Carcinoma Arising in a Thyroglossal Duct Cyst: Report of a Case and Review of the Literature. *Endocrine Surgery*, **17**, 295-298.

[32] Ohtsuki, N. and Kumoi, K. (2002) Papillary Carcinoma Arising in the Thyroglossal Duct Remnant. *Journal of Japan

Society for Head and Neck Surgery, **12**, 85-88. http://dx.doi.org/10.5106/jjshns.12.85

[33] Okabayashi, K., Kinoyo, T., Okuda, K., Nishiwaki, S. and Anodo, K. (2004) Case Report of a Papillary Thyroid Carcinoma Arising from a Thyroglossal Duct Cyst. *Journal of Japan Surgical Association*, **65**, 2589-2592.

[34] Hori, R. and Haji, T. (2005) Papillary Carcinoma Arising from the Lateral Branch Remnant of the Thyroglossal Duct. *Practica Otologica*, **98**, 421-425.

[35] Umiyama, T., Watanabe, H., Namba, M., Namba, G. and Suzaki, H. (2006) A Case Report of Papillary Carcinoma Arising from a Thyroglossal Duct Remnant. *Otolaryngology-Head and Neck Surgery* (*Tokyo*), **78**, 90-91.

[36] Kajikawa, H., Matushiro, N., Kamakura, T., Kitamura, T. and Okumura, S. (2008) A Case of Papillary Carcinoma Arising from Thyroglossal Duct. *Journal of Japan Society for Head and Neck Surgery*, **18**, 259-265. http://dx.doi.org/10.5106/jjshns.18.259

[37] Sato, K. and Takahashi, S. (2008) Clinical Analysis of 4 Cases of Thyroglossal Duct Cyst Papillary Carcinoma. *Practica Oto-Rhino-Laryngologica*, **101**, 479-484. http://dx.doi.org/10.5631/jibirin.101.479

[38] Sakamoto, K., Tomita, T., Imanishi, Y. and Ogawa, K. (2008) Study from Cases—A Malignant Tumor of Head and Neck. A Tumor of Anterior Neck. *Journal of Otolaryngology, Head and Neck Surgery*, **24**, 657-660.

[39] Kadokawa, Y., Shiomori, T., Nagatani, G., Mori, T., Ueda, N., Inaba, T., Wakasugi, T., Ohbuchi, T. and Suzuki, H. (2010) A Case of Thyroglossal Duct Carcinoma and Concomitant Warthin's Parotid Glands Tumors. *Practica Oto-Rhino-Laryngologica*, **103**, 575-579. http://dx.doi.org/10.5631/jibirin.103.575

[40] Uemura, A., Takahara, M., Nagato, T., Ueda, S., Hayashi, T. and Harabuchi, Y. (2013) A Case of Papillary Carcinoma of the Thyroglossal Duct. *Practica Oto-Rhino-Laryngologica*, **106**, 447-453. http://dx.doi.org/10.5631/jibirin.106.447

[41] Suzuki, S., Taniguchi, S. and Uchida, H. (1982) Report of a Case of Carcinoma Arising in a Thyroglossal Duct Remnant. *Practica Oto-Rhino-Laryngologica*, **75**, 722-727. http://dx.doi.org/10.5631/jibirin.75.2special_722

[42] Otsuka, K., Ikeda, E., Naito, M., Konishi, J., Yamada, M., Moriyama, S., Tsuji, H., Furutani, S., Kawakami, S. and Ono, K. (1996) Follicular Carcinoma Arising in a Thyroglossal Duct Remnant. *Journal of Japanese Society for Clinical Surgery*, **57**, 1585-1588.

[43] Shimizu, K., Kikkawa, A., Uchiyama, K., Ide, M., Shibuya, T. and Shoji, T. (1992) Clinical Features of 23 Operative Cases of Thyroglossal Duct Cysts Including One Squamous Cell Carcinoma with Literature Review. *Journal of the Japanese Practical Surgeon Society*, **53**, 504-509. http://dx.doi.org/10.3919/ringe1963.53.504

[44] Ahuja, A.T., King, A.D., King, W. and Metreweli, C. (1999) Thyroglossal Duct Cysts: Sonographic Appearances in Adults. *American Journal of Neuroradiology*, **20**, 579-582. http://.ajnr.org/content/20/4/579.full.pdf+html

[45] Ahuja, A.T., King, A.D. and Metreweli, C. (2000) Sonographic Evaluation of Thyroglossal Duct Cysts in Children. *Clinical Radiology*, **55**, 770-774. http://dx.doi.org/10.1053/crad.2000.0514

[46] Wadsworth, D.T. and Siegel, M.J. (1994) Thyroglossal Duct Cysts: Variability of Sonographic Findings. *American Journal of Roentgenology*, **163**, 1475-1477. http://dx.doi.org/10.2214/ajr.163.6.7992750

34

Surgical Excision of Clivus Chordoma with the Use of Coblator—A Case Report*

Saloni Shah[1], Roma Gandhi[1], Hemang Brahmbahtt[1], Rajesh Viswakarma[2]

[1]B.J. Medical College, Civil Hospital, Ahmedabad, India
[2]ENT Department, Civil Hospital, Ahmedabad, India
Email: drsaloni155@gmail.com

Abstract

Chordomas are dysembryogenic tumors originating from the notochordal process [1] [2]. They are aggressive tumours with unique diagnostic and management challenges. Primary therapy is complete surgical removal of the tumour as much as possible. The likelihood of recurrence is high in spite of complete surgical resection. A 52-year-old female patient presented with complaints of decreased vision in right eye, nasal bleeding, nasal blockage and difficulties in swallowing. CT scan and nasal biopsy were performed which confirmed the diagnosis of clivus chordoma. The CT scan showed extension into nasopharynx, nasal cavity and oropharynx pushing onto the soft palate. Surgical excision of the mass was performed with coblator by both intraoral and intra nasal approach [3]. On follow-up, nasal endoscopy and CT were done; the patient was relieved of the symptoms and was clinically better.

Keywords

Chordoma, Clivus, Nasopharynx, Oropharynx, Endoscopic Excision, Coblator

1. Introduction

Chordomas are tumors of notochordal origin that may affect the axial skeleton anywhere from the coccyx to the base of the skull, in either a midline or paramedian position. The cranial and caudal extremes of the spine are most often affected. The notochordal cells are preferentially left behind in the clivus and sacrococcygeal regions when the remainder of the notochord regresses during fetal life. Chordomas are rare, aggressive, slow-growing, invasive, and locally destructive tumors [1] [2].

35% to 40% of these tumors involve the clivus. These are rare tumors with an estimated incidence of 0.51 cases per million and approximately 1% of intracranial tumors [1] [2].

The clivus is the surface of a portion of occipital and sphenoid bones in the base of the skull. It is surrounded by the neurovascular structures of the brainstem, which includes both internal carotid arteries. Tumors of the

*Guided by Dr. Rajesh Viswakarma (Head of the ENT Department, Civil Hospital, Ahmedabad, India).

clivus can be benign or cancerous; they can be classified as chordomas or chondrosarcoma. Clival chordoma becomes symptomatic by locally invading surrounding cranial nerves and brain stem structures.

Although there is no racial predilection for chordomas, the incidence in males is 2-fold greater than in females (2:1), and the tumors are found primarily in adults, occurring rarely in patients younger than 30 years. The most common sites are the skull base, the sacrum, and the mobile spine [1] [2].

These tumors are difficult to manage because of their critical location and propensity to recur; they have been treated in the past years with combination of surgery and radiotherapy. No single surgical method has emerged as a standard of therapy for resection of these tumors, although numerous surgical approaches to the clivus are described. Surgical goal involves complete removal of tumor as much as possible. The role of adjuvant radiotherapy thereafter is still subject to debate. With the continued development of advanced microsurgical techniques in skull base surgery, more extensive dissections as well as combined approaches to the skull base have been advocated.

2. Pathology

Chordomas have 3 histological variants: classic, chondroid, and dedifferentiated. Classic chordomas appear as soft, gray-white, lobulated tumors composed of groups of cells separated by fibrous septa. They have round nuclei and an abundant vacuolated cytoplasm described as physaliferous. They are pathologically identified by their physaliferous features and immunoreactivity for S-100 and epithelial markers such as MUC1 and cytokeratins. Some studies have postulated that the notochord developmental transcription factor, brachyury, could be a novel discriminating biomarker for chordomas [1] [2].

Clivalchordoma patient presentation: most common headache, diplopia secondary to VI cranial nerve paresis and visual changes including blurring or sometimes loss of vision. The patient may present with multiple lower cranial nerve palsy symptoms such as facial numbness and asymmetry, dysphagia, hoarseness and speech problems. Finally, large tumors may cause brainstem compression and patients may present with long tract signs and ataxia [4]-[7].

We present a case report of a patient who presented initially with decreased vision in right eye, nasal blockage, nasal bleeding, decreased hearing and difficulty in swallowing and later was diagnosed to have a clival chordoma. We discuss the treatment modalities and present a systematic review of the literature.

3. Case Presentation

A 52-year-old Caucasian woman, living alone and previously in good health, was admitted on 25/6/13 at CHA with complaints of decreased vision in right eye and nasal blockage, one month before she was operated for nasal polyp in Bhuj general hospital. After the operation the patient again developed the complaints of nasal blockage and nasal bleeding associated with decreased vision and difficulty in swallowing.

On examination nasal mass was present in right nasal cavity with right side soft palate bulge. Cranial nerve examination was normal.

A computed tomography (CT) scan of paranasal sinuses showed large (55 × 43 × 76 mm) ill defined inhomogeneous enhancing soft tissue density mass filling posterior nasal cavity causing erosion of clivus, sphenoid sinus, ethmoid sinus and medial wall of left orbit, inferiorly extending in to oropharyngeal space.

Nasal endoscopy and biopsy was taken on 1/7/13 and sent for HPE which confirmed diagnosis of a chordoma in the clival region.

An endonasal endoscopic excision of the nasal mass was done with the help of coblator on 11/7/13.

PRE OPERATIVE IMAGES

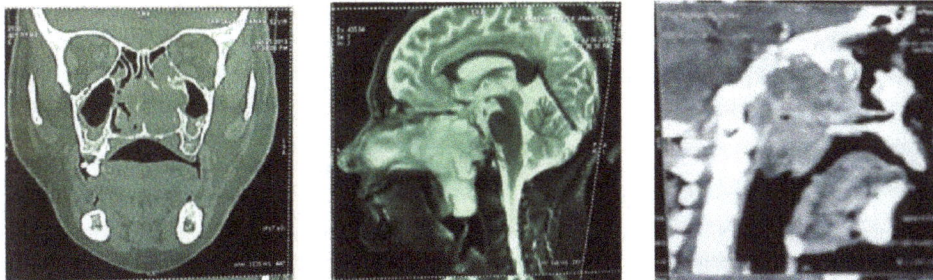

POST OPERATIVE IMAGES

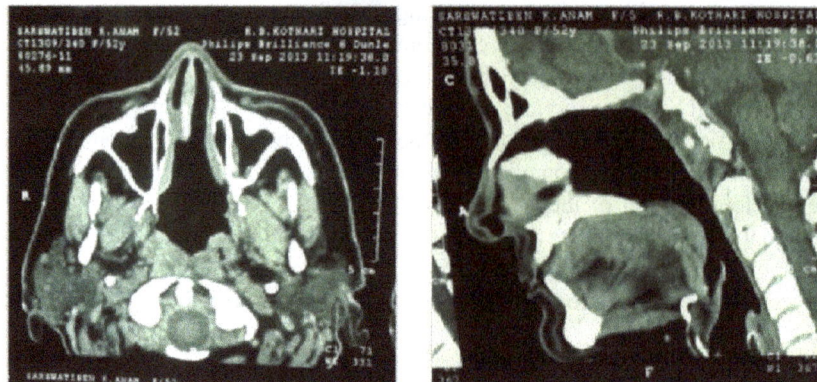

Post op the patient was followed. Patient was clinically better with complete relief of symptoms. Post op CT PNS was done on 23/9/13 which showed about 16.6 × 14.4 mm size abnormal enhancing lesion noted at left infratemporal fossa left lateral wall of nasopharynx? Residual mass lesion.

No adjunctive radiotherapy or any other therapy was used for this patient.

4. Discussion

Endoscopic approach to clivalchordomas comes with less morbidity to the patient as compared to conventional trans cranial approaches.

Clivalchordomas can be managed by a variety of conventional surgical approaches: transcranial, transsphenoidal, transoropharyngeal and maxillary osteotomy approaches.Transcranial approaches involve brain retraction and have increased risks of cerebral edema and hematoma, apart from carotid, basilar artery and optic nerve trauma. These complications can be greatly reduced with anterior (transnasal, transoral and transfacial) approaches. Currently, endoscopic surgery has opened a new avenue in the management of clivalchordomas, not only as a direct surgical access but also by providing an excellent visualization of the clivus and surrounding structures, especially the anterior dura and the basilar artery [3] [8].

Radiation therapy can reduce the risk of recurrence after surgery and prolong survival. For patients who are not candidates for surgery, radiation therapy is sometimes used as the primary treatment. Chordomas are resistant to radiation, meaning that very high doses of radiation are required to control these tumors. Because of their proximity to vital anatomy such as the brain and spinal cord, which cannot tolerate high doses of radiation, specialized forms of radiation are used to focus radiation on the tumor while avoiding surrounding tissue [8] [9].

5. Conclusion

Endonasal endoscopic surgery provided safe and reliable tumor resection for a lower clival lesion. We believe that this minimally invasive procedure should be considered as an alternative to traditional surgical treatment.

References

[1]   Adebayo, A., Clark, M. and Mansell, N.J. (2008) Cerebrospinal Fluid Rhinorrhea Secondary to Ecchordosis Physaliphora. *Skull Base*, **18**, 395-400. http://dx.doi.org/10.1055/s-0028-1087221

[2]   Gardner, W.J. and Tuner, O. (1941) Cranial Chordoma: A Clinical and Pathologic Study. *JAMA Surgery*, **42**, 411-425. http://dx.doi.org/10.1001/archsurg.1941.01210080211013

[3]   Jiang, W.H., Zhao, S.P., Xie, Z.H., Zhang, H., Zhang, J.Y. and Xiao, J.Y. (2009) Endoscopic Resection of Chordomas in Different Clival Regions. *Acta Otolaryngologica*, **129**, 71-83. http://dx.doi.org/10.1080/00016480801995404

[4]   Kitai, R., Yoshida, K., Kubota, T., Sato, K., Handa, Y., Kasahara, K. and Nakajima, H. (2005) Clival Chordoma Manifesting as Nasal Bleeding. A Case Report. *Neuroradiology*, **47**, 368-371. http://dx.doi.org/10.1007/s00234-005-1367-7

[5]   Koshiyama, H., Sakamoto, M., Fujiwara, K., Kim, Y.C., Teraura, T. and Koh, T. (1992) Chondroid Chordoma Presenting with Hypopituitarism. *Internal Medicine*, **31**, 1366-1369. http://dx.doi.org/10.2169/internalmedicine.31.1366

[6]   Macdonald, R.L., Cusimano, M.D., Deck, J.H., Gullane, P.J. and Dolan, E.J. (1990) Cerebrospinal Fluid Fistula Secondary to Ecchordosis Physaliphora. *Neurosurgery*, **26**, 515-519.
        http://dx.doi.org/10.1227/00006123-199003000-00022

[7]   Menezes, A.H., Gantz, B.J., Traynelis, V.C. and McCulloch, T.M. (1997) Cranial Base Chordomas. *Clinical Neurosurgery*, **44**, 491-509.

[8]   Raffel, C., Wright, D.C., Gutin, P.H. and Wilson, C.B. (1985) Cranial Chordomas: Clinical Presentation and Results of Operative and Radiation Therapy in Twenty-Six Patients.

[9]   Weber, A.L., Liebsch, N.J., Sanchez, R. and Sweriduk Jr., S.T. (1994) Chordomas of the Skull Base: Radiologic and Clinical Evaluation. *Neuroimaging Clinics of North America*, **4**, 515-527.

35

Klestadt's Cyst: Case Report

Kartik Parelkar, Smita Nagle, Mohan Jagade, Reshma Hanwate, Madhavi Pandare, Devkumar Rangaraja, Kiran Kulsange, Bandu Nagrale, Arpita Singhal

Department of ENT, Grant Govt Medical College & Sir J J Group of Hospitals, Mumbai, India
Email: kartikparelkar@ymail.com

Abstract

Klestadt's cyst, more commonly known as the nasolabial cyst, is an uncommon, non-odontogenic, and soft tissue cyst. It is classified as a fissural cyst, found outside the bone, and on the region corresponding to the nasolabial furrow and alar nose. Following its description first by Zukuerkandl in 1882, only 267 cases have been found in English literature. In spite of the low occurrence of nasolabial cysts, it is important to recognize the clinical characteristics of this lesion. The purpose of this report is to review the literature and discuss the histomorphology and etiology of this condition, and also its management by surgical excision. As per our experience, sublabial approach is the best for complete and scarless excision of this cyst.

Keywords

Klestadt's, Nasolabial Cyst, Non-Odontogenic

1. Introduction

The nasolabial cyst is a rare nonodontogenic cyst originating in maxillofacial soft tissues [1]. Following its description first by Zukuerkandl in 1882, only 267 cases have been found in English literature [2].

Rao revised the nomenclature and defined nasolabial cysts as lesions located entirely within soft tissue, different from nasoalveolar cysts, which caused maxillary bone erosion [3].

There are two main etiological theories having been proposed. One holds that the lesion arises from trapped nasolacrimal duct tissue [4], while the other affirms that it is an embryonic fissural cyst [5]. Klestadt [6] first postulated an embryologic origin for these cysts and considered that these lesions must originate from embryonic epithelium, entrapped in the developmental fissures between the lateral nasal and maxillary processes. Since then, many authors have classified this entity based on Klestadt's embryologic theory as a fissural cyst [7].

Klestadt's cyst presents at an extraosseous location in the region of the nasolabial fold and can cause swelling in the furrow, alar nose elevation and upper lip projection.

Though uncommon, management of this cyst is based on its correct diagnosis. Hence, we report this case of nasolabial cyst.

2. Case Report

A 45-year-old woman presented to our ENT department with a right sided nasal mass (**Figure 1**) which she had noticed since last 2 years. She had complaints of partial nasal obstruction on the same side.

There was no h/o epistaxsis, nasal trauma or any previous surgery. On examination the mass was visible in the right nasal vestibule; the furrow of the alar cartilage was lost partially.

The swelling was cystic in consistency and could be palpated bimanually through the nose and the oral cavity. Rest of the oral cavity and the nose appeared to be normal.

A CT (computed tomography) with contrast of the paranasal sinuses revealed a 2.3 × 2.1 cm round mass like lesion in the right anteroinferior nasal cavity. CT attenuation value measured 59 HU on plain scan and 73 HU on post contrast study, with homogenous enhancement. There was minimal scalloping of the adjacent maxillary bone but no obvious erosion (**Figure 2**).

After routine pre-anaesthetic workup and patients consent excision of the mass was planned. Asublabial incision of approximately 4 cms was made on the right side and the cyst was finely dissected from the surrounding tissue (**Figure 3** and **Figure 4**).

There was a small breach in the floor of the nose, the mucosa was reposited and sandwiched between a layer of betadine soaked gelfoam. The sublabial incision was sutured with vicryl 4 - 0. Postoperative period was insignificant. There is no evidence of recurrence 6months postoperatively.

The histopathological report stated that the cyst contained yellowish straw coloured fluid and it was lined by respiratory epithelium with squamous metaplasia and mucous glands in the fibrous stroma suggestive of a nasolabial cyst (**Figure 5**).

3. Discussion

Nasolabial cysts represent about 0.7% of all cysts in the maxillofacial region [2], and 2.5% of non odontogenic cysts [1]. Many authors believe that its prevalence is actually higher than presented in the literature; however, due to misdiagnosis, indexes remain low [1].

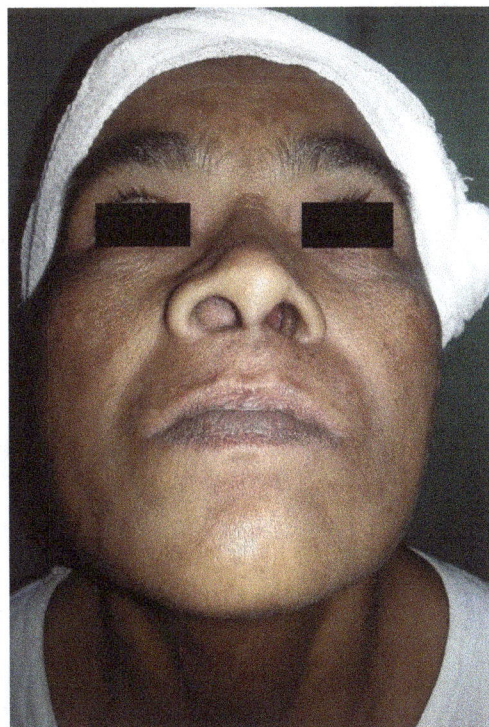

Figure 1. Right nasal mass.

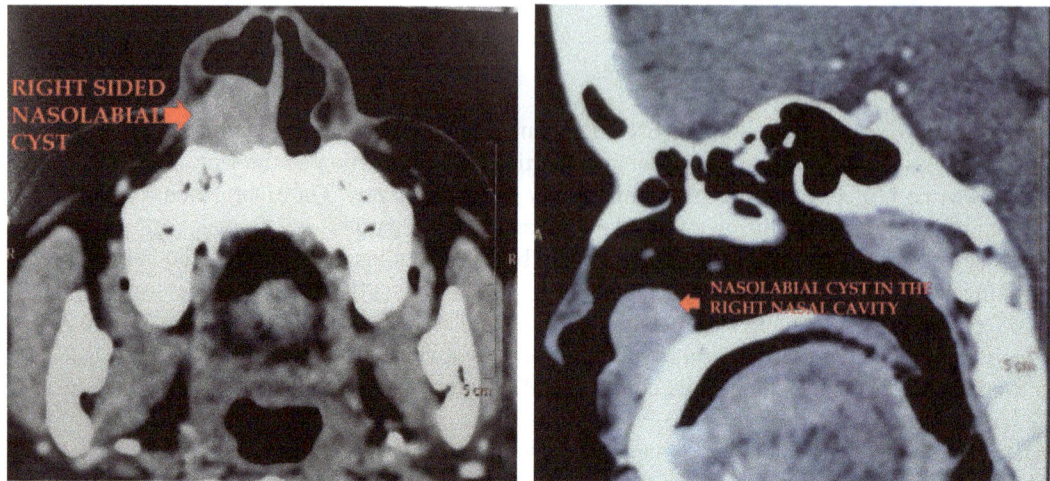

Figure 2. CT scan showing the nasolabial cyst in the right nasal cavity (axial and sagittal cuts respectively).

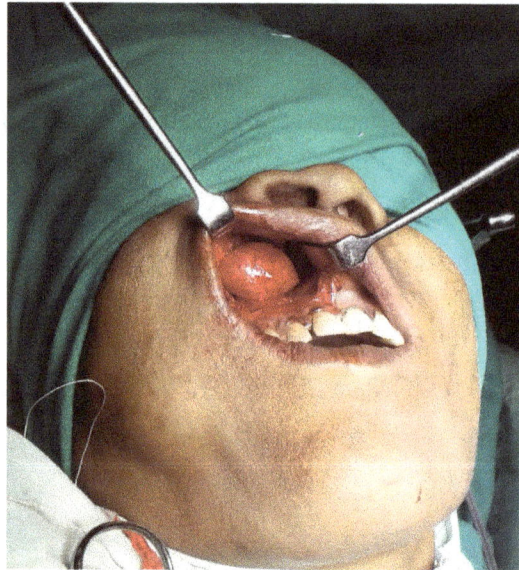

Figure 3. Intraoperative view after dissecting the cyst from the surrounding tissue.

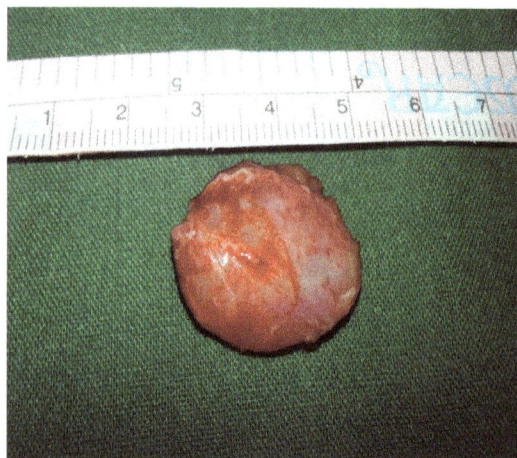

Figure 4. Excised nasolabial cyst specimen.

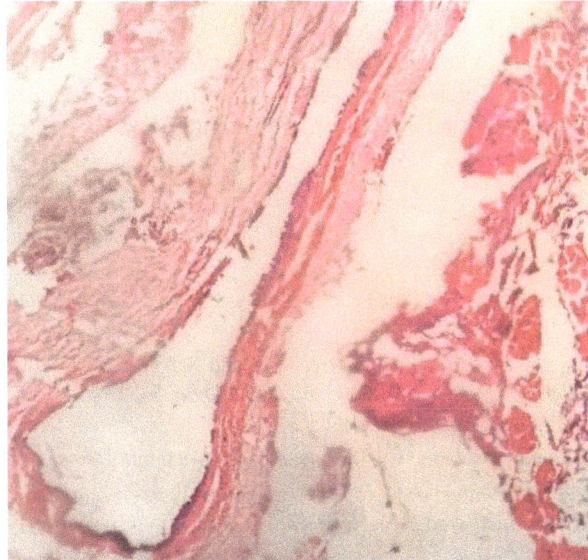

Figure 5. H & E stained slide showing ciliated columnar epithelial lining and fibrous stroma of the cyst wall.

These cysts are usually unilateral, but bilateral cases have been also reported, it has been estimated that approximately 10% of the cases are bilateral [8] [9]. There is a sex predilection of incidence in females (3.7:1) and age predilection in 2nd to 7th decade though it frequently occurs during middle age [1].

The clinical findings are fairly typical. Patients usually complain of a swelling adjacent to the nose, and sometimes the cyst may be observed on routine examination [10] [11]. The development of swelling in the maxillary buccal sulcus may reach great dimensions, causing discomfort with the use of dentures, breathing obstruction and facial asymmetry. In this report, the patient mainly complained about alar nose flaring, diminished nasolabial sulcus, and nasal mass which was actually the elevated floor of the nasal cavity.

Due to similar signs and symptoms, this lesion may be misdiagnosed as a dental or periodontal abscess, odontogenic cyst, tumor and choanal polyp [12].

The odontogenic cysts that should be excluded are periapical inflammatory lesions (granuloma, cyst or abscess) that have thinned out the bone. Careful examination of the adjacent teeth and testing its vitality can help to rule out this possibility. Orthopantomogram (OPG) will show evidence of non vital tooth with radiolucency. OPG in our patient was normal.

Dentigerous cyst also needs to be excluded. Usual radiographic appearance of dentigerous cyst is that of a well-demarcated radiolucent lesion attached at an acute angle to the cervical area of an unerupted tooth.

Another possible cyst of non-odontogenic origin is the epidermoid or epidermal inclusion cyst. As opposed to the normal pink or bluish coloration of a nasolabial cyst, this cyst is yellow hue in colour and patient may have a history of trauma or previous surgery.

Also neoplasm that needs to be excluded in this area is minor salivary gland tumor. As oppose to nasolabial cyst, minor salivary gland tumors are usually non fluctuant.

CT scan can help to exclude mass lesions causing bony erosion and most of the differentials. Though in the literature, rare cases of radicular absorption due to these cysts do exist. However, minimal scalloping of the maxillary bone as observed in our case was also observed by other authors [13] [14].

Histologically, the cyst may be lined by pseudostratified columnar epithelium which is sometimes ciliated often with goblet cells and mucous cells, or by stratified squamous epithelium [15].

Though marsupialisation has been done in some cases, surgical excision via the sublabial incision is the treatment of choice.

Because this cyst is usually closely related to the floor of the nose [16] [17] perforation of the nasal mucosa may be expected during its removal. When very small perforations are caused, they can be left untreated, as in our case. However, larger ones must be sutured.

Malignant transformation is rare and has been documented in only one case [18].

4. Conclusion

Klestadt's cyst is rare maybe due to its misdiagnosis and must be kept in mind in differential diagnosis of nasal vestibule, nasal base, and sublabial area lesions. Although uncommon in occurrence, it is imperative for the clinician to make an accurate diagnosis and provide appropriate treatment.

References

[1]   Mervyn, S. and Speight, P. (2007) Cysts of the Oral and Maxillofacial Regions. 4th Edition, Blackwell publishing limited, Singapore.

[2]   Patil, K., Mahima, V.G. and Divya, A. (2007) Klestadt's Cyst: A Rarity. *Indian Journal of Dental Research*, **18**, 23-26. http://dx.doi.org/10.4103/0970-9290.30918

[3]   Tiago, R.S., Maia, M.S., Nascimento, G.M., Correa, J.P. and Salgado, D.C. (2008) Nasolabial Cyst: Diagnostic and Therapeutical Aspects. *Revista Brasileira de Otorrinolaringologia*, **74**, 1. http://dx.doi.org/10.1590/S0034-72992008000100007

[4]   Precious, D.S. (1987) Chronic Nasolabial Cyst. *Journal of the Canadian Dental Association*, **53**, 307-308.

[5]   Wesley, R.K., Scannel, T. and Nathan, L.E. (1984) Nasolabial Cyst: Presentation of a Case with a Review of the Literature. *Journal of Oral and Maxillofacial Surgery*, **42**, 188-192. http://dx.doi.org/10.1016/S0278-2391(84)80032-4

[6]   Klestadt, W.D. (1953) Nasal Cyst and Facial Cleft Cyst Theory. *Annals of Otology, Rhinology, and Laryngology*, **62**, 84-89. http://dx.doi.org/10.1177/000348945306200108

[7]   Egervary, G. and Csiba, A. (1969) Bilateral Nasolabial Cyst. *Dental Digest*, **75**, 504-507.

[8]   Smith, R.A., Katibah, R.N. and Merrell, P. (1982) Nasolabial Cyst: Report of a Case. *Journal of the Canadian Dental Association*, **11**, 727-729.

[9]   Roed-Petersen, B. (1969) Nasolabial Cysts: A Presentation of Five Patients with a Review of the Literature. *British Journal of Oral Surgery*, **7**, 84-95. http://dx.doi.org/10.1016/S0007-117X(69)80002-8

[10] Campbell, R.L. and Burkes Jr., E.F. (1975) Nasolabial Cyst: Report of Case. *The Journal of the American Dental Association*, **91**, 1210-1213. http://dx.doi.org/10.14219/jada.archive.1975.0575

[11] Rao, R.V. (1955) Naso-Labial Cyst. *Journal of Laryngology & Otology*, **69**, 352-354. http://dx.doi.org/10.1017/S0022215100050799

[12] Werner, P.E., Lehman, R.H., Collentine, M.E. and Darling, R.J. (1968) Intraoral Presentation of a Nasal (Choanal) Polyp: Report of Case. *Journal of Oral Surgery*, **26**, 588-592.

[13] Balfour, R.S. (1977) Nasoalveolar Cyst. *J MD State Dent Assoc*, **20**, 92-94.

[14] Seward, G.R. (1962) Nasolabial Cysts and Their Radiology. *Dent Pract*, **12**, 154-161.

[15] Pereira Filho, V.A., Silva, A.C., Moraes, M., Moreira, R.W. and Villalba, H. (2002) Nasolabial Cyst: Case Report. *Brazilian Dental Journal*, **13**, 212-214. http://dx.doi.org/10.1590/S0103-64402002000300015

[16] Allard, R.H.B. (1982) Nasolabial Cyst. A Review of the Literature and Report of Cases. *Int J Oral Surg*, **11**, 351-359.

[17] Brandão, G.S., Ebling, H. and Souza, I.F. (1974) Bilateral Nasolabial Cyst. *Oral Surgery, Oral Medicine, Oral Pathology*, **37**, 480-484. http://dx.doi.org/10.1016/0030-4220(74)90124-8

[18] López-Ríos, F., Lassaletta-Atienza, L., Domingo-Carrasco, C. and Martinez-Tello, F.J. (1997) Nasolabial Cyst: Report of a Case with Extensive Apocrine Change. *Oral Surgery, Oral Medicine, Oral Pathology, Oral Radiology, and Endodontology*, **84**, 404-406. http://dx.doi.org/10.1016/S1079-2104(97)90039-1

36

Esthesioneuroblastoma, Thyroid Gland Carcinoma and Gastrointestinal Stromal Carcinoma

Plamen Nedev

Department of Neurosurgery and ENT Medical University Varna, Bulgaria and University Hospital, Clinic of Otorhinolaryngology "St. Marina", Varna, Bulgaria
Email: drnedev@avb.bg

Abstract

Olfactory neuroblastoma (esthesioneuroblastoma, ENB) is a rare tumor arising from the olfactory neuroepithelium. We report a case of ENB located in inferior nasal concha, combined with thyroid gland carcinoma and gastrointestinal stromal carcinoma in a 77-year-old man. The tumor was resected endonasally. When the final diagnosis of olfactory neuroblastoma was confirmed by histopathologic examination and immunohistochemical staining, the PET/CT examination was performed. The imaging revealed a small focus of a moderately increased cancer activity in the thyroid region. A gastrointestinal stromal carcinoma was detected one year after the resection of the thyroid gland. We discuss the clinical appearance of ENB, staging systems, diagnosis and management. During the endonasal surgery, ENB was removed entirely. Seven days after operation, in order to monitor the postoperative result, PET/CT was performed and a papillary thyroid cancer was detected. One year after the thyroid surgery, gastroendoscopy showed a neoplastic formation in the stomach. In conclusion, we state that when identified as aggressive tumors such as ENB, it is necessary to provide regular examinations in order to detect distant ENB metastases or other neoplastic localisations.

Keywords

Esthesioneuroblastoma, Olfactory Neuroblastoma, Thyroid Gland Carcinoma, Gastrointestinal Stromal Carcinoma (GIST)

1. Introduction

Olfactory neuroblastoma (esthesioneuroblastoma, ENB) is a tumor arising from the olfactory neuroepithelium.

Usually, the tumor mass originates from the superior nasal cavity meatus and it is presented as a nasal polyp that occupies superior turbinate, superior portion of nasal septum and cribriform plate. Its biological activity ranges from indolent growth to local recurrence and rapid widespread metastasis [1]. We report a rare case of olfactory neuroblastoma combined with thyroid gland carcinoma, treated successfully with surgical resections. One year after surgeries, the clinical examination of the patient showed gastrointestinal stromal carcinoma.

2. Case Report

2.1. History

A 77-year-old man has a history of obstruction in the left nasal cavity and recurrent hemorrhage. Those symptoms disturbed the patient for about 3 - 4 months. The patient does not report other symptoms as hypo- or anosmia, diplopia, facial pain, etc. In the previous examination an ENT specialist diagnosed a benign nasal polyposis and recommended operative treatment.

2.2. Physical Examination and Investigation

The anterior rhinoscopy examination confirmed a tumor mass obturating the left nasal cavity. The neoplasm had whitish-red color, smooth surface and soft consistency, resembling nasal polyposis. There were not neck lymphadenopathies. Coronal and axial CT scans examinations showed 5, 5 - 6 cm/4, 5 - 5 cm tumor mass in inferior and middle nasal meatus without lesions in the neighboring structures (**Figure 1**). The complete blood count was within normal limits.

2.3. Surgery 1

On the endoscopic examinations, polypoid-like mass with bleeding tendency was observed in the left inferior meatus. The tumor lesion arised from inferior nasal conchae. The formation had well defined margins. Other soft tissues and bone structures were not engaged. During surgery the neoplasm's consistency seems to be much easier to tear apart than a bening polyp. The hole tumor mass was removed completely. The diagnosis of esthesioneuroblastoma was determined byhystological analysis (**Figure 2**) and by use of special stains such as immunohistochemistry (**Figure 3**).

2.4. Postoperative Period

The postoperative period was normal; the patient was stable, with restored nasal breathing, without hemorrhage. Seven days after surgery, in order to monitor the postoperative result PET/CT was performed (**Figure 4** and **Figure 5**). The staging FDG PET/CT after the removal of the esthesioneuroblastoma in the nasal cavity revealed that there are no hypermetabolic lesions, indicative of local recurrence/residual tumor or distant metastases. There were not pathological activities in the lungs, axiles, abdominal organs and spine. However a small focus of moderately increased activity is noted in the thyroid region. This finding could be considered as second malignancy

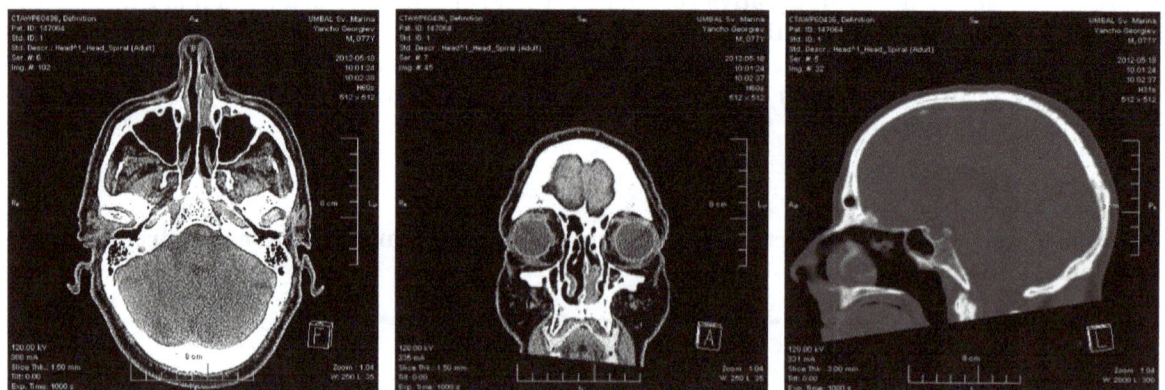

Figure 1. Axial, coronal and sagital CT scans showed 5, 5 - 6 cm/4, 5 - 5 cm tumor mass in left inferior and middle nasal meatus without lesions in the neighboring structures.

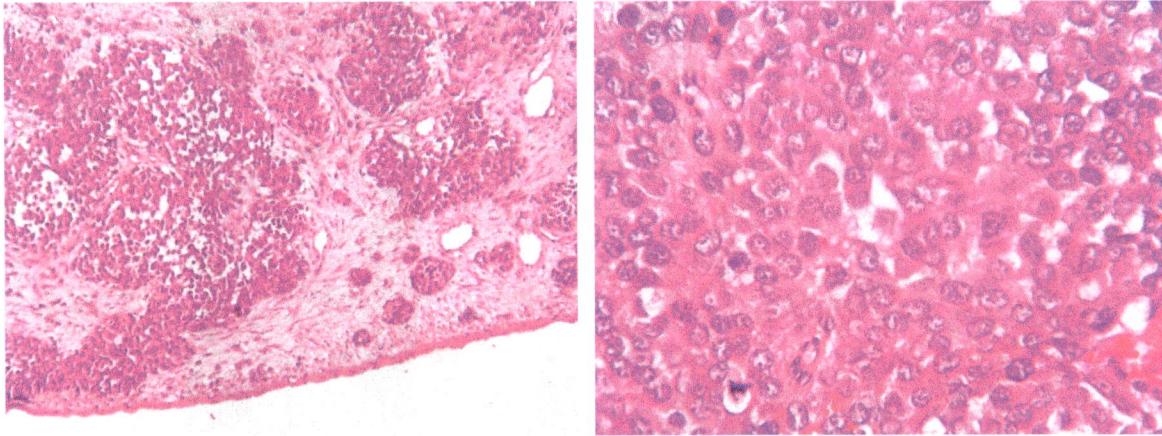

Figure 2. Hematoxylin and eosin stain showed proliferation of neoplastic cells containing uniform round nuclei and scant cytoplasm and cells with dispersed chromatin. Magnification times: 10×10 left hand photo; 40×10 right hand photo.

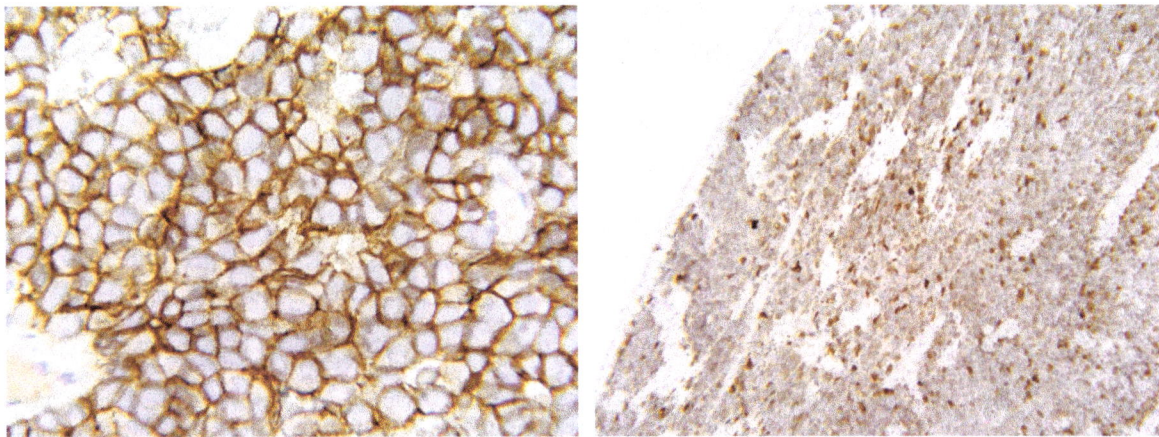

Figure 3. Immunohistochemisrty, hematoxylin and eosin stain 40×10, CD 56 (+); S-100 protein (+) GFAP, AE1/AE3 (−). Morphological diagnosis: esthesioneuroblastoma.

island in this patient. Further evaluation proved papillary thyroid cancer. The echographic examination visualized a node structure (5 - 8 mm), with irregular outlines.

2.5. Surgery 2

Second surgical procedure was performed. The intraoperative findings showed 8 mm node (SUV 3.3) in the right superior lobe of the thyroid gland. A partial thyroid resection was done. The histology confirmed papillary thyroid cancer (**Figure 6**).

2.6. Postoperative Care

The patient was discharged without additional courses of chemotherapy or radiation. Six months after the second surgery, the final histopathologic report showed no evidence of recurrent ENB. The echographic examination of the rest of the thyroid gland revealed no suspect formations and the imaging (PET/CT) showed no other cancer activities. One year later the patient had gastrointestinal complaints and the fibrogastroendoscopy showed a neoplasmic formation in the stomach. The histological results confirm gastrointestinal stromal tumor (**Figure 7**). The tumor was considered as inoperable and chemotherapy was recommended.

3. Discussion

In the literature there are only few ENB casesarised from ectopic regions such as maxillary sinus, sphenoid sinus,

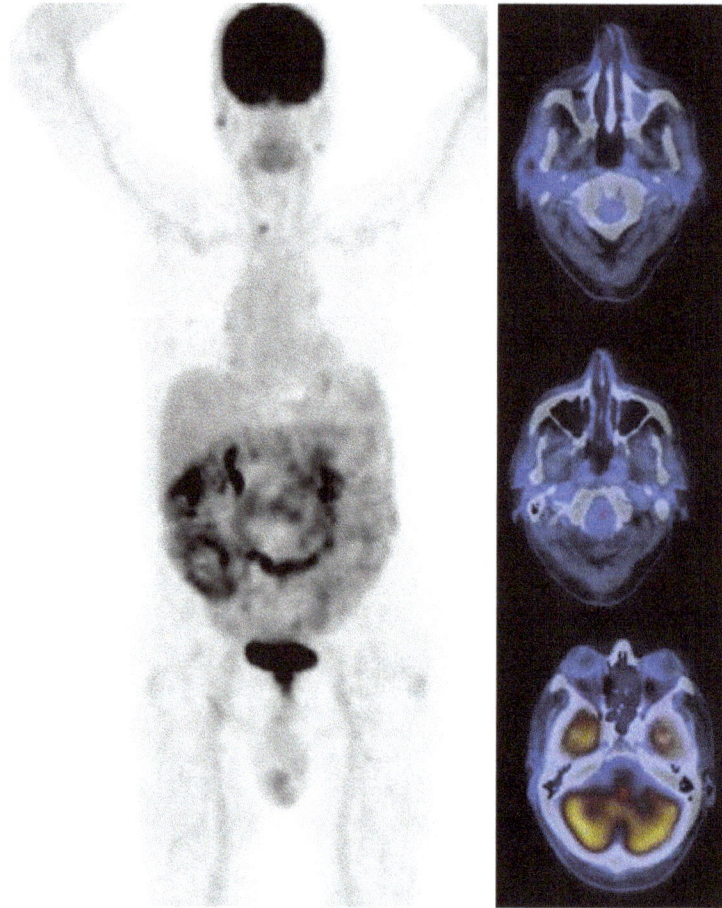

Figure 4. Staging FDG PET/CT performed after the removal of the ENB in the nasal cavity. There are no hypermetabolic lesions, indicative of local recurrence/residual tumors or distant metastases. A small focus of moderately increased activity is noted in the thyroid region.

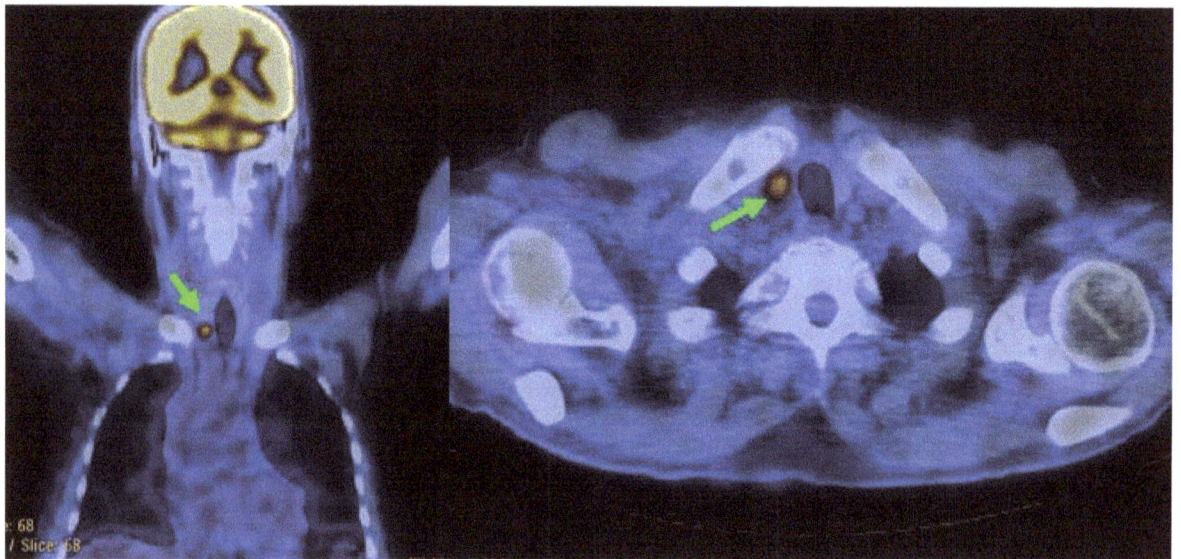

Figure 5. The noted focal uptake on FDG PET/CT is located in the right thyroid lobe. Due to the known high prevalence of malignancy in PET positive thyroid nodules the patient was referred for further evaluation which proved papillary thyroid cancer as a second malignancy in this patient.

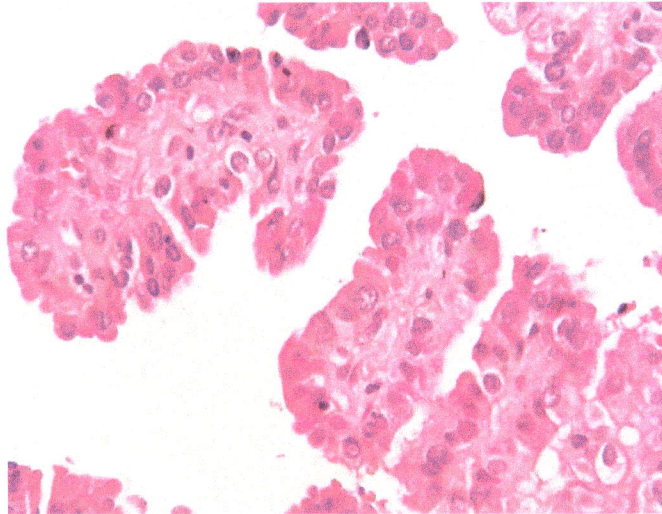

Figure 6. Hematoxylin and eosin stain 40 × 10. Papillary carcinoma of the thyroid gland.

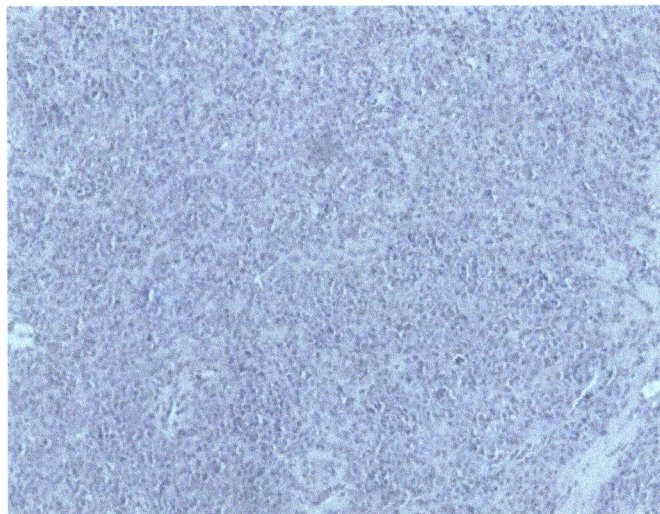

Figure 7. Hematoxylin and eosin stain showed proliferation of epitheloid monotonous cells with high N/C ratio, hyperchromatic nuclei, moderate nuclear and cellular polymorphism; high mitotic activity. Morphological diagnosis: gastrointestinal stromal carcinoma. Magnification times: 10 × 10.

etc. In 2007, Lee and Kim reported a primary olfactory neuroblastoma originating from the inferior meatus of the nasal cavity [2]. So far, we have not found reported case of ENB combined with thyroid gland carcinoma and GIST.

Esthesioneuroblastoma has been described by Berger and Luc in 1924 [3]. This neoplasm is relatively rare and it is known by various names: esthesioneuroepithelioma, esthesioneurocytoma, esthesioneuroblastoma, olfactory esthesioneuroma, intranasal neuroblastoma, and neural olfactory tumor [4]. The tumor can affect both children and adults, with a bimodal peak incidence between 11 and 20 years and between 51 and 60 years [5].

There are cases of 3-year-old [5] and 89-year-old man with ENB [2]. ENB is locally aggressive tumor that has an incidence of 3% to 6% of all intranasal tumors [6] and it metastasizes most commonly to cervical lymphnodes. Cervical lymph node metastasis (10% - 30%) and distant metastasis develop irrespective of tumour grade [7]. Distant metastases can be found in the lungs, the abdominal organs, thespinal cord or in the long bones.

The most common symptoms are nose bleeding, unilateral nasal obstruction, anosmia, facial pain and headache. Macroscopically ENB can be wrongly diagnosed as benign nasal polyp or malignant neoplasms such as: malignant lymphoma, sinonasal undifferentiated carcinoma, *etc.* Therefore any suspicious tissue should be subjected to histological analysis. One of the most important characteristics that can lead the surgeon to suspect a malignancy is the soft and easy to tear apart tumor mass tissue.

One of the most reliable histologic features is itslobular architecture. The circumscribed lobules or nests are made up of primitive neuroblastoma cells. They are usually located below an intact mucosa and in avascularized fibrous stroma. The tumor cells are small, round and blue [8]. The neoplastic cells form arosette- or pseudo-rosette-like pattern [9] [10]. The neoplastic ENB cells are characterized by uniform round nuclei, dispersed chromatin and scant cytoplasm. The final histopathological diagnosis can be established by light microscopy or by immunohistochemical staining and electron microscopy, depending on the tumor differentiation. The detailed analysis of ENB cytogenetic characterization is presented by Heidrun Holland *et al.* [11].

Thus, olfactory neuroblastomas can be detected, delineated and its characteristics suspected by CT and MRI, but definite diagnosis however is still based on histopathology [12]. Depending on the propagation of the tumor mass Dulgerov and Calcaterra [13] proposed a four-stage classification.

The clinical behavior of olfactory epithelium tumors depends on patient age and the clinical stage of the neoplasm. In this particular case the esthesioneuroblastoma was classified as Kadish stage A, because the tumor was confined to the nasal cavity and according TNM system the tumor was ranged as stage T1N0M0.

The treatment of ENB depends on the stage and the presence of metastases. It seems that so far the best results are obtained with a combination of surgical resection and radiotherapy, with or without chemotherapy [14].

Unfortunately, despite aggressive therapy, ENB has been noted to have a high local recurrence rate of 50% - 60% with 10% - 62% presenting as metastatic cases and 20% - 30% of those cases involving the CNS [15]. The patients with tumors of Kadish stage A have a 5-year survival rate ranging from 72% to 81% [5] [16] [17].

Survival according to treatment modalities was 65% for surgery plus radiotherapy, 51% for radiotherapy and chemotherapy, 48% for surgery, 47% for surgery plus radiotherapy and chemotherapy, and 37% for radiotherapy alone [16]. The histopathological grading according to Hyams and the presence of cervical lymph-node metastases emerged as prognostic factors [16] [18]. The disease-free actuarial survival and overall survival rates were 77% and 61% at 5 years and 53% and 42% at 10 years, respectively [19]. In 2015, Petruzzelli *et al.* published a retrospective analysis of 32 patients, where the estimated overall rate of survival at 10 years was 78% based on Kadish and T stage [20]. Esthesioneuroblastoma is an uncommon malignancy of the head and neck for which there is no defined treatment protocol [20].

In this case study we demonstrate that in some cases the diagnosis ENB might be unexpected because the tumor mass arises from the anterior end of the inferior nasal concha. The combination of ENB with thyroid gland carcinoma and GIST isextraordinary and we defined it as extremely rare.

In this particular case we did not recommended course of radiotherapy/chemotherapy because of the early stage of the ENB, its radical removal and the lack of regional or distant metastases. The thyroid gland carcinoma was removed radically as well. The GIST was considered as inoperable. Regardless of the course of chemotherapy the outcome was lethal 6 months after the diagnosis of gastrointestinal stromal tumor.

4. Conclusions

We presented a rare case of ENB with thyroid gland carcinoma as a second finding of cancer activity. The early stage of the tumors allowed applying surgical treatments. The thyroid gland carcinoma was found by PET/CT examination, which was applied in order to detect the presence of ENB possible metastases.

We cannot determine with certainty whether the thyroid gland carcinoma and gastrointestinal stromal tumor (diagnosed one year later) are metastatic from the ENB or whether they are primary cancer activities.

When identified as aggressive tumors such as ENB, it is necessary to provide regular examinations in order to detect distant ENB metastases or other neoplastic localisations.

References

[1]   Sampath, P., Park, M.C., Huang, D., Deville, C., Cortez, S. and Chougule, P. (2006) Esthesioneuroblastoma (Olfactory Neuroblastoma) with Hemorrhage: An Unusual Presentation. *Skull Base*, **16**, 169-173.
      http://dx.doi.org/10.1055/s-2006-939677

[2]   Lee, J.Y. and Kim, H.K. (2007) Primary Olfactory Neuroblastoma Originating from the Inferior Meatus of the Nasal Cavity. *American Journal of Otolaryngology-Head and Neck Medicine and Surgery*, **28**, 196-200.

[3]   Berger, L. and Luc, R. (1924) L'Estesioneuroepitheliome olfactif. *Buletin de L'Association francaise pour l'etudede de Cancer*, **13**, 410-421.

[4]   Arnol, P.M., Habib, A., Newell, K. and Anderson, K.K. (2009) Esthesioneuroblastoma Metastatic to the Thoracic Intradural and Extradural Space. *The Spine Journal*, **9**, 1-5.

[5]   de Santana Sarmento, D.J., *et al.* (2012) Aggressive Olfactory Neuroblastoma Invading the Oral Cavity: Report of a Rare Case and Review of the Literature. *Journal of Oral and Maxillofacial Surgery*, **70**, 252-257. http://dx.doi.org/10.1016/j.joms.2011.11.020

[6]   Bak, M. and Wein, R.O. (2012) Esthesioneuroblastoma: A Contemporary Review of Diagnosis and Management. *Hematology/Oncology Clinics of North America*, **26**, 1185-1207. http://dx.doi.org/10.1016/j.hoc.2012.08.005

[7]   Bragg, T.M., Scianna, J., Kassam, A., *et al.* (2009) Clinicopathological Review: Esthesioneuroblastoma. *Neurosurgery*, **64**, 764-770. http://dx.doi.org/10.1227/01.NEU.0000338948.47709.79

[8]   Yu, T., Xu, Y.K., Li, L., Jia, F.G., Duan, G., Wu, Y.K., Li, H.Y., Yang, R.M., Feng, J., Ye, X.H. and Qiu, Y.W. (2009) Esthesioneuroblastoma Methods of Intracranial Extension: CT and MR Imaging Findings. *Neuroradiology*, **51**, 841-850. http://dx.doi.org/10.1007/s00234-009-0581-0

[9]   Thompson, L.D. (2009) Olfactory Neuroblastoma. *Head and Neck Pathology*, **3**, 252-259. http://dx.doi.org/10.1007/s12105-009-0125-2

[10] Ferreira, M.C.F., Tonoli, C., Varoni, A.C.C., Gusmon, C.C., Alvarenga, M., Chagas, J.F. and Pascoal, M.B.N. (2007) Esthesioneuroblastoma. *Revista de Ciências Médicas Campinas*, **16**, 193-198.

[11] Holland, H., Koschny, R., Kruppd, W., Meixensberger, J., Bauer, M., Kirsten, H. and Ahnert, P. (2007) Comprehensive Cytogenetic Characterization of an Esthesioneuroblastoma. *Cancer Genetics and Cytogenetics*, **173**, 89-96. http://dx.doi.org/10.1016/j.cancergencyto.2006.09.024

[12] Gondim, J., Ramos Jr., F., Azevedo, J., Carrero Jr., F.P. and Tella Jr., O.I. (2002) Esthesioneuroblastoma: A Case Report. *Arquivos de Neuro-Psiquiatria*, **60**, 303-307. http://dx.doi.org/10.1590/S0004-282X2002000200024

[13] Dulguerov, P. and Calcaterra, T. (1992) Esthesioneuroblastoma: The UCLA Experience 1970-1990. *Laryngoscope*, **102**, 843-849. http://dx.doi.org/10.1288/00005537-199208000-00001

[14] Pickuth, D., Heywang-Kobrunner, S.H. and Spielmann, R.P. (1999) Computed Tomography and Magnetic Resonance Imaging Features of Olfactory Neuroblastoma: An Analysis of 22 Cases. *Clinical Otolaryngology*, **24**, 346-350. http://dx.doi.org/10.1046/j.1365-2273.1999.00295.x

[15] Shirzadi, A.S., Drazin, D.G., Strickland, A.S., Bannykh, S.I. and Patrick Johnson, J. (2013) Vertebral Column Metastases from an Esthesioneuroblastoma: Chemotherapy, Radiation, and Resection for Recurrence with 15-Year Follow-Up. *Case Reports in Surgery*, **2013**, 8 p.

[16] Dulguerov, P., Allal, A.S. and Calcaterra, T.C. (2001) Esthesioneuroblastoma: A Meta-Analysis and Review. *The Lancet Oncology*, **2**, 683-690. http://dx.doi.org/10.1016/S1470-2045(01)00558-7

[17] Kadish, S., Goodman, M. and Wang, C.C. (1976) Olfactory Neuroblastoma—A Clinical Analysis of 17 Cases. *Cancer*, **37**, 1571-1576. http://dx.doi.org/10.1002/1097-0142(197603)37:3<1571::AID-CNCR2820370347>3.0.CO;2-L

[18] Hyams, V.J. (1988) Olfactory Neuroblastoma. In: Hyams, V.J., Baksakis, J.G. and Michaels, L., Eds., *Tumors of the Upper Respiratory Tract and Ear*, Armed Forces Institute of Pathology, Washington DC, 240-248.

[19] Lund, V., Howard, D., Wei, W. and Spittle, M. (2003) Olfactory Neuroblastoma: Past, Present, and Future? *The Laryngoscope*, **113**, 502-507. http://dx.doi.org/10.1097/00005537-200303000-00020

[20] Petruzzelli, G.J., Howell, J.B., Pederson, A., Origitano, T.C., Byrne, R.W., Munoz, L., Emami, B. and Clark, J.I. (2015) Multidisciplinary Treatment of Olfactory Neuroblastoma: Patterns of Failure and Management of Recurrence. *American Journal of Otolaryngology*, in Press. http://dx.doi.org/10.1016/j.amjoto.2015.02.008

37

Parathyroid Adenoma Presenting as a Giant Cystic Neck Mass

Thomas Muelleman[1], Eric Rosenberger[1], Clinton Humphrey[1,2], Christopher G. Larsen[1,2]

[1]Department of Otolaryngology—Head and Neck Surgery, University of Kansas Medical Center, Kansas City, KS, USA
[2]Department of Otolaryngology—Head and Neck Surgery, St. Luke's Hospital, Kansas City, MO, USA
Email: tmuelleman3@kumc.edu, erosenberger@kumc.edu, chumphrey@kumc.edu, clarsen@kumc.edu

Abstract

We present a case report of a parathyroid adenoma, which presented as a giant cystic neck mass while providing thorough reviews of the pathophysiology of parathyroid adenomas and the differential diagnosis for large, cystic neck masses in adults. A 72 year old female presented to a tertiary academic medical center with a complicated past medical history and was found to have an asymptomatic central neck mass which measured 10.5 × 7.7 × 4.1 cm on ultrasound and extended from the retropharyngeal space with mass effect on the hypopharynx, esophagus, trachea, and right carotid space structures as well as the superior mediastinum. She had elevated calcium and parathyroid hormone (PTH) levels. She underwent surgical excision of this mass and had an uneventful postoperative period. Large cystic neck masses generate a wide differential diagnosis. In adults, it is important to consider the rare possibility of parathyroid adenoma, especially in patients who may not be able to communicate vague symptoms of hypercalcemia. This particular parathyroid adenoma is several orders of magnitude larger than an average parathyroid adenoma and its massive size served as a distraction for the proper diagnosis as large, cystic neck masses in adults are to be considered cancer until proven otherwise.

Keywords

Parathyroid Adenoma, Giant Parathyroid Adenoma, Large Cystic Neck Mass, Hypercalcemia

1. Introduction

Hyperparathyroidism is a relatively rare condition usually caused by an overproduction of parathyroid hormone (PTH) due to a single parathyroid adenoma [1]. Presenting symptoms are generally secondary to hypercalcemia and include vague symptoms such as constipation, lethargy, confusion, myalgia, nausea, bone pain, and kidney stones. Hypercalcemia is much more common, affecting 1% - 4% of the adult population, with most causes related to malignancy and secretion of parathyroid hormone-related protein (PTHrP). PTH levels will be low in cases of malignancy with elevated PTHrP [1]. Laboratory analysis demonstrating elevated levels of PTH and alkaline phosphatase combined with hypophosphatemia further refines the diagnosis towards a parathyroid adenoma. A 24-hour urine collection can rule out benign familial hypocalciuric hypercalcemia.

Parathyroid gland and parathyroid adenoma identification can occur via specific radiologic studies including the technetium-99 m sestamibi scan, but can also be found incidentally on thyroid ultrasound, MRI, and computed tomography of the neck [2]. Parathyroid adenomas generally appear as hypervascular soft tissue masses but have been described in case reports as cystic masses of several centimeters [3].

This case report illustrates a complex patient presenting for surgical resection due a giant cystic parathyroid adenoma, the size of which is the largest heretofore reported in the literature.

2. Case Report

A 72-year-old female presented from her assisted living facility for evaluation of asymptomatic hypercalcemia found on routine examination. Her past medical history was significant for mental retardation, schizoaffective disorder, diabetes mellitus, splenic lesions of unknown significance, and breast cancer. The patient was unable to offer any personal history, and her court appointed caretaker was unavailable. Review of systems revealed thirst, vague abdominal pain, and nausea. Medications at the time of otolaryngology consultation included bisphosphonate therapy (pamidronate), IV hydration, calcitonin, and IV furosemide.

Physical examination revealed a large central neck mass with significant tracheal deviation to the left without stridor or increased work of breathing. No evidence of dysphonia or dysphagia was present.

Her initial calcium level of 12.0 increased to 13.3 after admission, with PTH level of 169 (normal < 60 pg/ml). 24 hr urine calcium was not obtained secondary to inpatient therapy for hypercalcemia. Ultrasound and subsequent fine needle aspiration revealed a large, possible multi-lobed cystic mass of 7.7 × 4.1 × 10.5 cm. Fine needle aspiration (FNA) demonstrated dark fluid but found no evidence of malignancy. A slight decrease in serum calcium and PTH level occurred following FNA.

CT imaging of the neck with contrast demonstrated a complex cystic mass 8.2 × 5.6 × 10.5 cm with a 0.7 × 0.5 cm nodular and solid focus along the right lateral cyst border. The mass extended from the retropharyngeal space with mass effect on the hypopharynx, esophagus, trachea and right carotid space structures and extended into the superior mediastinum. No significant cervical lymphadenopathy was present. See **Figure 1** and **Figure 2**.

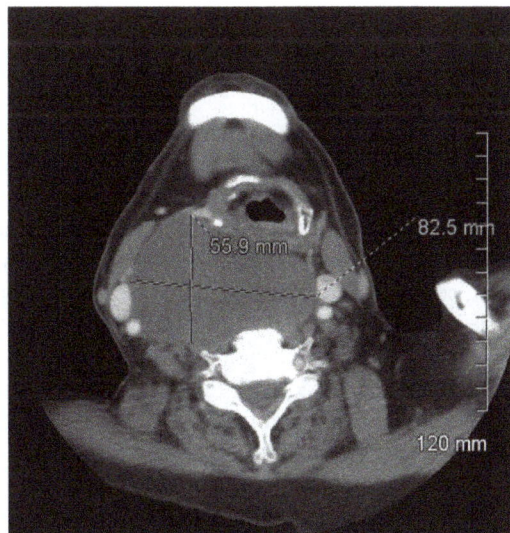

Figure 1. Computed tomography (CT) scan with contrast of neck. This axial slice demonstrates the patient's cystic neck mass and laryngeal deviation to the left.

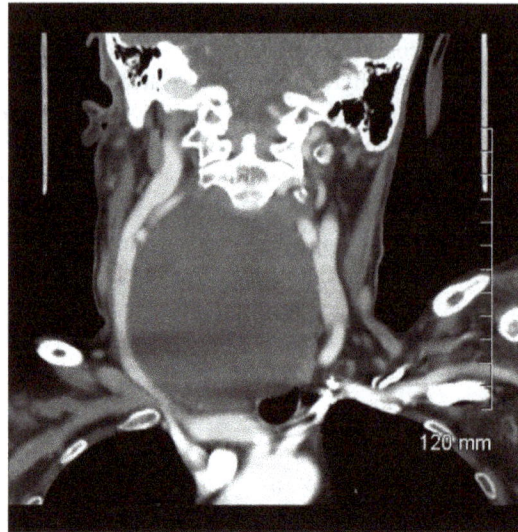

Figure 2. CT scan with contrast of neck. This coronal slice highlights the cystic parathyroid adenomas proximity to the great vessels laterally as well as the descending trachea, superior mediastinum, right lung pleura, and arch of the aorta inferiorly.

Surgical excision proceeded next. Division of the platysma immediately revealed a fibrous capsule surrounding a large, dark, fluid-filled cyst. Careful dissection of the capsule was aided by removal of approximately 100 ml of cyst fluid. The cyst was adherent to the right lateral tracheal wall and the posterior and superior border of the right thyroid lobe. The right recurrent laryngeal nerve was identified inferiorly and traced to the cricothyroid joint prior to cyst wall transection. Intraoperative PTH monitoring began at time of incision, 125, decreasing to 63, five minutes after cyst isolation, and decreased to 10, five minutes after case end. The wound was then copiously irrigated with saline and closed in three layers. Intraoperative frozen section and final pathology were consistent with parathyroid adenoma. See **Figure 3** [4].

The patient tolerated the procedure well and she was admitted to the hospital as an inpatient. Her incisions healed well and calcium levels remained stable after surgery. She was then discharged back to her assisted living facility. She continued to heal well and was seen in the postoperative clinic. She continues to follow with her primary care physician.

3. Discussion

The presentation of a large, cystic neck mass in an adult provokes a broad differential diagnoses based on mass location, characteristics, symptoms, and medical history. In the pediatric population, congenital anomalies such as thyroglossal duct cyst, lymphatic malformation, branchial cleft cyst, and vascular malformation are more likely than carcinoma. [5] In adults, cystic neoplasms are assumed to be cancer until proven otherwise and their differential diagnosis includes metastatic squamous cell carcinoma (especially HPV + tumors), metastatic papillary thyroid cancer, thyroid cysts, cervical thymoma, and more uncommonly, parathyroid adenoma [6].

Parathyroid adenomas average weight is between 0.5 and 5 g [7]. A recent large retrospective review reserved the term "giant parathyroid adenomas" for those adenomas with weight above the 95th percentile among all parathyroid adenomas, which they found to be >3.5 g [8]. Reports in the literature have highlighted giant parathyroid adenomas of smaller size than the adenoma highlighting in this case report [3] [9]-[13]. This patient's mass was likely able grow to this large size due to social factors. She was mentally retarded and unable to convey any knowledge of the mass. Caretakers likely did not notice the mass due to its soft and pervasive nature. The mass was eventually discovered secondary to workup for several vague complaints. Her complaints of thirst, abdominal pain, and nausea were likely secondary to underlying hypercalcemia. However, these symptoms cannot be attributed with certainty to hypercalcemia given the patient's mental status. Her laboratory levels of serum calcium and the concern for carcinoma in this patient were the two main factors that led to surgical excision [14].

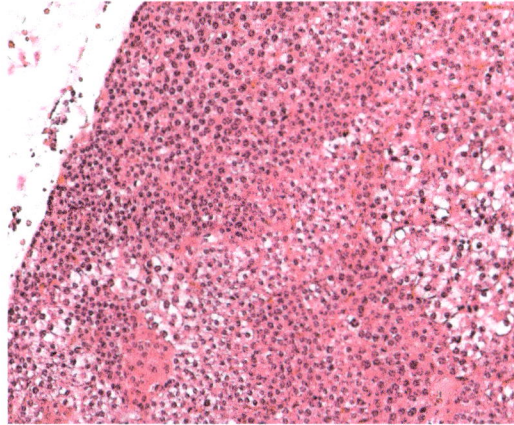

Figure 3. Histopathologic slides of a typical parathyroid adenoma. Parathyroid adenomas are characterized by uniform, polygonal chief cells with small, centrally placed nuclei. A few nests of larger oxyphil cells are present as well. Mitotic figures are rare. Adipose tissue is also rare [7].

4. Conclusion

This case report highlights a complicated patient with a massive cystic neck mass, ultimately confirmed to be a cystic parathyroid adenoma on final pathology. The general practitioner and otolaryngologist should maintain a high level of suspicion for patients with mental retardation who present with new symptoms, even if the patient is not able to accurately describe these symptoms. Also, the case serves as a reminder to include parathyroid adenoma in the differential diagnosis of a large cystic neck mass in an adult patient.

References

[1] Wysolmerski, J.J. and Insogna, K.L. (2008) The Parathyroid Glands, Hypercalcemia, and Hypocalcemia. In: Kronenberg, H.M., Schlomo, M., Polansky, K.S., Larsen, P.R., Eds., *Williams Textbook of Endocrinology*, 11th Edition, WB Saunders, St. Louis, 266.

[2] Ghervan, C., Silaghi, A. and Nemes, C. (2012) Parathyroid Incidentaloma Detected during Thyroid Sonography—Prevalence and Significance beyond Images. *Medical Ultrasonography Journal*, **14**, 187-191

[3] Asghar, A., Ikram, M. and Islam, N. (2012) A Case Report: Giant Cystic Parathyroid Adenoma Presenting with Parathyroid Crisis after Vitamin D Replacement. *BMC Endocrine Disorders*, **12**, 14. http://dx.doi.org/10.1186/1472-6823-12-14

[4] Romanidis, K., Karathanos, E., Nagorni, E., *et al.* (2014) Parathyroid Adenoma Detected with 99mTc-Tetrofosmin Dual-Phase Scintigraphy: A Case Report. *BMC Research Notes*, 7, 335. http://dx.doi.org/10.1186/1756-0500-7-335

[5] Acierno, S.P. and Waldhausen, J.H. (2007) Congenital Cervical Cysts, Sinuses and Fistulae. *Otolaryngologic Clinics of North America*, **40**, 161-176. http://dx.doi.org/10.1016/j.otc.2006.10.009

[6] Chen, A. and Otto, K.J. (2010) Differential Diagnosis of Neck Masses. In: Flint, P.W., Haughey, B.H., Lund, V.J., *et al.*, Eds., *Cummings Otolaryngology—Head and Neck Surgery*, 5th Edition, Mosby/Elsevier, Philadelphia, 1636-1642. http://dx.doi.org/10.1016/B978-0-323-05283-2.00117-8

[7] Anirban, M. (2015) The Endocrine System. In: Kumar, V., Abbas, A. and Aster, J., Eds., *Robbins and Cotran Pathologic Basis of Disease*, 9th Edition, Saunders, Philadelphia, 1073-1139.

[8] Spanheimer, P., Stoltze, A., Howe, J., Sugg, S., Lal, G. and Weigel, R. (2013) Do Giant Parathyroid Adenomas Represent a Distinct Clinical Entity? *Surgery*, **154**, 714-719. http://dx.doi.org/10.1016/j.surg.2013.05.013

[9] Garas, G., Poulasouchidou, M., Dimoulas, A., Hytiroglou, P., Kita, M. and Zacharakis, E. (2015) Radiological Considerations and Surgical Planning in the Treatment of Giant Parathyroid Adenomas. *The Annals of The Royal College of Surgeons of England*, 97, e64-e66. http://dx.doi.org/10.1308/003588415X14181254789682

[10] Ebina, K., Miyoshi, Y., Izumi, S., *et al.* (2015) A Case of Adolescent Giant Parathyroid Adenoma Presenting Multiple Osteolytic Fractures and Postoperative Hungry Bone Syndrome. *Clinical Case Reports*, **3**, 835-840. http://dx.doi.org/10.1002/ccr3.360

[11] Neagoe, R., Sala, D., Borda, A., Mogoanta, C. and Muhlfay, G. (2014) Clinicopathologic and Therapeutic Aspects of Giant Parathyroid Adenomas—Three Case Reports and Short Review of the Literature. *Romanian Journal of Morphology and Embryology*, **55**, 669-674.

[12] Haldar, A., Thapar, A., Khan, S. and Jenkins, S. (2014) Day-Case Minimally Invasive Excision of a Giant Mediastinal Parathyroid Adenoma. *The Annals of The Royal College of Surgeons of England*, **96**, e21-e23. http://dx.doi.org/10.1308/003588414X13946184900480

[13] Sisodiya, R., Kumar, S., Palankar, N. and Dinesh, B.V. (2011) Case Report on Giant Parathyroid Adenoma with Review of Literature. *Indian Journal of Surgery*, **75**, 21-22. http://dx.doi.org/10.1007/s12262-011-0306-6

[14] Morris, L. and Myssiorek, D. (2009) When Is Surgery Indicated for Asymptomatic Primary Hyperparathyroidism? *The Laryngoscope*, **119**, 2291-2292. http://dx.doi.org/10.1002/lary.20740

38

Large Ameloblastoma of Mandible: Our Experience with Intermaxillary Fixation

Anoop Attakkil, Vandana Thorawade, Rajesh Kar, Shobhna Chandran, Devkumar Rengaraja, Karthik Rao, Dnyaneshwar Rohe

Department of ENT, Grant Medical College & Sir J.J. Hospital, Mumbai, India
Email: fasttrack2317@gmail.com

Abstract

Ameloblastomas are benign dental tumors, constituting 15% of oral neoplasms, most frequent odontogenic tumor of the jaw. Patient presenting at a late stage usually presents with large swelling with facial deformity. We present a case of 50 years old male who presented with recurrent ameloblastoma on the left side of the mandible causing facial disfigurement and functional impairment. Adequate removal of the tumor required hemimandibulectomy and intermaxillary fixation was done without any bony reconstruction. We would like to focus on the excellent postoperative result with regard to facial symmetry and functional improvement obtained in this case, though the available management protocols differ and are more advanced in current scenario. This case report gives hope and guidance to the surgeons who face difficulty in managing the deforming benign bony tumors due to the unavailability of facility and funds to reconstruct.

Keywords

Ameloblastoma, Resection, Intermaxillary Fixation, Mandible

1. Introduction

WHO defines the solid/multicystic ameloblastoma as a slowly growing, locally invasive, epithelial odontogenic tumour of the jaws with a high rate of recurrence if not removed adequately, but with virtually no tendency to metastasize [1]. Ameloblastoma is the second most common odontogenic tumour which is generally slow growing but locally invasive. Its peak incidence is noted between 30 and 60 years of age, while the tumour is rare below the age of 20 years. It exhibits no gender predilection and occurs over a wide age range. The tumour occurs exclusively in the jaws, rarely in the sinonasal cavities [1]. Clinical presentation is usually swellings of the jaws which may be variably sized and associated with rare incidences of pain or paraesthesia. It may show unilocular or multilocular radiolucencies resembling cysts and they may reveal scalloped borders.

It spreads slowly by infiltration through the medullary spaces and may erode cortical bone leading to resorption of the cortical plate and may extend into adjacent tissues. Patients commonly present at a late stage when the tumor causes significant facial deformity or malocclusion and functional impairment. The treatment of choice is en bloc resection of the tumor owing to the high recurrence rate of the tumor following a simple curettage (75%) [2]. In case of large sized tumors, extensive surgical resection usually results in large tissue defects which lead to severe aesthetic and functional impairment. In huge ameloblastoma, the key to the treatment lies in attaining wide local resection of the tumor and reconstruction of the patient's appearance with minimal functional limitations. It demands the availability of well equipped plastic surgery reconstruction teams which often poses limitations for the surgeons to proceed with excision.

We presented a case of huge ameloblastoma which was involving the left half of the mandible causing facial deformity and malocclusion. Enbloc resection of the tumor was done and managed with primary closure and intermaxillary fixation postoperatively for two weeks. Our case report highlights the aesthetic quality and improvement of functions which is attained by this management accepting the fact that the advanced surgical reconstruction should be done where the faculty and facility are available. We have also tried to present a concise review of the relevant literature.

2. Case Report

A 45 years old male presented to our department, with a bulging mass on the left half of the face arising mandible, gradually enlarged over past 7 years to the present size without pain or inflammation. There was a large firm swelling over the left mandibular region which was non tender extending from the left angle of mouth anteriorly to the angle of mandible (**Figure 1**). Intraorally, the mucosal bulge was present on the left side of the floor of mouth with intact and smooth buccal mucosa. Malocclusion was present. He reported having undergone excision of tumor over the same site 25 years back. The treatment details were not available except for the histopathology report which suggested ameloblastoma. Computerised Tomography with three dimensional reconstruction showed a huge radiolucent region in the mandibular area on the left side including the body and ramus (**Figure 2**). Biopsy done from the mucosal side confirmed the diagnosis of ameloblastoma. A segmental mandibulectomy with wide local excision and reconstruction with bone graft and titanium plating to stabilise the mandible was planned.

Under general anaesthesia, an extra-oral surgical approach through a lip splitting incision was done and skin flap was raised exposing the mandible. The solid tumour was noted to involve the whole of left mandible measuring about 7 × 6 cm which was involving the body, ramus and head of condyle (**Figure 3**). Hemimandibulectomy was done with en bloc resection of the tumour. No bony reconstruction was done. Intermaxillary fixation

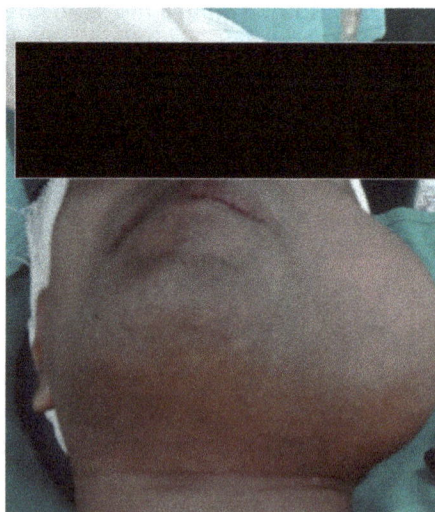

Figure 1. Large ameloblastoma on the left side of the face producing facial asymmetry.

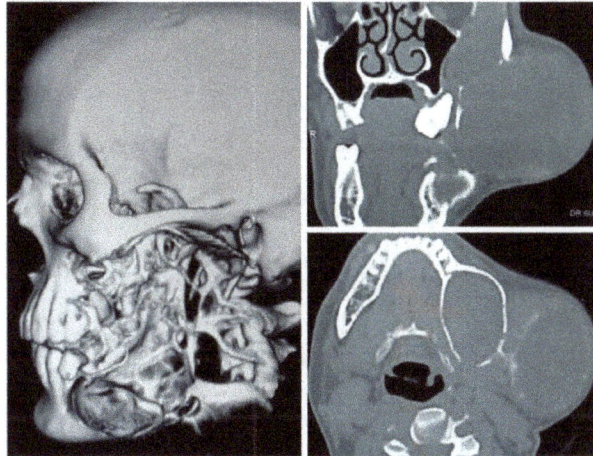

Figure 2. Three dimensional computerised tomography showing the enormous size and extent of ameloblastoma.

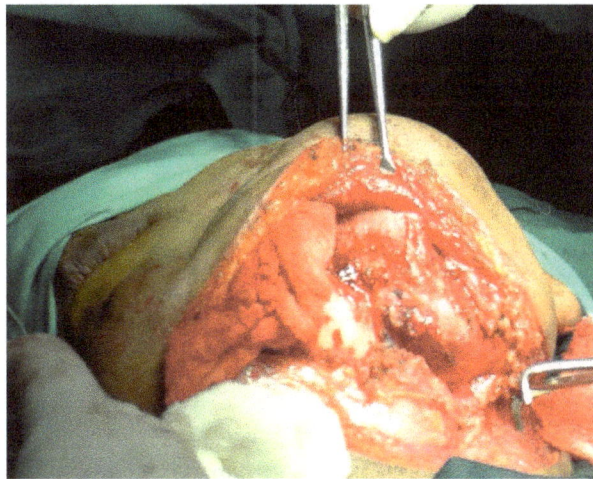

Figure 3. Intraoperative photograph after the exposure of tumor.

was done to prevent the deviation of the mandible. Patient was on Ryle's tube feeding. Postoperative period was uneventful. Histopathology was confirmatory for follicular ameloblastoma that showed islands of epithelial cells with a central mass of polyhedral cells surrounded by well organized single layer of cuboidal or tall columnar cells with nuclei placed at the opposite pole of basement membrane resembling pre-ameloblasts (**Figure 4**). Intermaxillary fixation was removed after 6 weeks. Negligible deviation of the jaw was noted with little compromise on chewing and swallowing. The jaw movements were satisfactory (**Figure 5**). Patient was evaluated after three months where he had no significant complaints except for the depression over his left cheek. Patient refused for the reconstruction of cheek defect. On follow-up evaluation one year later, he had no difficulty in swallowing, chewing and maintained good voice.

3. Discussion

The ameloblastoma is the second most common odontogenic tumor, first being odontoma. It arises from any number of residual epithelial elements of tooth development: reduced enamel epithelium, rests of Serres, rests of Malassez or the basal layer of the oral mucosa [3]. It can also develop from within a dental follicle or a dentigerous cyst.

Ameloblastoma is a benign, locally infiltrating tumor characterized by a slow growth pattern and can grow to enormous size. Typically an ameloblastoma present as painless slow growing mass that may cause facial asymmetry, displacement or loosening of teeth, malocclusion, and pathologic fractures due to expansion of bone and

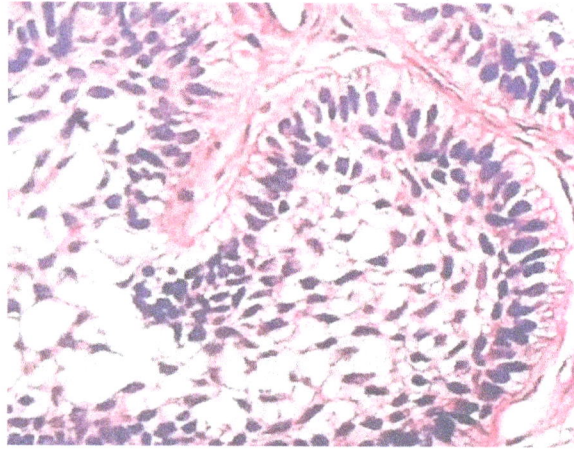

Figure 4. Histopathological features of follicular amelobalstoma demonstrated.

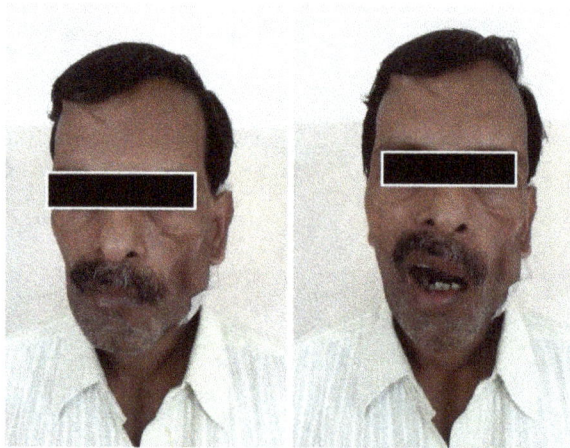

Figure 5. Showing the post operative picture after 3 months where the acceptable cosmetic & functional results can be appreciated.

invasion into soft tissue. Buccal and lingual cortical expansion is common even progressing to cortical perforation [3]. In our case, patient presented after 7 years when it caused facial deformity and malocclusion.

The lesion has a very wide age range with a peak occurrence in the third and forth decades and it has no sex predilection. The posterior mandible appears to be a preferred site [3]. Radiographically the lesion can appear as a unilocular or multilocular radiolucency with ill-defined borders making it difficult to determine the exact size of the lesion.

When the ameloblastomas grows into, or completely through the connective tissue layer of the lesion or recurs, en bloc resection is the advocated treatment with a 1.0 to 1.5 cm bony margin and one uninvolved overlying anatomic barrier margin is advocated. In a review of 60 mandibular ameloblastoma cases, there was no recurrence of those cases treated via en bloc resection as compared to enucleation and curettage in which the recurrence rate was as high as 25% to 50% [4].

Reconstruction of large defects of mandible had always been a challenge to the head and neck surgeons. The reconstruction aims in attaining accepted cosmetic results and structural integrity that restores the functions like chewing, speech and swallowing to a better extent. Literature review shows various surgical techniques described for reconstruction of mandible but the micro vascular flap reconstruction is the most preferred in current scenario. Vascularised bone flaps can be used to rebuild any defect extension, while bone grafts should have their use restricted to smaller defects, less than 5 cm in length [5].

The autogenous grafts can be taken from fibula, iliac crest, scapula and radial forearm. Fibula has been proposed as the choice for reconstruction owing to the acceptable bone length and thickness and minimal donor site morbidity [6]. In a comparative study done between vascularised iliac crest flap and vascularised free fibular flap, free fibular flap proved to be more superior with less complication rates and better cosmetic and functional results [7]. In a case series of 10 cases it was shown that vascularised fibula flap with simultaneous placement of integrated dental implants could attain better results than conventional methods [8].

Multiphasic approach was recently advocated where the reconstruction of the surgical defect with autogenous or revascularized autogenous bone graft followed by prosthetic restoration by endosseous implants [9]. Internal distraction osteogenesis of the mandible has been proposed which reduces the postoperative morbidity and causes distraction of soft tissue along with the bone but the increased duration of the treatment is the limitation [10].

In our case, the unavailability of better microvascular reconstruction facility limited our reconstruction plans. Besides, financial status of the patient was not good enough to afford the treatment. Hence wide local excision was done which eventually resulted in hemimandibulectomy followed by intermaxillary fixation. Though it cannot be considered as the acceptable method in the era of recent advances, the cosmetic and functional results obtained in our patient were worth reporting. The limitation of the availability of resources and facilities always poses a challenge to the head and neck surgeons to proceed with resection of such tumors. Aramany et al. reported a case series of 14 patients who were treated by use of immediate intermaxillary fixation after segmental resection of the mandible to eradicate cancerous lesions which has shown that use of intermaxillary fixation during the first 6 postoperative weeks will reduce the degree of deviation [11]. This will keep the muscles in neutral position and prevent deviation. Inter maxillary fixation in our patient done for six weeks gave proper occlusion and prevented the deviation of the jaw preserving the aesthetics and functional integrity. The swallowing, chewing and voice quality was remarkably better in the post operative period and patient was satisfied with the treatment.

4. Conclusion

En bloc tumour resection has been accepted as the treatment of choice in ameloblastoma. Huge ameloblastoma presenting with facial asymmetry had been always a challenge in reconstruction which requires the expertise in micro vascular reconstruction. Excellent results had been attained with microvascular reconstruction with free fibula. Our experience with en-bloc resection and internal maxillary fixation has provided good results in regard to the structural integrity and aesthetics. We reported this case to provide an insight to the head and neck surgeons to dare to proceed with the treatment of the benign tumors of mandible overcoming the limitations of the resources.

References

[1]   (2005) Pathology and Genetics of Head and Neck Tumours. IARC WHO Classification of Tumours Series Volume 9 of World Health Organization Classification of Tumours, World Health Organization, IARC Press, 296.

[2]   Turgut, M., Unsal, A. and Ozkara, E. (2012) Adenomatoid Ameloblastoma in the Mandible and Maxilla: Report of a Case. Indian Journal of Otolaryngology and Head & Neck Surgery, 63, 1-3. http://dx.doi.org/10.1007/s12070-011-0166-1

[3]   Chung, W.L., Cox, D.P. and Ochs, M.W. (2006) Odontogenic Cysts, Tumors, and Related Jaw Lesions. In: Bailey, B.J., Johnson, J.T. and Newlands, S.D., Eds., Head & Neck Surgery-Otolaryngology, Fourth Edition, Lippincott Williams & Wilkins, Philadelphia, PA, 1569-1575.

[4]   Eppley, B.L. (2002) Re: Mandibular Ameloblastoma: Analysis of Surgical Treatment Carried out in 60 Patients between 1977 and 1998. Journal of Craniofacial Surgery, 13, 400. http://dx.doi.org/10.1097/00001665-200205000-00007

[5]   Foster, R.D., Anthony, J.P., Sharma, A. and Pogrel, M.A. (1999) Vascularized Bone Flap versus Nonvascularized Bone Grafts for Mandibular Reconstruction: An Outcome Analysis of Primary Bony Union and Endosseous Implant Success. Head Neck, 21, 66-71. http://dx.doi.org/10.1002/(SICI)1097-0347(199901)21:1<66::AID-HED9>3.0.CO;2-Z

[6]   Disa, J.J. and Cordeiro, P.G. (2000) Mandible Reconstruction with Microvascular Surgery. Seminars in Surgical Oncology, 19, 226-234. http://dx.doi.org/10.1002/1098-2388(200010/11)19:3<226::AID-SSU4>3.0.CO;2-N

[7]   Yilmaz, M., Vayvada, H., Menderes, A., Demirdover, C. and Kizilkaya, A. (2008) A Comparison of Vascularised Fibular Flap and Iliac Crest Flap for Mandibular Reconstruction. Journal of Craniofacial Surgery, 19, 227-234

[8]   Chana, J.S., Chang, Y.M., Wei, F.C., *et al.* (2004) Segmental Mandibulectomy and Immediate Free Fibula Osteo Septo Cutaneous Flap Reconstruction with Endosteal Implants: An Ideal Treatment Method for Mandibular Ameloblastoma. *Plastic and Reconstructive Surgery*, **113**, 80-87. http://dx.doi.org/10.1097/01.PRS.0000097719.69616.29

[9]   Becelli, R., Carboni, A., Cerulli, G., Perugini, M. and Iannetti, G. (2002) Mandibular Ameloblastoma: Analysis of Surgical Treatment Carried out in 60 Patients between 1977 and 1998. *Journal of Craniofacial Surgery*, **13**, 395-400. http://dx.doi.org/10.1097/00001665-200205000-00006

[10]   González-Garcia, R., Rubio-Bueno, P., Naval-Gías, L., *et al.* (2008) Internal Distraction Osteogenesis in Mandibular Reconstruction: Clinical Experience in 10 Cases. *Plastic and Reconstructive Surgery*, **121**, 563-575.

[11]   Aramany, M.A. and Myers, E.N. (1977) Intermaxillary Fixation Following Mandibular Resection. *Journal of Prosthetic Dentistry*, **37**, 437-444. http://dx.doi.org/10.1016/0022-3913(77)90145-7

39

Roadmap of Otolaryngology—Head and Neck Surgery Clinic in a Tertiary Center: A Prospective Cohort Study of 1178 Patients

Ameen Z. Alherabi

Department of Ophthalmology & Otolaryngology—Head & Neck Surgery, Umm Al-Qura University and King Abdullah Medical City, Makkah, Saudi Arabia
Email: herabi@hotmail.com

Abstract

Objectives: An Otolaryngology—Head and Neck Surgery clinic is an integral part of any modern tertiary center outpatient department. The objective of this article is to present our experience in developing a local electronic Makkah Otolaryngology—Head and Neck DATABASE (MO-HND) and provide a roadmap for the development of Otolaryngology—Head and Neck Surgery clinics in other tertiary centers. Methods: This is a prospective audit of all patients attending our clinic over 3 months period (July to September 2014). The data were recorded using our MO-HND. Results: A total of 1178 patients were included. The mean age was 27.7 ± 6.7 years. Participants included 586 males (49.7%) and 592 females (50.3%). There were 1139 (96.6%) Saudi and 39 (3.4%) non-Saudi patients. The specialist clinic undertook most of the workload (66%). The majority of surgery bookings (94%) were carried out through a consultant clinic. Of all participants, 80% were diagnosed with general ENT conditions, 21% underwent a procedure in the clinic, and 29% required further investigations. The surgical conversion rate was 16.3%. Conclusion: Electronic DATABASES have become important tools for improving medical services. Primary and secondary level medical centers and hospitals should increase their role in alleviating pressure from tertiary and quaternary level hospitals. In turn, a model concentrated on subspecialty clinics and services should be developed.

Keywords

ENT, Otolaryngology, Head and Neck, Clinic

1. Introduction

An Otolaryngology—Head and Neck Surgery clinic is an integral part of any modern tertiary center outpatient department. The distribution of services and activities within such clinics is very much center-dependent. However, such services and activities are very different within primary, secondary, tertiary, or quaternary centers. In general, within tertiary centers, the general platform of these clinics is similar, but there are differences typically related to the specific geographical distribution of diseases and referral system [1]-[5].

The idea of developing an electronic DATABASE for ENT clinics was initiated by Neumann in 1967 [6]. Subsequently, this idea has evolved along with the development of the medical field and computer systems. There was scant specific literature in the field of otolaryngology specific DATABASES; but they all encouraged further development and pointed to many health related issues that could be improved using such DATABASES (e.g., services planning, clinics allocations, operating time allocation, equipment's needed, man power planning) [1]-[6]. Our first experience with electronic DATABASES was in 2009 with the head and neck oncology DATABASE in Makkah [1]. The purpose of this report is to present our experience in the development of our local electronic Makkah Otolaryngology—Head and Neck DATABASE (MO-HND) and provide a roadmap for the Otolaryngology—Head and Neck Surgery clinic in tertiary centers.

2. Methods

This prospective cohort study was conducted between July-September 2014following the creation and development of the Makkah Otolaryngology—Head & Neck DATABASE (MO-HND). The DATABASE was developed using Microsoft© Access 2009 (Microsoft Corporation) as a collaborative project between UMM AL-QURA University and the ministry of health hospitals in Makkah, Saudi Arabia. After obtaining ethical approval from the Institutional Review Board and administration, relevant patient demographics, diagnosis, therapy, and clinic information were included in the DATABASE (see **Figure 1**).

The inclusion criteria of this study were all patients of both genders and all age groups who attended the Otolaryngology—Head & Neck Surgery clinic at our hospital in Makkah. All relevant demographic data were recorded prospectively during the patient clinic encounter.

Data presented as means ± SD for continuous variables and as percentages for categorical variables. Group comparisons were conducted using a t-test for continuous variables and chi-squared test for discrete variables. A *p-value* was calculated using Fisher's Exact Test and a p-value of <0.05 was considered as statistically significant. Relative risk (RR) and 95% confidence intervals (CI) were also presented when appropriate. Data analysis was carried out using Microsoft© Excel 20013 (Microsoft Corporation, Seattle, WA) and SPSS© Version 17 (SPSS Inc., Chicago, IL).

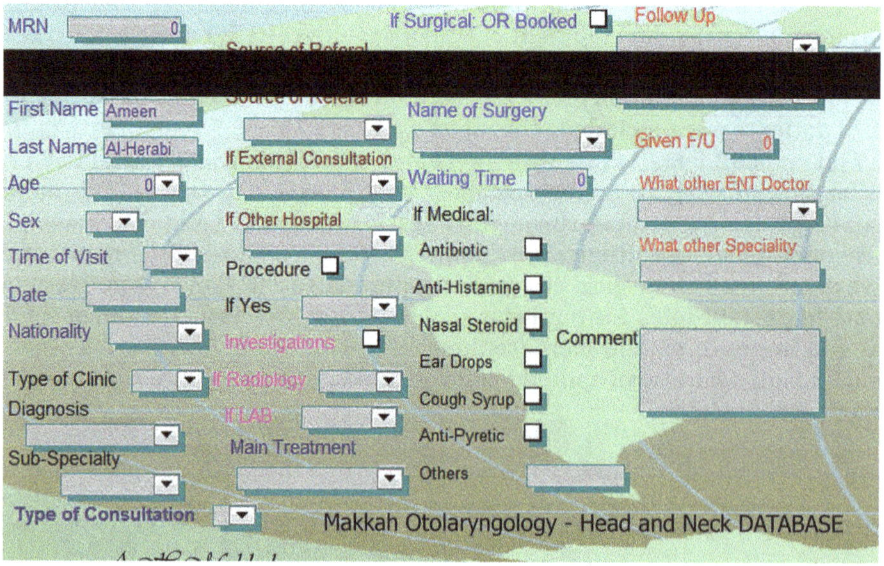

Figure 1. Makkah Otolaryngology—Head and Neck DATABASE (MO-HND) interface.

3. Results

A total of 1178 patients who met our inclusion criteria and presented to the Otolaryngology—Head and Neck Surgery clinic were included in this study. The mean age was 27.7 ± 6.7 years (age range = 5 days - 81 years). Age group distributions are shown in **Table 1**. There was a statistically significant trend toward younger age group presenting to the Otolaryngology—Head & Neck Surgery clinic, with age groups 0 - 50 years old representing 86.1% of total patients (chi-squared test = 58.4, p = 0.0001). There was no significant difference in the number (males 49.7%, females 50.3%) or ratio (male to female ratio = 1:1.01) of male and female participants (p = 0.93, RR = 1.005, 95% CI = 0.92 - 1.09).

There was a statistically significant difference between the number of Saudi (n = 1139, 96.6%) and non-Saudi (n = 39, 3.4%) patients (p = 0.0001, RR = 0.363, 95% CI = 0.33 - 0.38). Of non-Saudi patients, 12 (1.0%) were from Egypt, 10 (0.9%) from the Philippines, 8 (0.7%) from Pakistan, and 9 (0.8%) from other countries. There was also a statistically significant difference between the distribution of patients who attended the clinic during the morning shift (09:00 - 12:00) (n = 726, 61.6%) and afternoon shift (13:00 - 16:00) (n = 452, 38.4%) (p = 0.0001, RR = 0.791, 95% CI = 0.73 - 0.85).

There are three types of clinic in our outpatient Otolaryngology—Head & Neck Surgery structure: Consultant clinic, Specialist clinic, and Resident clinic. The distribution of patients' attendance at these clinics is shown in **Figure 2**. Analysis revealed that the Specialist clinic represented 780 (66%) of total patients (chi-squared test = 218.24, p = 0.0001). However, most OR booking was completed via a Consultant clinic (180 of 192 patients, 94%). Of the total patients, there was a significant difference between the number of follow-up (n = 731, 62%) and new patients (n = 447, 38%) (p = 0.0001, RR = 0.784, 95% CI = 0.72 - 0.85).

Patients' diagnoses were established after the patients were triaged by the ENT clinic nurse then examined by the clinic physician. Recording of diagnoses was based on the International Classification of Diseases (ICD-10) [7]. The distribution of patients' diagnoses according to subspecialty is shown in **Figure 3** and the distribution of specific patients diagnoses within each subspecialty is shown in **Table 2**.

Table 1. Age group distributions of 1178 patients attending Otolaryngology—Head and Neck Surgery clinic.

Age group	Frequency	Percentage (%)
0 - 18	446	37.9
19 - 50	568	48.2
>51	164	13.9
Total	1178	100

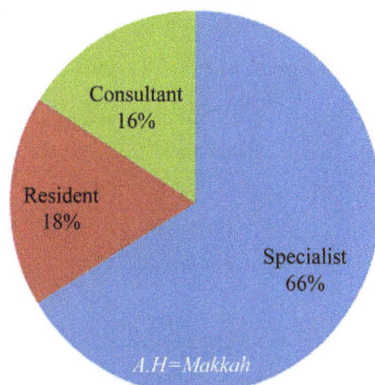

Figure 2. The distribution of all non-Saudi nationalities patients included in the ENT HAJJ clinic study.

Table 2. Diagnosis distributions of 1178 patients attending Otolaryngology—Head and Neck Surgery clinic.

Diagnosis sub-specialty	Number		Percentage (%)
	936		80
	Upper respiratory tract infection	205	17.4
	Allergic Rhinitis	160	14
	Adeno-tonsillar disease	139	12
	External & middle ear infectious & inflammatory disease	118	10
	Deviated nasal septum	82	7
	Wax	48	4
General	Nasal trauma/fracture	33	3
	Hearing loss	22	1.9
	Hoarseness	21	1.8
	Tracheostomy	20	1.7
	Reflux laryngitis	20	1.7
	Dizziness	19	1.6
	Epistaxis	17	1.4
	Foreign body	14	1
	Others	18	1.5
	96		8
Rhinology	Sino-nasal polyposis	66	5.6
	Naso-lacrimal disease	25	2
	Choanal atresia	5	0.4
	69		6
Otology	Mastoid & middle ear disease	65	5.6
	Bell's palsy	3	0.3
	Acoustic neuroma	1	0.1
	61		5
	Thyroid mass	31	2.6
	Head & neck mass/tumor	13	1
	Thyroglossal duct cyst	5	0.4
Head & Neck	Parotid gland disease	5	0.4
	Submandibular gland disease	3	0.25
	Laryngocele	2	0.2
	Glomus tumor	2	0.2
	13		1
Fascioplastic	Nasal deformity	11	0.8
	Flap reconstruction	2	0.2
	3		0.3
Pediatric	Subglottic stenosis	2	0.2
	Laryngeal papillomatosis	1	0.1
Total	1178		100

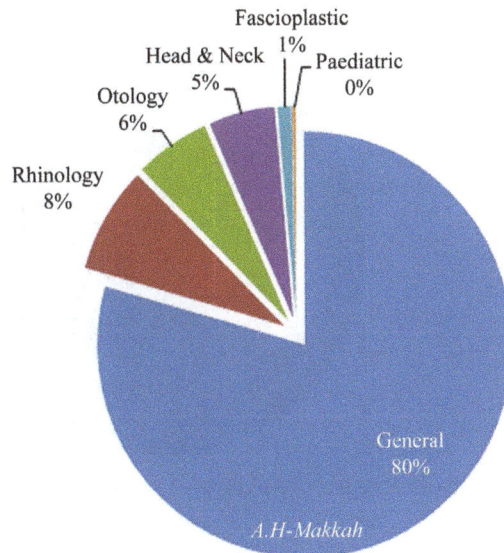

Figure 3. Diagnosis distributions of 1178 Otolaryngology—Head and Neck Surgery clinic patients according to subspecialty.

The source of referrals to the Otolaryngology—Head and Neck Surgery clinic is shown in **Figure 4**. Of the 1178 patients that attended the clinic, there was a significant difference between patients that had an in-clinic procedure (n = 250, 21%) and those who did not (n = 928, 89%) (p = 0.0001, RR = 0.553, 95% CI = 0.51 - 0.59). The distribution of specific procedures performed is shown in **Table 3**. There was also a significant difference between the number of patients who had a requested investigation (n = 341, 29%) and those who did not (n = 837, 71%) (p = 0.0001, RR = 0.652, 95% CI = 0.60 - 0.70). The distribution of the specific requested investigations is shown in **Table 4**.

Additionally, the number of patients booked for surgery (n = 192, 16.3%); widely known as surgical conversion rate (SCR), and those primarily assigned to medical therapy (n = 986, 83.7%) differed significantly (p = 0.0001, RR = 0.495, 95% CI = 0.45 - 0.53). The distribution of detailed types of medical therapy is shown in **Table 5**. The reason there are a total of 1491 medical therapies is that some patients were given more than one medication. For the 192 patients booked for surgery, the surgical waiting time ranged from 1 - 9 months (average = 7.2 months). The future plans for all clinic patients are shown in **Figure 5**. For the 858 (73%) patients receiving follow-up, the wait time ranged from 1 - 28 weeks (average = 6.1 weeks).

4. Discussion

The MO-HND is our institutional model for ENT patients' data management. The primary intention is for it to act as a system that provides useful patient demographic statistics to assist future service planning and monitoring. There is scant literature that outlines comprehensive descriptive statistics of a modern Otolaryngology—Head and Neck Surgery clinic in a tertiary center [1]-[3] [5].

A total of 1178 patients were seen in our Otolaryngology - Head and Neck Surgery clinic. Patients' average age was 27.7 years old (86.1% of patients were between 0 - 50 years old), and it is clear that younger age groups predominate. Age-related findings contrast those reported in Boiza *et al*.'s [8] study in Spain, which indicated that of 1516 ENT attending patients, 57.86% were over 65 years old. Of these patients, 61.2% were seen for an ear disorder. These findings clearly demonstrate geographic variance related to the health care system. In addition, in the current study there was an equal gender distribution, which differs from Alherabi's [9] study that reported that of 1047 patients, 63.3% were male and 36.7% were female. However, in that study the ENT clinic setup occurred during HAJJ time (pilgrimage). Regarding patients' nationalities, in our study, there were 1139 (96.6%) Saudi and 39 (3.4%) non-Saudi patients. This differs from a study by Alherabi [9], which reported that out of 1047 patients, 31.6% were non-Saudi. However, once again, the ENT clinic setup in that study occurred during HAJJ. Egypt, the Philippines, and Pakistan represented most of the non-Saudi country nationalities, which are also the predominant countries of origin of hospital staff. Furthermore, the daily operation of the clinic was

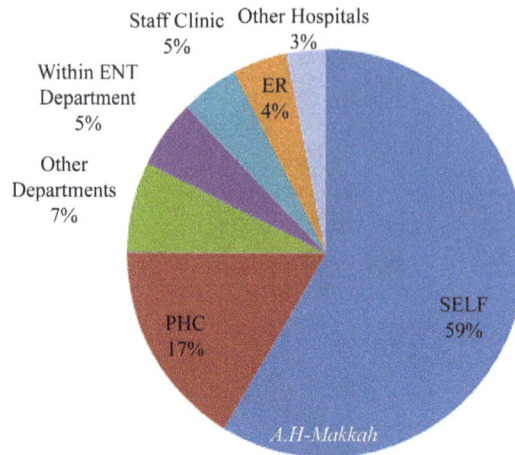

Figure 4. Source of referrals of 1178 patients attending Otolaryngology—Head and Neck Surgery clinic according to subspecialty (PHC: Primary Health Care).

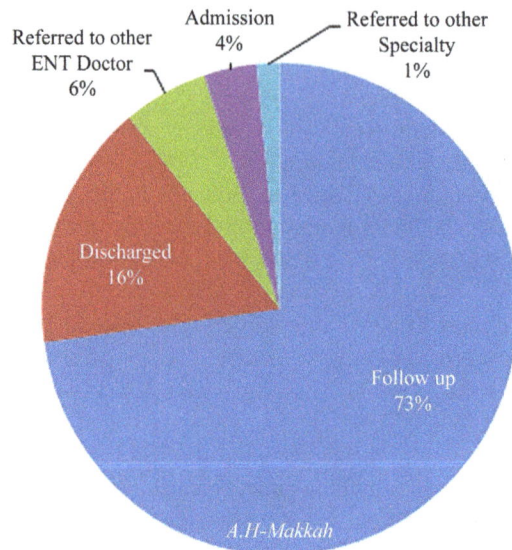

Figure 5. Future plans for 1178 Otolaryngology—Head and Neck Surgery clinic patients.

Table 3. Distribution of procedures for 1178 patients attending Otolaryngology—Head and Neck Surgery clinic.

		Number	Percentage (%)
	NO	928	79
	YES	250	21
Procedures	Ear Debridement	88	35.2
	Endoscopy	86	34.4
	Wound care	36	14.4
	FB removal	22	8.8
	Epistaxis cautery	12	4.8
	Others	6	2.4
	Total	250	100

Table 4. Distributions of requested investigations for 1178 patients attending the Otolaryngology—Head and Neck Surgery clinic.

			Number	Percentage (%)
Investigation		NO	837	71
		YES	341	29
	Radiology	Plain X-ray	118	34.5
		CT	54	16
		MRI	6	1.8
		U/S	6	1.8
	Audiology	Audiogram	70	20.6
		Tympanogram	21	6
	Laboratory Blood Work		66	19.3
	Total		341	100

Table 5. Surgical and medical therapy distributions of 1178 patients attending the Otolaryngology—Head and Neck Surgery clinic.

		Number	Percentage (%)
Surgical		192	16.3
		986	83.7
Medical	Antibiotic	388	26
	Anti-histamine	306	20.5
	Nasal steroid	272	18.2
	Anti-pyretic	260	17.5
	Ear drops	106	7.1
	Nasal saline wash	76	5
	Cough syrup	36	2.5
	Others	47	3.2
	Total	1491	100

not equally distributed between the morning shift (09:00 - 12:00), where 726 (61.6%) patients attended, and the afternoon shift (13:00 - 16:00) where 452 (38.4%) attended. This represented an increased patient load of 37.6%, which is comparable to Alherabi [9] study that reported a 30.4% increase in patient load in the morning.

Although the service model in our hospital is consultant-based, 66% of patients in the outpatient clinic were seen by specialist clinics and represent a major operational workforce. Resident's clinics saw 18% of all patients and were mainly for screening, preadmission, or postoperative clinics. Consultants saw only 16% of patients; however, 94% of the operative booking was completed through a consultant clinic. Consequently, this reflects a surgical filtration process in decision making from a junior to more senior level clinic. A study by Koay *et al.* [10] about a nurse-led preadmission clinic for elective ENT surgery admission showed that using a standard proforma for clerking was appropriate for nurses. Although a number of unnecessary investigations were requested, all clerking notes were well kept. Additionally, 440 patients (96.9%) underwent their operations without complications. Thus, it was concluded that a nurse-led preadmission clinic is effective in the management of elective ENT operating lists [10]. In another study, Daniel and colleagues, 11 addressed the question of "Is a doctor needed in the adult ENT pre-admission clinic?" Here, it was concluded that designing a preadmission protocol that could easily be used by nurses could eliminate most changes made by doctors. Thus, it was recommended that all ENT departments consider implementing nurse-led preadmission clinics [11]. Dexter et al. also advised the introduction of a proforma, and advice on handwriting significantly increased the quality of case notes [12]. In our Otolaryngology—Head and Neck Surgery clinic we found that there was a significant circulation of patients, as 62% were follow-ups and 38% were new patients.

Examining the distribution of services within the Otolaryngology—Head and Neck Surgery clinic showed that a significant 80% of cases were diagnosed with a general ENT condition. Although the hospital is considered a tertiary center, only 20% of total cases were true tertiary-level cases. This represented a major burden to providing a specialized service to a system overwhelmed with primary- or secondary-level cases. Of the 80% of patients that attended the clinic with a general condition it was found that 31.4% were simple upper respiratory tract infection (URTI) and allergic rhinitis cases that could have been easily managed in a primary health care center. Although many of their cases were referred as emergency or semi-emergency cases, many of them were not. Congruently, Herve et al. [13] conducted a study in France where they examined 1237 patients in a similar clinic and found that most cases were not true emergencies (53%) and that the predominant pathological cases managed were acute external and middle ear otitis, epistaxis, vertigo, and facial injuries. Emergency care was more justified when a general practitioner or another emergency unit referred the patients. A study by Wheatley et al. [2] from England reported that 75% of patients seen in an open access clinic could have waited until the next day to be seen. Furthermore, when Timsit et al. [5] examined 20,563 patients in an ENT adult emergency clinic, they found that only 10% of the consultations appeared to be real medical emergencies. Subsequently, Mylvaganam et al. [14] were able to reduced patient waiting times from 70 minutes to 35 minutes and reduce inappropriate referrals from 7% to 2% by establishing an ENT emergency clinic.

Of the 20% of cases representing true subspecialty level cases, the majority were related to Rhinology (8%), Otology (6%), and Head and Neck (5%). These subspecialties will represent the future planned subspecialty clinics in our modern Otolaryngology—Head and Neck Surgery department. Of the 8% patients that attended the clinic with a rhinologic diagnosis, 66 (5.6%) had nasal polyposis, which was a significant number and represents an important condition affecting the Makkah community. Furthermore, of the 6% (n = 96) of patients that attended the clinic with an otologic diagnosis, 65 (5.6%) had mastoid and middle ear disease. Likewise, this number is significant and reflects a condition affecting our community.

In addition, 5% of patients (n = 61) attended the clinic with a head and neck diagnosis. In a 2009 study conducted by our group [1] to address the head and neck oncology experience in Makkah, 44 patients concluded all oncological services of head and neck cancer patients including surgery, radiotherapy, and chemotherapy should be provided in one oncology center. Thus, these should be managed through one standard channel (the head and neck oncology board) to achieve standard patient care, adequate follow up, and surveillance [1]. Another issue regarding caring for head and neck cancer patients in a general ENT clinic was raised by Ali and colleagues [15], who stated that unwarranted fears about cancer are best dealt with by the referring clinician. Other clear benefits from a specialized ENT-head and neck clinic include rapid patient access to specialist management and the development of subspecialty skills [3].

In the current study, 31 patients (2.6%) were found to have a thyroid-related problem. Overall, the most common head and neck cancers identified in Saudi Arabia were thyroid and nasopharyngeal cancers. [1] This clearly differs from western statistics presented in a study of 881 patients that indicated that laryngeal and oral cancer represented 47.8% of all head and neck cancers [16]. A study by Morinaka et al. addressing the magnitude of thyroid disease in an ENT clinic found that 1.8% of 6348 outpatients had thyroid-related problems [4]. In our clinic, fascioplastic and pediatric otolaryngology cases were the minimal burden, representing 1% and 0.3% of cases.

The sources of referral represented a surprising result, since it could be expected that most referrals to a tertiary center would come from at least secondary-level institutions or centers. However, it was found that 76% of all referrals came from primary health care centers or simple patient self-referral.

While hospitals were thought to be the main source of referrals to tertiary hospitals, only 7% of the total consultations came from other departments within our hospital, and only 3% came from other hospitals. García et al.

[17] showed that internal medicine and pediatric departments were the most frequent source of referrals. An audit from Ireland demonstrated that out of 3.3 million outpatients attendees, 20% were directed towards ENT services. Here, the researchers concluded that there were poor compliance rates with their newly introduced standardized referral form [18].

Of all patients that attended the clinic, 21% (n = 250) of patients underwent a procedure. However, only 34 patients had emergency-related procedures; namely, foreign body removal and epistaxis cautery. In Mori's Japanese study, it was demonstrated that out of 2184 outpatient surgeries, myringotomy, coagulator ablation of the nasal mucosa, removal of a foreign body in the external auditory canal, and insertion of a ventilation tube accounted for 90% of the total number of procedures performed on outpatients [19].

Of all patients that attended the clinic, 29% (n = 341) has received a request for further investigation. The most common requests were plain X-rays (34.5%) and audiological tests (26.6%). Ayshford *et al.* showed that of 1155 patients seen by one ENT surgeon, 76% of patients required an investigation (audiometry, endoscopy, microscopy of the ear, a minor procedure or X-ray) [20]. In the current study, the SCR was 16.3%. A British report addressing SRC within all surgical specialties after general practitioner referral showed that ENT SRC ranged from 23% - 29% [21]. As a true reflection of the availability of resources including operative time, manpower, and surgical beds, our average elective surgery waiting time was 7.2 months. Similarly, a report from New Zealand showed the children had to wait for 7 months for their elective tonsillectomies [22]. The Royal College of Surgeons of England has published clear guidelines for the management of surgical waiting lists that led to the recommendation to create a preadmission clinic for elective ENT surgery [10] [11] [23].

As for medical therapy, antibiotics were prescribed in 26% of cases. A previous study by our group showed that antibiotics were prescribed to 94.7% of patients that attended the ENT clinic during Hajj time [9]. In a US study by Gaur *et al.*, it was reported that of 1952 pediatric patients diagnosed with viral infections, 33.2% received antibiotics. In addition, antibiotic use was greater among those who worked in non-teaching (39.6%) than teaching hospitals (32.5%) [24]. A 1995 Canadian study showed that 74% of 39,145 children diagnosed with respiratory infections received antibiotics [25]. Follow-up was undertaken in 73% of cases, and only 16% were discharged. In a study by Fishpool *et al.* addressing the frequency of attendance at an ENT emergency clinic, it was reported that insisting patients seen more than twice in an ENT emergency clinic be reviewed by a consultant and introducing management guideline reduced excess clinic appointments by 70% [26].

Limitations of this study include any cross sectional descriptive study limitations like only three months sample size; although generated reasonable patient sample size. Which; will also, needs a longitudinal follow of its recommendations to confirm validity and practicability in a mass scale and provide a map for health administrators to monitor and plan future resources.

Implications of findings for future research of this study represent first step in the scientific ladder to generate further studies with higher level of evidence and more question-focused research.

5. Conclusion

Creating and benefiting from electronic patient DATABASES are becoming important parts of improving medical services for continuous monitoring and auditing health services provided. Primary and secondary level medical centers and hospitals should increase their role to help alleviate pressure from tertiary and quaternary level hospitals. In turn, this should be used to develop a model and concentrate on subspecialty clinics and services.

Acknowledgements

Great thanks to Dr. Riham Malabari, Dr. Mohammad Alessa, Dr. Turki Kamal, Dr. Omar Bahathiq, and Dr. Rakan Yamani for their help in data collection and entry.

Disclosure of Benefits

The author has not disclosed any affiliation or financial involvement with organizations or entities with a direct financial interest in the subject matter or materials discussed in the manuscript. No funding was received for this work from any organization.

References

[1]   Al-Herabi, A.Z. (2009) Head and Neck Oncology Experience in Makkah, Saudi Arabia. *Saudi Medical Journal*, **30**, 1316-1322.

[2]   Wheatley, A.H., Temple, R.H., Camilleri, A.E. and Jones, P.H. (1999) ENT Open Access Clinic: An Audit of a New Service. *Journal of Laryngology and Otology*, **113**, 657-660. http://dx.doi.org/10.1017/S0022215100144767

[3]   Banfield, G. and McCombe, A. (1997) Establishing a New ENT-Head and Neck Clinic. *Journal of the Royal Army Medical Corps*, **143**, 153-154. http://dx.doi.org/10.1136/jramc-143-03-05

[4]   Morinaka, S. (1995) On the Frequency of Thyroid Diseases in Outpatients in an ENT Clinic. *Auris Nasus Larynx*, **22**, 186-191. http://dx.doi.org/10.1016/S0385-8146(12)80057-5

[5]   Timsit, C.A., Bouchene, K., Olfatpour, B., Herman, P. and Tran Ba Huy, P. (2001) Epidemiology and Clinical Findings in 20,563 Patients Attending the Lariboisiere Hospital ENT Adult Emergency Clinic. *Ann Otolaryngol Chir Cervicofac*, **118**, 215-224.

[6]   Neumann, H. (1967) Electronic Data Documentation in the ENT Clinic. *Archiv für klinische und experimentelle Ohren-, Nasen-und Kehlkopfheilkunde*, **188**, 532-541. http://dx.doi.org/10.1007/BF01278578

[7]   World Health Organization (2007) International Classification of Diseases (ICD-10). 10th Revision.

[8]   Calvo Boizas, E., Rodrguez Gutierrez, A. and Gomez Toranzo, F. (1999) Care for Elderly Patients at an ENT Clinic. Descriptive Study. *Acta Otorrinolaringológica Española*, **50**, 56-59.

[9]   Alherabi, A.Z. (2009) Road Map of an Ear, Nose, and Throat Clinic during the 2008 Hajj in Makkah, Saudi Arabia. *Saudi Medical Journal*, **30**, 1584-1589.

[10] Koay, C.B. and Marks, N.J. (1996) A Nurse-Led Preadmission Clinic for Elective ENT Surgery: The First 8 Months. *Annals of the Royal College of Surgeons of England*, **78**, 15-19.

[11] Daniel, M. and Banerjee, A.R. (2004) Is a Doctor Needed in the Adult ENT Pre-Admission Clinic? *The Journal of Laryngology & Otology*, **118**, 796-798. http://dx.doi.org/10.1258/0022215042450715

[12] Dexter, S.C., Hayashi, D. and Tysome, J.R. (2008) The ANKLE Score: An Audit of Otolaryngology Emergency Clinic Record Keeping. *Annals of the Royal College of Surgeons of England*, **90**, 231-234. http://dx.doi.org/10.1308/003588408X261537

[13] Herve, J.F., Wiorowski, M., Schultz, P., Chambres, O., Lannoy, L., Rakotobe, H., *et al.* (2004) ENT Resident Activity in the Strasbourg Hospital ENT Emergency Clinic. *Annales d Oto-Laryngologie et de Chirurgie Cervico-Faciale*, **121**, 33-40.

[14] Mylvaganam, S., Patodi, R. and Campbell, J.B. (2009) The ENT Emergency Clinic: A Prospective Audit to Improve Effectiveness of an Established Service. *The Journal of Laryngology & Otology*, **123**, 229-233. http://dx.doi.org/10.1017/S0022215108003022

[15] Ali, S. and Bingham, B.J. (2005) Unfounded Worries about Cancer in Patients Attending a Routine Otolaryngology Clinic. *Journal of the Royal Society of Medicine*, **98**, 415. http://dx.doi.org/10.1258/jrsm.98.9.415

[16] Altumbabic, H., Salkic, A., Ramas, A., Burgic, M., Kasumovic, M. and Brkic, F. (2008) Pattern of Head and Neck Malignant Tumours in a Tuzla ENT Clinic: A Five Year Experience. *Bosnian Journal of Basic Medical Sciences*, **8**, 377-380.

[17] Cano, F.J.G., Del Hoyo, A.S., López, M.Z., Nicolás, J.L.L., Torre, I.M. and López, J.A.P. (2001) Descriptive Epidemiology of Hospital Interconsultations Carried out at the ORL Service for a Year in the San Millan-San Pedro Hospital Complex. *Anales Otorrinolaringológicos Ibero-Americanos*, **28**, 487-500. (In Spanish)

[18] Oosthuizen, J.C., McShane, D., Kinsella, J. and Conlon, B. (2014) General Practitioner ENT Referral Audit. *Irish Journal of Medical Sciences*, **184**, 143-146.

[19] Mori, Y. (2013) Office Surgery in a Private ENT Clinic: A Statistical Analysis of 2,814 Outpatient Surgeries. *Nippon Jibiinkoka Gakkai Kaiho*, **116**, 703-708. (In Japanese) http://dx.doi.org/10.3950/jibiinkoka.116.703

[20] Ayshford, C.A., Johnson, A.P. and Chitnis, J.G. (2001) What Is the Value of ENT Specialist Outreach Clinics? *The Journal of Laryngology & Otology*, **115**, 441-443. http://dx.doi.org/10.1258/0022215011907965

[21] Jones, R. (2013) Does Growth in GP Referral Link Directly to Growth in Inpatient Demand? *Healthcare Analysis & Forecasting*, **3**, 1-4.

[22] Donn, A.S. and Giles, M.L. (1991) Do Children Waiting for Tonsillectomy Grow out of Their Tonsillitis? *The New Zealand Medical Journal*, **104**, 161-162.

[23] The Royal College of Surgeons of England (1991) Guidelines for the Management of Surgical Waiting Lists.

[24] Gaur, A.H., Hare, M.E. and Shorr, R.I. (2005) Provider and Practice Characteristics Associated with Antibiotic Use in

Children with Presumed Viral Respiratory Tract Infections. *Pediatrics*, **115**, 635-641.
http://dx.doi.org/10.1542/peds.2004-0670

[25] Wang, E.E., Einarson, T.R., Kellner, J.D. and Conly, J.M. (1999) Antibiotic Prescribing for Canadian Preschool Children: Evidence of over Prescribing for Viral Respiratory Infections. *Clinical Infectious Diseases*, **29**, 155-160. http://dx.doi.org/10.1086/520145

[26] Fishpool, S.J., Stanton, E., Chawishly, E.K. and Hicklin, L.A. (2009) Audit of Frequent Attendees to an ENT Emergency Clinic. *The Journal of Laryngology & Otology*, **123**, 1242-1245. http://dx.doi.org/10.1017/S0022215109990478

40

The Value of High Antistreptolysin O Titre as an Indicator of Tonsillectomy in Upper Egypt

Essam A. Abo El-magd[1], Mona Abdel Meguid[2], Abd El Rahman El Tahan[1]

[1]Department of Otolaryngology, Faculty of Medicine, Aswan University, Egypt
[2]Department of Clinical Pathology, Faculty of Medicine, Al Azhar University, Asuit, Egypt
Email: esamali801@yahoo.com

Abstract

Background: In this study, we aimed to evaluate the benefit of performing of tonsillectomy in patients with raised serum ASO titre only in absence or presence of group A beta heamolytic streptococci (GABHS) in throat swab. Materials and methods: In this prospective cohort study, 196 patients below the age of 14 were suffering from non-specific streptococcal infections, without fulfilling the clinical parameters used for the diagnosis of chronic tonsillitis 156 patients had a raised ASO titre above 200 iu/ml. Throat swab culture was performed in all patients. Results: The results showed that out of the 156 patients, 52 had positive throat swab for GABHS. All of the patients underwent tonsillectomy. Follow-up of the patients for one year after the operation, 88% of the first group with high ASO titre and positive throat swab showed improvement of symptoms; 25% of the second group with high ASO titre and negative throat swab showed improvement of symptoms. Conclusion: Our study shows that isolation of GABHS from the patients tonsils by throat swab along with high ASO titre may be an indication of tonsillectomy in absence of any other indications.

Keywords

GABHS, Non Specific Strept Infection, ASO Titre, Throat Swab Culture, Tonsillectomy

1. Introduction

A raised ASO titre level is one of the most relevant retrospective serological indices of antecedent GABHS infection. A single titre of more than 200 iu/ml is considered as a raised value. Serum ASO titre is raised when there is an infection of any organ of the body by GABHS, so the increased serum ASO titre should not be the only deciding criterion for tonsillectomy if GABHS is not present in the palatine tonsils [1]. GABHS is the most common bacteria that cause acute tonsillitis. Streptococcal infection can lead to rheumatic fever. The incidence of rheumatic fever in untreated cases of tonsillitis is 3% and in treated cases, the incidence falls to 0.3%. It has been estimated that rheumatic heart disease constitutes 25% to 40% of all cardiovascular diseases in third world countries [2]. Recurrent tonsillitis is the most common indication of tonsillectomy. Recurrent infections are further defined as [3]:

1) 7 or more attaches for one year or;
2) 5 attaches per year for 2 years or;
3) 3 attaches per year for 3 years.

Clinical parameters used for the diagnosis of chronic tonsillitis were as follows [2]:

1. Recurrent attaches of tonsillitis;
2. Tender, atrophic or hypertrophic tonsils with persistent sore throat;
3. Congested anterior pillar;
4. Palpable jugulodigastric lymph node;
5. Expression of cheesy material from crypts on applying pressure on the tonsils.

In cases of infrequent recurrent tonsillitis and sings of chronic tonsillitis cannot be detected, it is difficult to take the decision of tonsillectomy. Patients complaining of non-specific manifestations such as anorexia and failure to thrive, myalgia and arthralgia, recurrent upper respiratory tract infection and recurrent otitis media may get benfite from tonsillectomy. Colonization of the tonsils by GABHS is also an important indication of tonsillectomy. To establish the carrier state of GABHS in tonsils, different investigations have been advocated the following [1]:

1. Throat swab culture;
2. Fine needle aspiration from the core of the tonsil;
3. Serum antistreptlysin O titre;
4. Core culture of the dissected tonsil after tonsillectomy.

2. Materials and Methods

We designed a prospective cohort study, recruiting 196 children suffering from repeated sore throat and upper respiratory tract infection, post-streptococcl arthralgia and arthritis (arthritis after pharyngeal infection with beta hemolytic streptococcal in patients had no other criteria of rheumatic fever) and any other non specific strept infection manifestation. The study was conducted in the ENT department of Qena university hospital, south valley university. Egypt from January 2012 to December 2012. One hundred and fifty six patients who showed raised ASO titre above 200 iu/ml were included in this study. Throat swab were cultured from pyogenic organisms from the surface of the tonsil using sterile swab sticks. Then the swab was immediately inoculated into nutrient agar, blood agar and McConkeys agar plates. Identification of the bacteria was done after isolation as per the standard procedure. A detailed history of each patient was taken which include the chief complaint, history of present illness and past illness. The onset, duration and progress of the symptoms were taken. After complete clinical examination, blood and urine examination were done. Blood examination included complete blood picture, bleeding time, prothrombin time and concentration, partial thromboplastin, ESR and CRP. Urine was examined for sugar and albumen. All the patients underwent tonsillectomy under general anesthesia by dissection method. Consent for all these procedures were obtained from the guardians. Patients who had an acute tonsillitis, peritonsillar abscess or suspected neoplasm were excluded from this study. Follow up the patient-for one year as regard clinical improvement of symptoms. Statistical analysis was done using Chi square method.

3. The Results

This study consisted of 85 female and 71 male. The youngest patient was 4 years and the oldest was 14. From those 156 patients 52 patients showed GABHS in throat swab culture while 104 patients had negative throat swab culture.

Of the 104 patients with elevated ASO titre and negative swab for GABHS:

1. 60 patients were complaining of recurrent sore throat and 18 patients improved after tonsillectomy (30%);
2. 44 patients were complaining of post streptococcal arthritis and 11 patients improved after tonsillectomy

(25%).

Of the 52 patients with elevated ASO titre and positive throat swab for GABHS:

1. 30 patients had recurrent sore throat, of those patients 26 were improved after tonsillectomy (86.6%);

2. 22 patients had recurrent post streptococcal arthritis, 18 patients were improved after tonsillectomy (81.8%)

As regard to major complaint of the study participants in **Table 1**, the results showed repeated sore throat found in 55 patients, while other complaints like anorexia and failure to thrive and repeated upper respiratory tract infections present only in 30 patients.

According to number of episodes of sore throat after tonsillectomy during one year follow-up in the first group, **Table 2** showed that, more than 2/3 of patients (70%) have three or more attacks per year.

On the other hand there are 3 or more attacks of post streptoccal arthritis after tonsillectomy in 3/4 (75%) of patients (**Table 3**).

Regarding number of attacks of sore throat and arthritis after tonsillectomy in the second group with positive throat swab, **the majority of them (86.6%) and (81.8%) have less than 3 attacks per year respectively** (**Table 4** and **Table 5**).

According the result showed in **Table 6**, the majority of patients (84.6%) of group B versus (27.8%) of patients of group A improved after tonsillectomy.

4. Discussion

A high ASO titre indicates the presence of a recent streptococcal infection [4]. A rise of ASO antibody generally takes place from one to four weeks after streptoccal infection and after that the titre returns to the previous level

Table 1. Characteristics of 196 patients.

Number of patients (196)	Complaint
55 patients	Repeated sore throat
46 patients	Non specific arthragia and myalgia
35 patients	Repeated otitis media
30 patients	Anorexia and failure to thrive
30 patients	Repeated upper respiratory tract infection

Table 2. Number of episodes of sore throat after tonsillectomy during one year follow up in the first group.

Number of attacks of sore throat	Number of patients	Percentage
>three attacks per year	42	70%
<three attacks	18	30%

Table 3. Number of attacks of post streptoccal arthritis after tonsillectomy.

Number of attacks after 1 year	Number of patients	Percentage
>three attacks per year	33	75%
<three attacks per year	11	25%

Table 4. Number of attacks of sore throat after tonsillectomy in the second group with positive throat swab.

Number of attacks of sore throat	Number of patients	Percentage
>three attacks per year	4	13.4%
<three attacks per year	26	86.6%

Table 5. Number of attacks of post streptococcal arthritis.

Number of attacks of arthritis	Number of patients	Percentage
>three attacks per year	4	18.2%
<three attacks per year	18	81.8%

Table 6. Comparison between the group with high titre and negative throat swab (group A) versus the second group with high titre and positive throat swab (group B).

Groups	Number of improved cases	Percentage
Group A 104 patients	29	27.8%
Group B 52 patients	44	84.6%

(p < 0.001).

within two or three months. Throat swab culture is positive in 80% of streptococcal infections but may be negative in cases of chronic infection. Antigen detection test is very sensitive, but it is very costly and not available in all the centers. ASOT titre test is the most widely used test. It is more popular because of its availability in our country, less cost and reasonable sensitivity. Very few studies have been reported regarding the value of ASO tire as an indicator of tonsillectomy. So, comparative discussion is limited. Indication of tonsillectomy depends mainly on clinical diagnosis. History of five or more episode of tonsillitis per year for at least one year, disabling episodes of sore throat prevent normal functions and sore throat due to tonsillitis [1] On examination **1)** tender, atrophic or hypertrophic tonsils with persistent sore throat; **2)** presence of congested anterior pillar; **3)** palpable jugulodigastric lymph node; **4)** expression of cheesy material from crypts on applying pressure on the tonsils [2]. In our study these clinical finding were not conclusive but the patients were complaining and the tonsils were accused. Of 104 patients with high ASO titre above 200 iu/ml and negative throat swab, 60 patients had recurrent sore throat more than three times per year which were disabling episodes with bad effect on normal daily life. After tonsillectomy only 18 patients improved with percentage of 30%. The remaining 44 patients had recurrent attacks of arthritis only 11 patients improved after tonsillectomy with a percentage of 25%. Reactive arthritis has been defined as a sterile inflammatory arthritis occurring in conjunction with bacterial infection at a site distant from the joints. Previous reports have postulated the relationship between streptococcal tonsillitis and reactive arthritis. It has thus been termed post-streptococcal reactive arthritis rather than acute rheumatic fever [5]. 52 patients with high ASO titre and positive throat swab, 30 patients had recurrent sore throat and 26 patients improved after tonsillectomy with a percentage of 86.6%. The remaining 22 patients had recurrent attacks of arthritis, 18 patients improved after tonsillectomy with a percentage of 81.8. In comparison between the first group with high ASO titr and negative throat swab (104) and the second group with high ASO titre and positive swab (52), the improved rate was 27.4% in the first group and 84.4% in the second group with a p value of 0.001 which is statistically significant. Our results are in line with Hombrom *et al.* 2012 [1] who concluded that one should perform throat swab culture along with ASO titre before doing tonsillectomy in absence of any other indications. Viswanathan *et al.* 2000 [2], reported that there were significant reduction of sore throat attacks after tonsillectomy within one year after operation. They concluded that tonsillectomy had a significant role in preventing or reducing recurrent streptococcal throat infection. This observation is very important, since incidence of rheumatic fever and rheumatic reactivation can be reduced by prevention of streptococcal infection. Motanoski *et al.* [6] showed that patients who had under gone surgery have lower infection rate with GABHS. Paradise *et al.* [7] also found that throat infection was markedly reduced in the first 2 years after tonsillectomy. Kobayashi *et al.* [8] suggested that a reactive arthritis induced by tonsillitis and cured by tonsillectomy. Other studies investigated the link between arthritis and tonsillectomy. The effect of tonsillectomy on rheumatoid arthritis was reported as a decrease in the degree of pain and amelioration of the disease [9] [10].

5. Conclusion

From the results of this study, it is evident that one should perform throat swab culture with ASO titre before doing tonsillectomy in absence of any other indications. A high ASO titre only is not an indicator of tonsillectomy. A high ASO titre with positive throat swab culture can be considered as an indication of tonsillectomy.

References

[1] Hembrom, R., Roychaudhuri, B.K. and Saha, A.K. (2012) Evaluation of the Validity of High ASOT only as an Indicator of Tonsillectomy. *Indian Journal of Otolaryngology and Head & Neck Surgery.*

[2] Viswanathan, N. and Sasikumaran, S. (2000) Effect of Tonsillectomy on ASO-Titre. *Indian Journal of Otolaryngology and Head & Neck Surgery*, **52**, 329-331.

[3] Dhingra, P.L. (2010) Diseases of Ear Nose and Throat. Fourth Edition, Elsevier, India, 382.

[4] Satoshi, F., Hanwa, Y., *et al.* (1988) Streptococcal Antibody: As an Indicator of Tonsillectomy. *Acta Oto-Laryngologica*, **454**, 286-291.

[5] Deighton, C. (1993) Beta Haemolytic Streptococci and Reactive Arthritis in Adults. *Annals of the Rheumatic Diseases*, **52**, 475-482. http://dx.doi.org/10.1136/ard.52.6.475

[6] Motonoski, G.M., *et al.* (1968) Epidemiology of Streptococcal Infections in Rheumatic and Non Rheumatic Families. *American Journal of Epidemiology*, **87**, 226.

[7] Paradise, J.L., Bluestone, C.D., Bachman, R.Z., *et al.* (1984) Efficacy of Tonsillectomy for Recurrent Throat Infection in Severly Affected Children; Results of Parallel and Non Randomized Clinical Trials. *The New England Journal of Medicine*, **310**, 674-683. http://dx.doi.org/10.1056/NEJM198403153101102

[8] Kobayashi, S., Tamura, N., Akimoto, T., *et al.* (1996) Reactive Arthritis Induced by Tonsillitis. *Acta Oto-Laryngologica*, **523**, 206-211.

[9] Kataura, A. and Tsubota, H. (1996) Clinical Analysis of Focus Tonsil and Related Diseases in Japan. *Acta Oto-Laryngologica*, **523**, 161-164.

[10] Kawano, M., Okada, K., *et al.* (2003) Simultaneous, Clonally Identical T Cell Expansion in Tonsil and Synovium in Patients with Rheumatoid Arthritis and Chronic Tonsillitis. *Arthritis & Rheumatism*, **48**, 2483-2488. http://dx.doi.org/10.1002/art.11212

Permissions

The contributors of this book come from diverse backgrounds, making this book a truly international effort. This book will bring forth new frontiers with its revolutionizing research information and detailed analysis of the nascent developments around the world.

We would like to thank all the contributing authors for lending their expertise to make the book truly unique. They have played a crucial role in the development of this book. Without their invaluable contributions this book wouldn't have been possible. They have made vital efforts to compile up to date information on the varied aspects of this subject to make this book a valuable addition to the collection of many professionals and students.

This book was conceptualized with the vision of imparting up-to-date information and advanced data in this field. To ensure the same, a matchless editorial board was set up. Every individual on the board went through rigorous rounds of assessment to prove their worth. After which they invested a large part of their time researching and compiling the most relevant data for our readers.

The editorial board has been involved in producing this book since its inception. They have spent rigorous hours researching and exploring the diverse topics which have resulted in the successful publishing of this book. They have passed on their knowledge of decades through this book. To expedite this challenging task, the publisher supported the team at every step. A small team of assistant editors was also appointed to further simplify the editing procedure and attain best results for the readers.

Apart from the editorial board, the designing team has also invested a significant amount of their time in understanding the subject and creating the most relevant covers. They scrutinized every image to scout for the most suitable representation of the subject and create an appropriate cover for the book.

The publishing team has been an ardent support to the editorial, designing and production team. Their endless efforts to recruit the best for this project, has resulted in the accomplishment of this book. They are a veteran in the field of academics and their pool of knowledge is as vast as their experience in printing. Their expertise and guidance has proved useful at every step. Their uncompromising quality standards have made this book an exceptional effort. Their encouragement from time to time has been an inspiration for everyone.

The publisher and the editorial board hope that this book will prove to be a valuable piece of knowledge for researchers, students, practitioners and scholars across the globe.

List of Contributors

Anoop Attakkil, Vandana Thorawade, Mohan Jagade, Rajesh Kar, Dnyaneswar Rohe and Reshma Hanowate, Devkumar Rangaraja, Kartik Parelkar
Department of ENT, Grant Medical College & Sir J.J. Hospital, Mumbai, India

Augusto Peñaranda and Juan Manuel García
Departamento de Cirugía, Grupo Implante Coclear, Fundación Santa Fe de Bogotá, Bogotá, Colombia

Sandra Martínez
Centro de Estudios e Investigación en Salud, CEIS, Fundación Santa Fe de Bogotá, Bogotá, Colombia

María Leonor Aparicio, Clemencia Barón
Grupo Implante Coclear, Fundación Santa Fe de Bogotá, Bogotá, Colombia

Masahiro Takahashi, Yasuhiro Arai, Naoko Sakuma, Daisuke Sano, Goshi Nishimura, Takahide Taguchi and Nobuhiko Oridate
Department of Otorhinolaryngology Head and Neck Surgery, Yokohama City University School of Medicine, Yokohama, Japan

Satoshi Iwasaki
Department of Otorhinolaryngology, International University of Health and Welfare, Mita Hospital, Tokyo, Japan

Shin-Ichi Usami
Department of Otorhinolaryngology, Shinshu University School of Medicine, Nagano, Japan

Kartik Parelkar, Smita Nagle, Mohan Jagade, Vandana Thorawade, Poonam Khairnar, Anoop Attakil, Madhavi Pandare, Rajanala Nataraj, Reshma Hanwate and Rajesh Kar
Department of ENT, Grant Government Medical College & Sir J J Group of Hospitals, Mumbai, India

Andrew M. Vahabzadeh-Hagh, Jayson Fitter and Dinesh K. Chhetri
Department of Head and Neck Surgery, UCLA David Geffen School of Medicine, Los Angeles, USA

Catherine Yim
Radiological Sciences, UCLA David Geffen School of Medicine, Los Angeles, USA

Reshma Hanwate, Vandana Thorawade, Mohan Jagade, Anoop Attakil, Kartik Parelkar, Madhavi Pandare, R. V. Natraj and Rajesh Kar
Department of ENT, Grant Government Medical College & Sir J J Hospital, Mumbai, India

Motohiro Sawatsubashi, Daisuke Murakami and Shizuo Komune
Department of Otolaryngology—Head and Neck Surgery, Graduate School of Medical Sciences, Kyushu University, Fukuoka, Japan

R. V. Nataraj, Mohan Jagade, Reshma Chavan, Rajesh Kar, Madhavi Pandare, Kartik Parelkar, Arpita Singhal and Kiran Kulsange
Department of Ear, Nose & Throat and Head & Neck Surgery, Grant Government Medical College, Mumbai, India

Anant Chouhan, Bhuvnesh Kumar Singh and Praveen Chandra Verma
Department of ENT, JLN Medical College, Ajmer, India

Kufre Robert Iseh, Mohammed Abdullahi, Daniel Jiya Aliyu, Stanley Amutta, Stephen Semen Yikawe and Joseph Hassan Solomon
Department of ENT, Usmanu Danfodiyo University Teaching Hospital, Sokoto, Nigeria

Eric W. Cerrati
Department of Otolaryngology, New York University, New York, USA

Teresa M. O. March, David Binetter, Yelena Bernstein and Milton Waner
Vascular Birthmark Institute of New York, Lenox Hill and Manhattan Eye, Ear and Throat Hospitals, New York, USA

Pavol Surda and Jonathan Hobson
Ear, Nose and Throat Department, Warrington and Halton Hospitals, Warrington, UK

Sai Spoorthi Nayak, Ehrlson De Sousa and Saumyata Neeraj
Department of ENT, Goa Medical College, Goa, India

Btissaam Belhoucha, Youssef Rochdi, Hassan Nouri, Lahcen Aderdour and Abdelaziz Raji
Department of ENT, CHU Med VI, Marrakech, Morocco

Zahra Essaadi and Mona Khouchani
Department of Oncology and Radiotherapy, CHU Med VI, Marrakech, Morocco

Carlos Yanez, Sandra Velázquez and Nallely Mora
American British Medical Center, Mexico City, Mexico

A. Ravindran, A. Amirthagani, Prince Peterdhas, S. Nagarajan, P. Palanivel, Rekha Salini and A. S. Jagan
Department of Otorhonolaryngology, Thanjavur Madical College, Thanjavur, India

Nobuhiro Uwa, Tomonori Terada, Kosuke Sagawa, Takeshi Mohri and Masafumi Sakagami
Department of Otolaryngology, Hyogo College of Medicine, Nishinomiya, Japan

Hiroyuki Hao, Yoshitane Tsukamoto and Seiichi Hirota
Department of Surgical Pathology, Hyogo College of Medicine, Nishinomiya, Japan

Takashi Daimon
Department of Biostatistics, Hyogo College of Medicine, Nishinomiya, Japan

Hiroshi Doi
Department of Radiology, Hyogo College of Medicine, Nishinomiya, Japan

Yohei Sotsuka
Department of Plastic Surgery, Hyogo College of Medicine, Nishinomiya, Japan

Guillaume van Eys
Department of Genetics and Cell Biology, University of Maastricht, Maastricht, The Netherlands

Marie-Luce Bochaton-Piallat
Department of Pathology and Immunology, University of Geneva-CMU, Geneva, Switzerland

Kartik Parelkar, Vandana Thorawade, Mohan Jagade, Smita Nagle, Rajanala Nataraj, Madhavi Pandare, Reshma Hanwate, Bandu Nagrale, Kiran Kulsange, Devkumar Rangaraja and Arpita Singhal
Department of ENT, Grant Government Medical College & Sir J.J. Group of Hospitals, Mumbai, India

Aslan Ahmadi, Hengameh Hirbod, Mostafa Cheraghipoor and Farzad Izadi
Department of Ear Nose & Throat, Hazrate Rasool Hospital, Tehran, Iran

A. Ravindran, A. Amirthagani, Prince Peter Dhas, S. Nagarajan, Senthil Kumar, Satheesh Kumar and Venkatesh
Department of Otorhonolaryngology, Thanjavur Madical College, Thanjavur, India

Lobna El Fiky and Badr Eldin Mostafa
Otolaryngology Department, Ain Shams University, Cairo, Egypt

Ali Kotb
Neurosurgery Department, Ain Shams University, Cairo, Egypt

Asil Tahir
Department of Otolaryngology/Head & Neck Surgery, Leighton Hospital, Crewe, UK

Prince Peter Dhas, Ravindran Ambika, Amirthagani Arumugam and Jagan Somasundaram
Department of ENT, Thanjavur Medical College, Thanjavur, India

Produl Hazarika, Seema Elina Punnoose and John Victor
Department of ENT, NMC Specialty Hospital, Abu Dhabi, UAE

Sreekala
Department of Pathology, NMC Specialty Hospital, Abu Dhabi, UAE

Nirmali Dutta
Department of Radiology, NMC Specialty Hospital, Abu Dhabi, UAE

Kejun Zhang, Binquan Wang, Yanli Zhang, Nasha Cheng, Changsheng Wang, Chunming Zhang, Wei Gao and Ganggang Chen
Department of Otolaryngology, Head and Neck Surgery, First Hospital, Shanxi Medical University, Taiyuan, China

Daniel López-Campos
ENT Service, University Hospital of the Canary Islands, Tenerife, Spain

Daniel López-Aguado and Eugenia M. Campos-Bañales
Department of Otorhinolaryngology, La Laguna University, Tenerife, Spain

José Luis de Serdio-Arias
ENT Service, University Hospital Nuestra Señora de Candelaria, Tenerife, Spain

Mar García-Sáinz
Pharmacology and Pharmacotherapy Service, University Hospital of the Canary Islands, Tenerife, Spain

Matthew M. Kwok and Paul Goodyear
Department of Otolaryngology/Head and Neck Surgery, Western Health, Melbourne, Australia

Nagula Parusharam and Kamreddy Ashok Reddy
Department of E.N.T., Kakatiya Medical College, MGM Hospital, Warangal, India

Lokesh Rao Magar
Department of Pathology, Kakatiya Medical College, MGM Hospital, Warangal, India

Jadi Lingaiah
Department of ENT & HNS, Chalmeda Anand Rao Institute of Medical Sciences, Karimnagar, India

Jayanto Tapadar
Plastic Surgery, Smayan Hospital, Varanasi, India

Preeti Tiwari
Trauma Centre, Institute of Medical Sciences, Banaras Hindu University, Varanasi, India

Tatiana G. T. Santos
University of Catholic Medical School, Brasilia, Brazil

Alessandra Ramos Venosa and Andre Luiz Lopes Sampaio
Department of Otolaryngology, University Hospital of Brasilia, Brasilia, Brazil

Produl Hazarika Seema E. Punnoose and Sanjay Arora
Department of ENT, NMC Specialty Hospital, Abu Dhabi, UAE

Ramagowdanapura Sadashivan Diesh
Department of Cardiothoracic Surgery, NMC Specialty Hospital, Abu Dhabi, UAE

Raghavendra K. Itgampalli
Department of Radiology, NMC Specialty Hospital, Abu Dhabi, UAE

Rohit Singh
Department of ENT & Head-Neck Surgery, Kasturba Medical College, Manipal, India

Ai Suzuki
Department of Otorhinolaryngology, Yokosuka City Hospital, Yokosuka, Japan
Department of Otorhinolaryngology, Yokosuka Kyosai Hospital, Yokosuka, Japan

Kazumasa Suzuki, Yoshiaki Mori, Yoshifumi Fujita and Takashi Hatano
Department of Otorhinolaryngology, Yokosuka Kyosai Hospital, Yokosuka, Japan

Nobuhiko Oridate
Department of Otorhinolaryngology — Head and Neck Surgery, Yokohama City University School of Medicine, Yokosuka, Japan

Saloni Shah, Roma Gandhi and Hemang Brahmbahtt
B.J. Medical College, Civil Hospital, Ahmedabad, India

Rajesh Viswakarma
ENT Department, Civil Hospital, Ahmedabad, India

Kartik Parelkar, Smita Nagle, Mohan Jagade, Reshma Hanwate, Madhavi Pandare, Devkumar Rangaraja, Kiran Kulsange, Bandu Nagrale and Arpita Singhal
Department of ENT, Grant Govt Medical College & Sir J J Group of Hospitals, Mumbai, India

Plamen Nedev
Department of Neurosurgery and ENT Medical University Varna, Bulgaria and University Hospital, Clinic of Otorhinolaryngology "St. Marina", Varna, Bulgaria

Thomas Muelleman and Eric Rosenberger
Department of Otolaryngology — Head and Neck Surgery, University of Kansas Medical Center, Kansas City, KS, USA

Clinton Humphrey
Department of Otolaryngology — Head and Neck Surgery, University of Kansas Medical Center, Kansas City, KS, USA
Department of Otolaryngology — Head and Neck Surgery, St. Luke's Hospital, Kansas City, MO, USA

Christopher G. Larsen
Department of Otolaryngology — Head and Neck Surgery, University of Kansas Medical Center, Kansas City, KS, USA
Department of Otolaryngology — Head and Neck Surgery, St. Luke's Hospital, Kansas City, MO, USA

Anoop Attakkil, Vandana Thorawade, Rajesh Kar, Shobhna Chandran,Devkumar Rengaraja, Karthik Rao and Dnyaneshwar Rohe
Department of ENT, Grant Medical College & Sir J.J. Hospital, Mumbai, India

Ameen Z. Alherabi
Department of Ophthalmology & Otolaryngology — Head & Neck Surgery, Umm Al-Qura University and King Abdullah Medical City, Makkah, Saudi Arabia

Essam A. Abo El-magd and Abd El Rahman El Tahan
Department of Otolaryngology, Faculty of Medicine, Aswan University, Egypt

Mona Abdel Meguid
Department of Clinical Pathology, Faculty of Medicine, Al Azhar University, Asuit, Egypt

www.ingramcontent.com/pod-product-compliance
Lightning Source LLC
Chambersburg PA
CBHW080247230326
41458CB00097B/4082